Topics in Palliative Care
Volume 5

Series Editors
Russell K. Portenoy, M.D.
Eduardo Bruera, M.D.

TOPICS IN PALLIATIVE CARE

Volume 5

Edited by

Eduardo Bruera, M.D.
University of Texas
M.D. Anderson Cancer Center
Houston, Texas

Russell K. Portenoy, M.D.
Beth Israel Medical Center
New York, New York

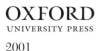

OXFORD
UNIVERSITY PRESS

2001

OXFORD
UNIVERSITY PRESS

Oxford   New York
Athens   Auckland   Bangkok   Bogotá   Buenos Aires   Calcutta
Cape Town   Chennai   Dar es Salaam   Delhi   Florence   Hong Kong   Istanbul
Karachi   Kuala Lumpur   Madrid   Melbourne   Mexico City   Mumbai
Nairobi   Paris   São Paulo   Shanghai   Singapore   Taipei   Tokyo   Toronto   Warsaw

and associated companies in
Berlin   Ibadan

Published by Oxford University Press Inc.,
198 Madison Avenue, New York, New York, 10016
http://www.oup-usa.org

Library of Congress Cataloging-in-Publication Data
Topics in palliative care / edited by Eduardo Bruera, Russell K. Portenoy
p. cm.—(Topics in palliative care: v. 5)
Includes bibliographical references and index.
ISBN 0-19-513220-3
1. Cancer—Palliative treatment.
I. Bruera, Eduardo.
II. Portenoy, Russell K.
III. Series.
[DNLM: 1. Palliative Care.   2. Neoplasms—drug therapy.
3. Pain—drug therapy.
WB   310   T674   1997]   RC271.P33T664   1997
616.99′406—dc20   DNLM/DLC   for Library of Congress   96-22250

9   8   7   6   5   4   3   2   1

Printed in the United States of America
on acid-free paper

To our wives,
Susan and Maria,
whose love and support
make our work possible.

Preface to the Series

Palliative Care, a series devoted to research and practice in palliative care, was created to address the growing need to disseminate new information about this rapidly evolving field.

Palliative care is an interdisciplinary therapeutic model for the management of patients with incurable, progressive illness. In this model, the family is considered the unit of care. The clinical purview includes those factors—physical, psychological, social, and spiritual—that contribute to suffering, undermine quality of life, and prevent a death with comfort and dignity. The definition promulgated by the World Health Organization exemplifies this perspective.°

> Palliative care is the active total care of patients whose disease is not responsive to curative treatment. Control of pain, of other symptoms, and of psychological, social and spiritual problems is paramount. The goal of palliative care is the achievement of the best possible quality of life for patients and their families.

Palliative care is a fundamental part of clinical practice, the "parallel universe" to therapies directed at cure or prolongation of life. All clinicians who treat patients with chronic life-threatening diseases are engaged in palliative care, continually attempting to manage complex symptomatology and functional disturbances.

The need for specialized palliative care services may arise at any point during the illness. Symptom control and psychological adaptation are the usual concerns during the period of active disease-oriented therapies. Toward the end of life, however, needs intensify and broaden. Psychosocial distress or family distress, spiritual or existential concerns, advance care planning, and ethical concerns, among many other issues, may be considered by the various disciplines that coalesce in the delivery of optimal care. Clinicians who specialize in palliative care perceive their role as similar to those of specialists in other disciplines of medicine: referring patients to other primary caregivers when appropriate, acting as primary caregivers (as members of the team) when the challenges of the case warrant this involvement, and teaching and conducting research in the field of palliative care.

°World Health Organization. Technical Report Series 804, Cancer Pain and Palliative Care. Geneva: World Health Organization, 1990:11.

With recognition of palliative care as an essential element in medical care and as an area of specialization, there is a need for information about the approaches used by specialists from many disciplines in managing the varied problems that fall under the purview of this model. The scientific foundation of palliative care is also advancing, and similarly, methods are needed to highlight for practitioners at the bedside the findings of empirical research. Topics in Palliative Care has been designed to meet the need for enhanced communication in this changing field.

To highlight the diversity of concerns in palliative care, each volume of Topics in Palliative Care is divided into sections that address a range of issues. Various sections address aspects of symptom control, psychosocial functioning, spiritual or existential concerns, ethics, and other topics. The chapters in each section review the area and focus on a small number of salient issues for analysis. The authors present and evaluate existing data, provide a context drawn from both the clinic and research, and integrate knowledge in a manner that is both practical and readable.

We are grateful to the many contributors for their excellent work and their timeliness. We also thank our publisher, who has expressed great faith in the project. Such strong support has buttressed our desire to create an educational forum that may enhance palliative care in the clinical setting and drive its growth as a discipline.

New York, N.Y.   R.K.P.
Houston, TX   E.B.

Contents

IV   Research Outcomes in Palliative Care

V   Opioid Tolerance: Reality or Myth?

VI   Pain and Other Symptoms: Treatment Challenges

Contributors

AKIRA AKABAYASHI, M.D.
School of Public Health
Department of Biomedical Ethics
Kyoto University Graduate School of
 Medicine
Kyoto, Japan

MARIELA BERTOLINO, M.D.
Unidad de Cuidados Paliativos
Hospital Tornu-Fundación FEMEBA
Ciudad de Buenos Aires, Argentina

TAMI BORNEMAN, R.N., B.S.N.
Nursing Research and Education
City of Hope National Medical Center
Duarte, California, USA

WILLIAM BREITBART, M.D.
Department of Psychiatry
Memorial Sloan-Kettering Cancer Center
New York, New York, USA

CARLEEN BRENNEIS, R.N.,
 M.H.S.A.
Regional Palliative Care Program
Grey Nuns Community Hospital and Health
 Centre
Edmonton, Alberta, Canada

EDUARDO BRUERA, M.D.
Department of Symptom Control and
 Palliative Care
University of Texas, M.D. Anderson Cancer
 Center
Houston, Texas, USA

CARLOS CENTENO, M.D., Ph.D.
Centro Regional de Medicina Paliativa y
 Tratamiento del Dolor
Hospital Los Montalvos
Salamanca, Spain

S. ROBIN COHEN, Ph.D.
Division of Palliative Care
Department of Oncology
McGill University
Royal Victoria Hospital
Montreal, P.Q., Canada

FRANCO DE CONNO, M.D.
Division of Pain Therapy and Palliative
 Care
National Cancer Institute
Milan, Italy

BETTY FERRELL R.N., Ph.D.,
 F.A.A.N.
Nursing Research and Education
City of Hope National Medical Center
Duarte, California, USA

JOSEPH J. FINS, M.D.
Weill Medical College of Cornell University
 and
New York Presbyterian Hospital—Weill
 Cornell Medical Center
New York, New York, USA

MARCOS GÓMEZ-SANCHO, M.D.,
 Ph.D.
Palliative Care Unit
Hospital El Sabinal
Las Palmas de Gran Canaria, Spain

PETER LAWLOR, M.D.
Edmonton Regional Palliative Care
 Program
Grey Nuns Community Hospital and Health
 Centre
Edmonton, Alberta, Canada

LAURIE LYCKHOLM, M.D.
Division of Hematology Oncology
Medical College of Virginia
Richmond, Virginia, USA

CINZIA MARTINI, M.D.
Division of Pain Therapy and Palliative Care
National Cancer Institute
Milan, Italy

DIANE E. MEIER, M.D.
Palliative Care Program
Mount Sinai School of Medicine
New York, New York, USA

SEBASTIANO MERCADANTE,
M.D.
Pain Relief and Palliative Care
Società Assistenza Ammalato Oncologico
   Terminale
Anesthesia and Intensive Care Unit and
Pain Relief and Palliative Care Unit
La Maddalena Clinic for Cancer
Palermo, Italy

R. SEAN MORRISON, M.D.
Palliative Care Program
Mount Sinai School of Medicine
New York, New York, USA

LEIA PHIOANH NGHIEMPHU,
M.D.
Department of Medicine
Beth Israel Medical Center
New York, New York, USA

JOSE PEREIRA, M.D.
Edmonton Regional Palliative Care Program
Grey Nun's Community Health Centre and
   Hospital
Edmonton, Alberta, Canada

RUSSELL K. PORTENOY, M.D.
Department of Pain Medicine and Palliative
   Care
Beth Israel Medical Center
New York, New York, USA

NARINDER RAWAL, M.D.,
   Ph.D.
Department of Anesthesiology and Intensive
   Care
Örebro Medical Centre Hospital
Örebro, Sweden

MAGNUS SJÖBERG, M.D., Ph.D.
Department of Anesthesiology and Intensive
   Care
Kungälv's Hospital
Kungälv, Sweden

THOMAS J. SMITH, M.D.
Division of Hematology Oncology
Medical College of Virginia
Richmond, Virginia, USA

WENDY M. STEIN, M.D.
Jewish Home for the Aging
Eisenberg Village
Reseda, California, USA

YOSUKE UCHITOMI, M.D.,
   Ph.D.
Psycho-Oncology Division
National Cancer Center Research Institute
   East
Chiba, Japan

RAYMOND VOLTZ, M.D.
Department of Neurology
Klinikum Grosshadern
University of Munich
Munich, Germany

ROBERTO WENK, M.D.
Programa Argentino de Medicina Paliativa-
   Fundación FEMEBA
San Nicolas, Argentina

I

CULTURAL ISSUES IN PALLIATIVE CARE

1

Models for the Delivery of Palliative Care: The Canadian Model

CARLEEN BRENNEIS AND EDUARDO BRUERA

The notion of palliative care, providing comfort to the dying, is not new to Canada or other countries. However, the context of the delivery of care has changed considerably since the mid-1970s. In the second half of the twentieth century in North America, care of the terminally ill moved from the home into the hospitals. The success of medical technology shifted the focus in hospitals to prolonging life and avoiding death. This change moved the medical care of the patient from the family physician and home nurse into a field of specialties, where until recently, palliative care was not recognized.[1-3] Beginning with the pioneering work of Dame Cicely Saunders at St. Christopher's Hospice in England in 1967, a focus on quality of life and symptom management has occurred throughout the hospice movement.

The first palliative care programs in Canada were established in Montreal and Winnipeg in 1975 (The Royal Victoria and St. Boniface Hospitals). The initial growth focused on hospital-based programs with some of the world's earliest specialty units within tertiary teaching hospitals. Canada is known internationally for the development of palliative care units and consultation teams within hospitals.[4-5] Since the palliative care units were under the auspices of host institutions, minimal standards of care were ensured.[6] Programs generally grew out of existing hospital-based programs and spread into the community through outpatient clinics and some home-based care.[2,6] In Canada, the connection to teaching hospitals and funding from the public health care system provided for a stronger academic base than most British and American programs, which maintained a strong hospice focus.[5] This chapter describes the growth of palliative care services delivery in Canada and uses the Edmonton Regional Palliative Care Program as an example.

Definition of Palliative Care

Palliative care was defined by the Palliative Care Foundation in 1981 along with the first guidelines on palliative care developed by National Health and Welfare.[7] The 1989 definition and guidelines by Health and Welfare Canada reflected more of a continuum of care with curative treatment and strengthened the notion of the interdisciplinary team. These updated guidelines reflected the increase of palliative care in the home.[2,8,9] The World Health Organization (WHO)'s definition of palliative care developed in 1990 again underscored the value of psychosocial, spiritual as well as physical care, yet continued to suggest palliative care be provided to patients not receiving active anti-disease therapy.[6,10] The Canadian Palliative Care Association (CPCA)'s, the national representative for hospice and palliative care in Canada, definition from the Standards Committee (1995) suggests palliative care is provided as primary, secondary, and tertiary roles throughout the trajectory of illness. In September 1998, the CPCA Board of Directors approved a short definition: "Hospice palliative care is aimed at relief of suffering and improving the quality of life for persons who are living with or dying from advanced illness or are bereaved."[11]

Palliative Care Development

In part because of the Report to Cancer 2000 Task Force by Expert Panel on Palliative Care (1991), there has been an ongoing debate about the types of palliative care services that should be created over the last several years. Impetus for these discussions have been:

1. Increasing burden of suffering based on the aging population and increasing cancer prevalence. This expands the population for palliative care. The number of people over 75 years of age is expected to increase by 158% from 1981 to 2021 (2.4% annually).[12] Across Canada, there is a projected increase in mortality with as many as 70,000 Canadians dying of cancer per year by 2000. Cancer has become more chronic yet 50% of patients will die of this disease following months or years of treatments. Cancer is characterized by aspects of physical, emotional, and spiritual suffering.[5] The Report to Cancer 2000 Task Force (1991) recommended reallocation of cancer resources to palliative care services, increased education and research, and a major shift of resources to home care. To a large extent, this reallocation of resources has not occurred.

2. Regionalization of health care service as a response to diminishing resources. The result of regionalization in most areas is an amalgamation and decrease in the number of acute care beds. As care shifts to the community, increased resources must move with the care to provide enhanced home care, respite, and other care options.[5,13,14] Part of the move to the community is to save the "hotel" and other costs associated with acute care beds. However, as yet there are no Canadian studies showing the cost of community care to be cheaper. And,

if the cost to the caregivers is included (cost shifted), costs savings are much less.[15–17]

3. Emphasis on community-based care as a response to individual choices. The literature is replete with an increased focus for community-based care. Palliative care is seen to be a model of care that works well for community care. Providing options of care for seniors, and informing and including patients in decision making has also enhanced focus on the option of maintaining quality of life and choosing end-of-life care at home. The proportion of patients who chose a home death, and have maintained their choice over time, is not well-documented.[(15,18–20)] Canada has had a long history of high use of acute care beds for palliative patients. The move toward more people dying at home requires a substantial shift in our socialization and learned expectation.

4. Increased medical provision of palliative care sometimes referred to as high tech. Increased options for care fuels the controversy between the potential for futile or depersonalized care, and patients' rights to access active symptomatic treatment.[2,21] There has been significant knowledge gained in symptom management and the use of this knowledge is not widespread beyond palliative care specialists, underscoring the need for more broadly targeted education.[4,21–23]

5. Public concern over care of the dying, as seen in the euthanasia debate and increasing discussion of advanced directive legislation. During the 1990s, there was strong public demand for more information and control related to health care issues, requiring improved communication between health care professionals and the public.[3]

6. The ongoing call for sensitive and standardized data collection to assess if palliative care services are making a difference for patients and families.[24–30] The lack of common definitions, measurement, and outcomes does not assist people who work in palliative care to clearly describe palliative care to other health professionals or to the public. The definition of palliative care, that which is offered when all else fails, is still prevalent with the public and with health care workers. Canada has begun to address this issue through a process of national consensus of definitions and identification of outcomes.[6,31]

Jurisdiction for Health Care

Canada has a publicly funded health care system. The Canada Health Act,[32] is federal legislation that facilitates reasonable access to health services without financial or other barriers through public administration, comprehensiveness, universality, portability, and accessibility. However, *comprehensiveness* describes health services provided by hospitals and medical practitioners, and it is up to the law of each province to define similar or additional services. Therefore, home care coverage varies from province to province and within regions of most provinces. Costs for medications and other services are provided through private insurance or provincial programs. Consequently, community-based palliative care can vary in the access to services and in the range of services. Patients may incur variable costs in medications, supplies, availability of home care and medical services, and family assistance such as respite.[9]

The Constitution of Canada defines health care as a provincial jurisdiction in Canada. In practice, responsibility for health care is shared between the federal and provincial governments. The federal government impacts health care through legislation, regulations, and activities of its various departments, and control of financial resources for funding of health care. The provinces have the authority over health care but do not have significant resources to fund it. Therefore the creation of standards is often the interplay between national bodies, such as the CPCA, the federal government Department of Health, and the provinces.[14] Consequently, a primary focus for the CPCA, founded in 1991, is the development of standardized principals of practice. In 1995, a working document including proposed definitions, statements of philosophy, principles of practice and model guidelines of practice was published as part of the process for consensus.[6] A second document outlining the status of consensus was completed in 1999.[31] Using the Delphi technique, the workgroup reached consensus on over 70 of the 101 items. Further national consensus building will continue, with completion anticipated by 2001. The process and result of gaining consensus on 13 principle functions will assist Canada in utilizing a common terminology, and ensuring that palliative care programs are aware of and choose to include these areas in model development.

Health Canada has provided some financial support of the CPCA. The CPCA promotes palliative care awareness, education, and research, advocating at a national level for policy, resource allocation, and support for caregivers. It organizes a national conference every second year and publishes a directory. There are provincial palliative care associations in each province. The *Journal of Palliative Care*, published by the Centre for Bioethics Clinical Research Institute of Montreal, a legacy of the Palliative Care Foundation from the 1980s, is a peer reviewed journal available internationally.

Programs of Care

Accurate statistical data about the number and type of programs, facilities, number of patients, and costs of palliative care in the literature for Canada are scarce.[14] The Canadian Palliative Care Foundation completed surveys in 1981 and 1986 and the McGill Palliative Care Service completed surveys in 1990. Further surveys have been completed by the CPCA in 1994 and 1997 in the Canadian Directory of Services Palliative Care. The information from these surveys must be viewed with caution since they are based on self-reporting. Not all programs may have provided information and the definitions are not standardized.[14,28] In 1997, for the first time, descriptor codes for common terminology were used in the directory.

Palliative care programs increased by over 300% between 1981 and 1986 (116 verses 359). The number of programs then decreased to 345 by 1990, and increased to 432 in 1994. The shift to community-based programs, rather than hospital-based programs, was noted during these time periods.[33] Programs that were based in hospitals increasingly had assigned palliative care beds (266 in 1981 to 767 in 1990). An increase was noted in long-term care facilities and the presence of a broader variety of professionals on the team.[28] Although there are over 600 palliative care services listed in the 1997 directory, the impact of regionalization, with the consolidation of acute care beds and the networking of services within an area, makes it difficult to determine if there is increased growth or an increase in reporting.

The number of programs and surveys does not assist us in knowing the access Canadians have to palliative care, particularly in rural settings. It is generally believed that a small minority of patients, 5%, has access to palliative care services.[13–14] The majority of terminally ill patients die in acute care facilities.[3,19,34]

There is currently a highly variable range of palliative care services development. Four provinces provide guidelines outlining components, or principles of palliative care services. Saskatchewan's guidelines outline a planning procedure and 12 core components for provision of services.[35] Some provinces, such as Manitoba, have specifically identified palliative care as a core health care service that every region must offer. In general, the literature discusses the need for a range of options depending on the needs of the person and his or her family at a particular point in time.[3,33,35] The Report of the Special Senate Committee on Euthanasia and Assisted Suicide (1995) recommended that palliative care programs become a top priority in restructuring the health care system and that there be an integrated approach to palliative care: "The delivery of care, whether in the home, in hospices or institutions, with the support of volunteers, must be coordinated to maximize effectiveness."[14] The Invitational Symposium reinforced the need to be flexible in allowing for episodes of heavy care, with lighter care in between. No one setting is the answer, and there are limits to what can be provided in the home. At the same time, a person may be able to stay home comfortably without the aid of any formal services. An interdisciplinary practice model including volunteers is promoted.[9]

A subcommittee update to the 1995 Special Senate Committee on Euthanasia and Assisted Suicide, released in June 2000, states that in the 5 years since the tabling of the report, little progress has been made in the area of quality end of life care. The new report recommends the federal government, in collaboration with provinces, develop a national strategy for end-of-life care.[36]

Provinces in Canada are in different stages of regionalization of health care services. Palliative care services, which require collaboration for continuity of care, can serve as a model of program of care across sectors. In her report to *Health Canada*, Kristianson (1997) recommends a mixed model, structured as a continuum of care weighted toward home care: ". . . Development of this model would require vigorous home supports, home substitutes for family caregivers respite, day hospices, trained family physicians who are affiliated with home care services. Long term hospice setting in extended care settings, and intensive specialized palliative care units in tertiary care teaching hospitals. Tertiary units would treat patients with complex symptoms and transfer to less intensive settings if stable. The model would include two consultative services: (a) a centralized, consultative service accessible by telephone or written consultation, and (b) a mobile palliative team to provide consultation to rural and remote communities."[2] Some individuals would continue to be cared for in settings where they have received the majority of their care (for example, pediatric settings, renal dialysis units, pediatric, medical units).

Communities with large specialized populations (e.g., persons with acquired immunodeficiency syndrome [AIDS]) may create specialized units. Canada's large rural geography underlines the need for programs to have outreach components. Kristianson and others emphasized that this continuum of care requires infrastructure.

At the Invitational Symposium on Palliative Care: Provincial and Territorial Trends and Issues in Community-Based Programming (1997), provinces generally reported that models were emerging utilizing generic services complemented by specialized services. Model development includes essential components of palliative care such as pain and symptom management, interdisciplinary team, medical consultation, psychosocial/counselling care, spiritual care, volunteer, and bereavement programs.

Four underpinnings in model development are: accessibility, continuity of care, education mandate, and research-based practice. An example of a program utilizing a mixed model in Edmonton, Alberta is presented.

Edmonton Regional Palliative Care Program

The Regional Palliative Care Program for the Capital Health Region in the Edmonton area began in July 1995 following 18 months of planning. Prior to 1995, palliative care consultation was available at two sites, the Misericordia Hospital and the Edmonton General Hospital. Both programs extended into the community through either a home program (distinct from home care) or an outpatient clinic. Palliative home care services have existed in Edmonton since 1985.

The World Health Organization, in its description of planning for services, recommended four types of information to be gathered for service development: (1) number of local deaths to estimate the need, (2) information about the area to define what is changing, (3) information about resources in the area, and (4) data about the adequacy of the resources to meet the need.[10] In Edmonton, the need for a coordinated, integrated palliative care program was based upon 78% of oncology patients dying in acute care hospitals, with an average of more than 20,000 patient days per year. Access to palliative care services was inconsistent and inequitable. In 1992, 290/1341 (22%) of the cancer patients who died that year accessed one of the two available services. The need to develop accessible, cost effective, quality palliative care services within the Edmonton region was identified.

The program was designed in the midst of health care reform in the province of Alberta. Alberta was one of the earliest provinces to restructure health care into regional health authorities and significantly decrease resources for health care. Acute care beds were decreased by 30% (2731 beds in December 1992 verses 1910 beds in January 1999). A community-based program that would decrease the need for acute care beds was a timely and supported proposal for the region. In addition, in 1993, the Alberta government produced guidelines titled *Palliative Care: A Policy Framework*. The document assigned responsibility for palliative care services to the regions, and emphasized a community-based approach within a continuum of care.[37] The region had a clear mandate to provide palliative care services.

The model chosen for the program fit well with the provincial guidelines and is similar to the mixed model described by Kristianson.[2] A community-based model based on a continuum of care shifts the focus of care from acute care to the home and hospice settings. Patients and their families should have access to palliative care services regardless of their care setting. The primary site of care is the home with palliative home care and family physician support. Clearly, a goal of the program is to increase the participation of the family physicians in palliative care and to provide these physicians with adequate support.

An essential component to the acceptance of a regionalized integrated palliative care service was to involve key stakeholders in the planning and implementation of the program. Stakeholders, with the authority to approve changes, were involved in the planning of the program, and formed the basis of the ongoing Regional Palliative Care Advisory Committee (Fig. 1.1). Overall administrative support for the stakeholders to be involved and implement change within their own areas proved essential to the process.

Agreed upon definitions of palliative care and its philosophies were supported (Tables 1.1, 1.2). The goal of the program was to (1) increase access to palliative care services, (2) decrease the number of deaths in acute care facilities and (3) increase participation of the family physician in the care of the terminally ill, and provide the physicians with adequate support. The structure of the program should support patients moving freely within the various components of the regional program.

Program structure

A centralized coordinating office was established with responsibilities to: (1) coordinate the delivery of care, (2) develop standards and common assessment tools (3) identify and advocate for funding, (4) provide education for professionals and the public, (5) coordinate research, (6) educate and support volunteers, (7) identify, coordinate, and encourage the development of bereavement

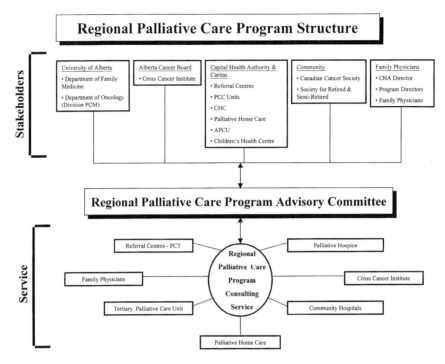

Figure 1.1. Regional palliative care program structure.

Table 1.1. Philosophy guiding the regional palliative care program

- Palliative care specialists (physicians and nurses), by offering support to primary caregivers (family doctors and interdisciplinary caregivers in the community and continuing care) and specialists when appropriate, will assist these people to provide quality palliative care through adherence to sound standards of practice.
- Every individual has the right to participate in informed discussions about the health care resource options that may help to optimize the quality of his or her life during the course of living with a life-threatening illness, especially when dying, and to choose the best possible options based on that information.
- Palliative care strives to meet the physical, psychological, social, and spiritual needs of patients and families, with sensitivity to their personal, cultural, and religious values, beliefs and practices, through patient-directed supportive interventions by an interdisciplinary team of appropriately trained professionals and volunteers.
- Care should be delivered in a patient-focused, family-centered environment.
- A patient or family-driven program contributes to successful achievement of health care outcomes.
- The program will promote interdependence, with each participating organization having both autonomy and accountability for delivering quality, cost-effective palliative care within a coordinated network of services.

Data from Ref. 47.

Table 1.2. Regional palliative care program: criteria for admission

Palliative Care Is:

Active total care offered to a patient with progressive disease and his or her family when it is recognized that the illness is no longer curable, in order to concentrate on the quality of life and the alleviation of distressing symptoms in the framework of a co-ordinated service. Palliative care neither hastens nor postpones death. It provides relief from pain and other distressing symptoms and integrates the psychological and spiritual aspects of care. In addition, it offers a support system to help relatives and friends cope during the patient's illness and bereavement.

(Medical/Nursing/Midwifery Advisory Committee—United Kingdom)

Based upon this definition, all people admitted to the program will:

- be experiencing progressive disease where the focus of care is on comfort, not cure, and improving his or her quality of life
- require active care to alleviate distressing symptoms related to physical, psychosocial, and spiritual needs

Approximately 85%–90% of these people will have a cancer diagnosis.

Admission Criteria to Specific Areas:

Home

- above criteria
- expected length of stay on the program of approximately 3-4 months
- do not require acute or tertiary care
- the ability to provide services within financial resources
- desire for the person or family to be cared for at home

Continuing Care (Hospice)

- above criteria
- cannot be managed at home
- do not require acute or tertiary care
- expected length of stay of approximately 2 months
- over 18 years
- accepting of no code status

Acute Care

- for management of acute medical problems (that is, pathological fracture, bleed, acute respiratory distress)
- anticipated short stay

Tertiary Palliative Care Unit

- severe symptom problems for which management has not been successful in any of the other settings, and requiring intensive management
- expected length of stay of approximately 2 weeks
- over 18 years
- accepting of no code status

Data from Ref. 47.

services, (8) manage the data and identify outcomes, and (9) provide consult teams (nurse or physician) to assist primary caregivers in providing care in the home, the hospice, and continuing care and community hospitals. The regional office liaises with the various levels of palliative care services to coordinate the delivery of services.

To increase access and provide quality palliative care services, multiple points of entry into palliative care were needed in order to address needs along a continuum of care. Four levels of care were identified to provide a continuum of care for patients and families in the region. Criteria of admission for palliative care overall and for each level of care were identified. The criteria have proved invaluable in describing the patient population, and the need for various levels of care given the complex needs of palliative care patients (Table 1.2). In all levels of care, access to consultants is available. However, to provide the shift of care from acute care to the community, increased resources were required in home care and palliative hospice.

Components of care

The following are the major components of the Edmonton Regional Palliative Care Program:

1. Palliative home care services: Palliative care services in the home were already available in the region. Increased funding was allocated to home care for increased delivery of palliative care at home, including 24-hour care. Some respite is provided in the home. Family physicians provide primary medical care for palliative patients in the community. Referrals can be made to a volunteer community day hospice program (Pilgrim's Hospice), or other day and respite programs in the region. Accessible transportation and level of acuity are barriers to patients' using these services.

2. A total of 57 palliative hospice beds in 3 continuing care centers were allocated from existing continuing care level services. The hospices received increase resources for nursing, interdisciplinary teams, and medications. Each of the three hospices has a dedicated nurse manager and 24-hour registered nurse coverage. Enhanced interdisciplinary teams include social work, pastoral care, pharmacy and rehabilitation. Respite care is available in the hospice if a bed is available.

3. Four full-time salaried teams of a consultant nurse and physician were established in order to provide community consultation. An automatic consultation occurs upon admission to a hospice bed. The consultants also serve as the access for palliative hospice beds, triaging, and coordinating admissions.

4. Each referral centers for acute care have nurse and physician teams available for consultation throughout the hospitals. Increased funding was provided to ensure equitable services to both referral centers. Community consultants provide coverage at the community hospitals.

5. The tertiary palliative care unit (14 beds), which existed previous to the regional program, could now focus on admitting patients with the most severe symptoms for which management has not been successful in any other setting.

6. Palliative care codes for physician reimbursement were added in 1994 in Alberta, allowing family physicians to be compensated for longer visits (including the home) required for palliative care assessment, and for family and interdisciplinary formal discussion.

7. A centralized training and support program for volunteers was designed in the first year of operation. Volunteers are members of their own site's volunteer program, with a centralized support and training base. Volunteers in this region do not provide physical care, but provide a multitude of services for patients, families, and staff.

8. A bereavement model was designed utilizing focus groups and staff input. The model outlines the need to identify persons at high risk for complicated bereavement, to provide equitable access to bereavement follow-up through information and telephone, and to identify community resources for bereavement.

9. To provide seamless care for palliative patients, strong links are required with the cancer agency to ensure that discharged patients, or patients no longer receiving curative therapy, are linked to regional palliative resources. A community liaison nurse based at the cancer agency is responsible for assessing all patients discharged who are receiving no further curative treatment. The nurse provides a palliative assessment, utilizing symptom assessment tools used throughout the region, and ensures the patient has a family physician caring for them. The nurse encourages patients to discuss with her or his family physician the physician's ability to provide home visits and on-call coverage 24 hours per day. The nurse maintains and distributes a list of family physicians able to care for palliative patients if the patient is not already linked to a physician. In addition, an interdisciplinary outpatient clinic for consultation of pain and symptom control is available for outpatients at the cancer agency.

10. To provide common language, decrease duplication, and ensure a complete assessment, common patient assessment tools are used by all sites. The following common tools are utilized; the Edmonton Symptom Assessment System,[38] the Mini Mental State Examination,[39,40] the CAGE Questionaire[41,42] and the Edmonton Staging System for cancer pain.[43] All data from the above assessments are entered into a palliative care database.

The program is designed to be evidenced-based and outcome-driven. Guidelines are set on best available research findings. Handbooks of palliative care guidelines are written for family physicians,[44,45] nurses[46] and family caregivers.[47] Outcomes of criteria of admission, availability of consultants, numbers of deaths per setting, and average length of stay were set out at the beginning of the program. The outcomes of the program for each year are compared to the data available during program planning (1992/1993) every year in the annual report of the program.

11. Education: A primary role of the program is to educate both health professionals and the public about palliative care. A model of care based on primary caregivers providing palliative care, with consultant support as necessary, requires initial and ongoing education for nursing, interdisciplinary staff, and family physicians. The average family physician will see 1–2 cancer deaths per year. In the Edmonton region, there are approximately 840 family physicians registered, with approximately 1300 cancer deaths per year. If one supports the continuum of care for patients, allowing physicians to follow their patients during the terminally ill phase, these physicians will require education and support in palliative care.[48,49] Attending physicians are encouraged to provide primary medical care for their patients in the hospice setting.

Consultants provide initial orientation to new staff working directly in any of the palliative care sites. Ongoing inservices, palliative care rounds and city wide rounds, community bus rounds (biweekly),[50] workshops, annual retreat for palliative care staff, and an annual palliative care conference (350 registrants in 1998) are provided. Standardization of teaching material is occurring, with the availability of audiovisual teaching aids and handouts about common palliative care topics.

12. Research: All physicians work within the Division of Palliative Medicine and therefore have clear expectations for education and research. The tertiary palliative care unit is designed as both an intense clinical, educational, and research unit for all disciplines. Family medicine residents rotate to the unit for 2 weeks, also going out into the community with the community consultants. There is an accredited conjoint Postgraduate Program in Palliative Medicine (College of Family Physicians and Royal College of Physicians and Surgeons of Canada), based on the tertiary unit. This unit frequently trains physicians from many settings for varying lengths of time. Because of common standards and ethics reviews, research studies are now easier to expand beyond the tertiary unit into other palliative care settings.

13. A palliative care database, created prior to the start of the program for the tertiary unit, was adapted to allow data entry from all levels of care. A dedicated database was considered essential for program planning and quality control. Patient demographics, clinical data (diagnosis, symptom assessment, Edmonton Staging Symptom (ESS), CAGE Questionnaire Mini Mental State Examination (MMSE), comfort assessment, and data describing the movement of patients through the program (referred from, discharged to, hospice preference site) are recorded. The referring physician is listed to gather information on the number and type of physicians referring patients. A data manager is responsible for quality control and reporting. All areas of the program, except home care, are presently entering data (acute care collects patients referred for palliative care consultation only). Home care began data entry in 1999.

Outcomes

An increase in access to palliative care services as measured by palliative care consultation was significant. During 1992, 290/1341 (21%) patients accessed a palliative care consult team compared to 1110/1326 (84%) in 1996 and 1070/1229 (87%) during 1997 ($p < 0.0001$ overall). The numbers of cancer patients access-

Table 1.3. Number of cancer deaths by site of death in the Edmonton Region (Capital Health Authority)

Place of death[b]	1992/1993[a] (%)	1994/1995[a] (%)	1996/1997[a] (%)	p
Acute care facilities[c]	1119 (86)	877 (71)	633 (49)	<0.0001
Palliative hospices	0	0	378 (30)	<0.0001
Continuing care centers[d]	53 (4)	96 (8)	38 (3)	<0.0001
Home	126 (10)	259 (21)	227 (18)	<0.0001
Other	6 (—)	8 (1)	3 (—)	=0.299
Total	1304 (100)	1240 (100)	1279 (100)	

[a] Based on fiscal year of April 1–March 31.
[b] Data from Alberta Cancer Registry except for Palliative Hospices data from Edmonton Regional Palliative Care data base. Data from the Alberta Cancer Registry are provisional as some deaths may be registered in subsequent years.
[c] All acute care hospitals in Capital Health Region, tertiary palliative care unit, and cancer center.
[d] Includes all continuing care level facilities such as nursing homes and auxiliary hospitals.

ing services were gathered from the records of the existing palliative care services in 1992, and from the program database in 1996 and 1997.

The total number of cancer deaths per year is reported from the Alberta Cancer Registry by site of care. Cancer deaths occurring in acute care facilities decreased significantly between 1992/1993 and 1996/1997. Table 1.3 describes the number and location of cancer deaths in acute care (tertiary, community, and cancer hospitals), palliative hospices, continuing care facilities (all levels including nursing home, and auxiliary) and in the home between 1992/1993 and 1996/1997. Primarily the shift in care was to palliative hospices and to the home.

Average length of stay in acute care also decreased significantly over the same time period (Table 1.4). The cancer center is a separate region from the acute care facilities in the Edmonton region and is therefore reported separately. The decrease in acute care deaths and in length of stay significantly decreased the number of acute care patient days.

The corresponding decrease in costs for palliative care in the use of palliative hospice beds at $161.70/day (1996/1997) and home care (costs not available) versus acute care medical beds $508/day (Department of Finance, Capital Health Authority) is significant, given the shift of care to hospice. However, further research is required to show actual cost savings realized, particularly costing of care in the home (including the shift of care to family caregivers).

Another indicator for the program is the number of physicians who consulted the program each year. During 1996/1997, 372 distinct physicians referred patients to consultants. Family physicians represented 77% (287) of all physicians referring. Of the 840 family physicians registered in the Edmonton region, 35% referred to the program. In 1996, 240/268 (89%) of palliative care cancer patients discharged from the cancer center chose to stay with their family physician, when asked if they wanted to change, or had no designated physician. For the 28 patients who requested a new family physician, one was found within 24

Table 1.4. Length of stay and number of patient days of last hospitalization before death in the Edmonton Region (Capital Health Authority)

	1992/1993[a]	1996/1997[a]	1997/1998[a]	p
Acute Care Hospital[b]				
Total number of deaths (%)[c]	825 (63%)	403 (32%)	373[d]	<0.0001
Mean length of stay in days (± SD)[e]	27 ± 16	15 ± 7	16 ± 7[f]	<0.0001
Total number of patient days	22,608	6,085	6,036	N/A
Cancer Center[g]				
Total number of deaths (%)[c]	130 (10%)	95 (7%)	115[d]	0.02
Mean length of stay in days (± SD)[e]	15 ± 21	9 ± 10	11 ± 11[h]	<0.005
Total number of patient days	1,958	875	1,275	NA

[a] Based on fiscal years April 1–March 31.
[b] Data from Capital Health Authority: Evaluation, Information, and Research.
[c] Percentage of cancer deaths in acute care over total number of cancer deaths in region.
[d] p value not possible for 1997/1998 because the proportion of acute care deaths over total number of deaths is not available.
[e] SD, Standard deviation.
[f] p < 0.0001 for 1992/1993 versus 1997/1998.
[g] Data from Cross Cancer Institute, Health Records (cancer center).
[h] p = 0.059 for 1992/1993 versus 1997/1998.

hours from the list of 150 physicians who volunteered to take care of new patients.[51]

A survey of family physicians was completed in 1999. A return of 39% (327/840) was received following two mail outs. Of the returned surveys, 72% (234) had referred to the program, and 35% (113) had cared for a patient in a hospice setting. There was strong agreement (6 or 7 on 7-point likert scale) that the palliative care physician consult improves patient care (83%), and helps a patient be cared for in their preferred setting (82%).

Outcomes by level of care

The establishment of outcome criteria prior to the initiation of the program was helpful in describing the direction, effect, and changes expected throughout all areas in the health care system in the region for palliative care. The collection and data entry of clinical data about the patient's symptoms assists us in monitoring the clinical status of the patient population.

Table 1.5 describes clinical outcomes for the levels of care. Specific data for home care patients are not available for the time period reported. Clinical data from consultant referrals do occur in the home (47%), but refer to a more severe population within the home, since a consultation had been requested. The outcomes for each level of care are discussed below:

1. The tertiary palliative care unit, as one of two sites to access palliative care in 1992, cared for 168 patients that year. The change expected in a regionalized

Table 1.5. Clinical outcomes[a] by site of care for patients discharged November 1, 1997–October 31, 1998

Site of care	TPCU[b]	Acute care[c]	Hospice[d]	Consultant[e]	Chi square
Number of Patients	163	664	499	924	
Age (mean ± SD)[f]	61.5 ± 13.9	68.6 ± 14.3	72.3 ± 12.6	70.6 ± 13.1	
CAGE[g]	26 (34/129)	11 (69/605)	N/A	21 (128/604)	$p < 0.0001$
Pain Stage 2 (ESS)[h]	64 (81/126)	34 (207/603)	N/A	N/A	$p < 0.0001$
Pain %[i]	57 (89/156)	32 (207/603)	36 (145/407)	54 (326/566)	$p < 0.0001$
Activity %	70 (107/154)	77 (483/624)	59 (254/431)	85 (471/564)	$p < 0.0001$
Nausea %	24 (37/152)	11 (69/636)	15 (55/368)	20 (115/571)	$p < 0.0001$
Depression %	43 (64/148)	28 (159/573)	29 (113/391)	36 (177/497)	$p = 0.0004$
Anxiety %	53 (81/152)	31 (178/583)	31 (125/403)	41 (199/490)	$p < 0.0001$
Drowsiness %	53 (81/154)	45 (282/621)	49 (204/417)	56 (308/548)	$p = 0.0026$
Appetite %	66 (121/152)	70 (431/617)	60 (257/428)	70 (386/551)	$p < 0.0001$
Wellbeing %	61 (89/147)	50 (270/540)	46 (184/404)	68 (256/379)	$p < 0.0001$
Shortness of Breath %	29 (45/153)	30 (132/630)	22 (88/393)	32 (177/560)	$p < 0.0001$
MMSE %[j]	40 (57/143)	39 (239/606)	58 (152/324)	28 (139/503)	$p < 0.0001$

[a] Data from Regional Palliative Care Program.

[b] Tertiary Palliative Care Unit.

[c] Patients referred for palliative consultations in tertiary referral centres: Royal Alexandra and University of Alberta Hospitals.

[d] Includes 57 palliative hospice beds.

[e] Patients referred for palliative consultation in community and community hospitals. Unique data for palliative home care not available.

[f] Mean ± standard deviation.

[g] Percentage of patients with positive CAGE Questionaire (≥2/4), indicating risk for chemical coping.

[h] Pain Stage: percentage of patients with pain stage 2 or 3, indicating poor prognosis for pain management, as measured by the Edmonton Staging System (ESS) for cancer pain.

[i] Score ≥ 5 for 0–10 ESAS (Edmonton Symptom Assessment Scale) indicating severe symptom for patient. First ESAS completed at site.

[j] Abnormal Mini-Mental Stage Examination (MMSE) ≤ 80% of answers correct. First MMSE completed at site. Indicator for cognitive impairment.

program, with enhanced community palliative care, was that the unit would care for more patients, address complex symptoms, and then discharge the patient to the most appropriate setting, resulting in a shorter length of hospital stay. Slightly fewer patients would die on the tertiary unit, since other options for palliative care would exist.

In 1997, the number of patients and the length of stay did not decrease. However, as options for admission to the most appropriate setting of care existed, the acuity of the patients admitted to the unit was higher. There will continue to be a subset of patients on the unit with higher acuity and poor coping mechanisms who will remain on the unit, as no other site of care can provide acute enough management (Table 1.5). The patients are younger (average age 62 versus 72 in the hospices) with a higher incidence of stage 3 pain (72%) indicating a poorer prognosis for pain management. Positive CAGE Questionaire scores are higher (26% versus 14% for acute care consultants), indicating poor coping mechanisms on this unit.

The patients on the tertiary unit have significantly higher scores of all symptoms measured by the ESAS. Table 1.5 outlines the first measurement of ESAS scores at the different levels of care. Because of the large number of corrections of comparison, the correction factor of Bonferroni was used. A score of 0.004 was accepted as significant.

2. Acute Care Hospitals: Palliative care nurse/physician consult teams in the two large referral hospitals provided consultation for 656 cases in 1997. These consultants tend to see patients earlier in their illness trajectory and provide skilled advice in symptom management, communication and discharge planning. In 1996/1997, 36% of patients were discharged home, 18% to hospice, 8% to the tertiary unit, 18% to other sites and 20% died.[47]

3. Palliative Hospice: The largest shift of care was the transfer of patients into the palliative hospices, the majority coming from the home (41%) and from acute care (38%). The average length of stay was much shorter than anticipated (42 verses 66 days). With a median length of stay of 22 days, half the patients were staying for short periods, increasing the acuity for the hospices. There were increased admissions, family conferences and preparation for death. Occupancy of the hospice beds was 92% in 1996/97.[52] This number allows for rapid admission to the hospices as required. As expected, incidence of cognitive impairment is highest in this setting (Table 1.5), and is often listed as a primary reason for admission.

4. Home: A small shift of care has occurred in cancer deaths occurring at home, much lower than the planned 40% (126 versus 227, an increase of 8% from 1992 to 1996). Further enhancements to palliative home care continue to occur in delivery of care. Access to lab and medication (community pharmacies available 24 hours/day, and will courier medications) have been resolved. It is unclear to what extent the availability of hospice bed influences patient and family choices for a home death. Hinton (1994)[17] describes how the availability of hospice beds permitted more confident perseverance at home, where people received 90% of the palliative care. However, further research is needed to determine to what extent patients and families prefer a home death in a regionalized system of palliative care, with palliative hospice available, as they move within a continuum of care.

Consultants are available to visit patients in the community. Consultants also support home care case managers through telephone consultation and education. Beginning February 1, 1999, the Alberta government introduced a palliative care drug plan that provides immediate medication coverage for those patients (primarily under 65 without health insurance) who do not have a drug plan.

Discussion

The outcomes outlined at the beginning of the program have generally been met in the first 3 years of operation. Access to palliative care, as measured by palliative care consultation, increased significantly, to 87% of cancer patients. The program is not exclusive to oncology (Table 1.2); patients with other diagnosis who require active palliative care to alleviate their symptoms are cared for and admitted to the program. In 1996/1997, 8.2% of patients' primary diagnoses were other than cancer. This does not include home care, which has a higher proportion of other diagnoses. However, the cancer population is used to determine outcomes because it is a population that is definable and most prevalent. The definition of palliative care, particularly in acute care facilities is not consistent. The population seen by the program is definable, but not every palliative care patient requires consultation and is therefore not recorded in the program database.

Data are collected from the Information Office for the region, the Capital Health Authority, on overall cancer deaths in acute care facilities. Data are also collected from the Cross Cancer Institute given that the Edmonton cancer center has inpatient oncology beds. (Table 1.4). Table 1.3 shows a discrepancy in the number of cancer deaths reported by the Alberta Cancer Registry and the Capital Health Authority for both the 1992/1993 and 1996/1997. This difference noted is 955 and 498 for the 1992/1993 and 1996/1997 period from the Capital Health Authority, verses 1119 and 633 for 1992/1993 and 1996/1997 for the Alberta Cancer Registry. The difference is most likely because of different methodologies of definition of cause of death (admission and discharge summaries verses death certificates). However, using either data source, a large and significant decrease in the number of cancer deaths has occurred in acute care facilities.

The model of care utilizing the family physician as the primary caregiver, with consultant support, is the most common and realistic in a regionalized model of care. However, involvement of the family physicians throughout the continuum of care, when care is shifted to the community, results in increased involvement of family physicians in both simple and complex cases. Issues of reimbursement, education, and a willingness to provide home or hospice visits and 24-hour coverage need to be addressed. Involvement of 35% of the family physicians per year, and more than 600 distinct physicians since the program began 3.5 years ago suggests family physicians are providing palliative care. Ongoing and creative methods of education are required, given that the average family physicians will only see 1–2 patients per year with a cancer death population of approximately 1300/year. Data collection is ongoing in determining what percentage of physicians follow patients into hospice settings. Determination of family physicians willing to care for new patients and measurement of physician satisfaction with palliative consultant and care options must be ongoing indicators of the program. Initial family and physician satisfaction was positive following 1 year of operation.[53] The survey of family physicians completed in 1999 supported the role of physician consultants in improving patient care.

Patient and family satisfaction data are collected at some settings within the program, but there is need for a unified measurement of satisfaction from both

patients and family. This very important indicator will add to the overall outcomes of the program.

A primary outcome of any program is the clinical outcome of care. In palliative care, this is a comparison of symptom management from prior to initiation of the program to the present. Issues of access and site of death, although
important, are put into context by the clinical indicators of good symptom
management. Unfortunately, this comparison is not possible since data collection on symptom management in the acute care facilities, where most of the
deaths were occurring in 1992/1993, did not occur. Today, measurement of
symptom distress is recorded on patients referred to consultants in acute
care, but not on every palliative care patient. The other issue for palliative
care is the interpretation of symptom measurement in a population where
clinical deterioration is the expected course.[24,29,54] This issue can only be
confirmed in prospective studies assessing physical and psychological symptom
management.

The criteria for admission and model design for the Edmonton area program
has attempted to clearly articulate the patient population and options for
care, based on patient need and preference (Table 1.2). This assists any type
of program in planning for resources and measuring outcomes, particularly in
palliative care, where definitions and standards of care are still developing
consensus. As recent literature in Canada and elsewhere discusses the need
for palliative care earlier in the illness trajectory[54,55] and to increase access of
palliative care beyond oncology,[6] the Edmonton area program continues to
discuss and define its mandate in relation to this particular community and
patient population.

Conclusion

The Edmonton Regional Palliative Care Program is one example of model development in a regionalized program using both generic services complemented by
specialized services. Other programs throughout Canada have developed to meet
the needs of their communities. Many programs have begun the process of
regionalized program of care only in the last few years. The process and results
of consensus building toward national definitions and standards in palliative care
continue to influence the direction and comprehensiveness of palliative care services in Canada.

Acknowledgment

The authors greatly appreciate the statistical and editorial assistance from Catherine Neumann, M.
Sc., Division of Palliative Medicine, University of Alberta.

References

1. Doyle D, Hanks G, MacDonald N. Introduction. In: Doyle D, Hanks G, MacDonald N, eds. *Oxford Textbook of Palliative Medicine*. New York: Oxford University Press, 1998:3–8.
2. Kristianson L. Generic versus specific palliative care services. Final report. Health Care and Issue Division Systems for Health Directorate. *Health Canada*, 1997.
3. Wilson DM, Anderson MC, Fainsinger RL. Social and health trends influencing palliative care and the location of death in twentieth-century Canada. Final Report. *Health Canada. National Health and Research Development Program, 1998.*
4. Doyle D, Hanks G, MacDonald N. The provision of palliative care. In: Doyle D, Hanks G, MacDonald N, eds. *Oxford Textbook of Palliative Medicine*. New York: Oxford University Press, 1998:3–8.
5. Report to Cancer 2000 task force. The Expert Panel on Palliative Care, 1991.
6. Ferris FD, Cummings I, eds. *Palliative Care: Towards a Consensus in Standardized Principles of Practice. First Phase Working Document*. Ottawa Ontario: Canadian Palliative Care Association, 1995.
7. Report of the working group on special services in hospitals. *Palliative Care Services in Hospitals, Guidelines*. Ottawa, Ontario: National Health and Welfare Canada, 1981.
8. Report of the subcommittee on institutional program guidelines. *Guidelines for Establishing Standards. Palliative-Care Services*. Ottawa, Ontario: Health and Welfare Canada, 1989.
9. LaPerriere B. Proceedings of the invitational symposium on palliative care: provincial and territorial trends and issues in community-based programming. *Health Canada. Health System and Policy Division*. 1997.
10. World Health Organization. *Palliative Cancer Care: Policy Statement Base on Recommendations of a WHO Consultation*. Leeds, February 1987. Copenhagen. World Health Organization, 1989.
11. Canadian Palliative Care Association. Board of Directors. *Avisco* 1999; Spring 27:2.
12. Task Force on the Allocation of Health Care Resources of the Canadian Medical Association (Watson J, chair). Health, a need for redirection. Ottawa: Canadian Medical Association, 1983.
13. Scott JF. Palliative care 2000: mapping the interface with cancer control. *J Pall Care* 1992; 8(1):13–16.
14. Of Life and Death. Report of the Special Senate Committee on Euthanasia and Assisted Suicide. Ottawa: *Senate of Canada*. 1995.
15. Chochinov HM, Kristianson L. Dying to pay: the cost of end-of-life care. *J Pall Care* 1998; 14(4):5–15.
16. Emanuel EJ. Cost savings at the end of life. What do the data show? *JAMA* 1996; 274(24):1907–1914.
17. Goodwin PJ. Economic factors in cancer palliation—methodological considerations. *Cancer Treat Reviews* 1993; 19:59–65.
18. Hinton J. Can home care maintain an acceptable quality of life for patients with terminal cancer and their relatives? *Pall Med* 1994; 8:183–196.
19. McWhinney IR, Bass MJ, Orr V. Factors associated with location of death (home or hospital) of patients referred to a palliative care team. *Can Med Assoc J* 1995; 152(3):361–367.

20. Cantwell P, Turio S, Brenneis C, et al. Predictors of home death in palliative care cancer patients. *J Pall Care* 2000; 16(1):23–28.

21. Downing GM, Braithwaite DL, Wilde JM. Victoria BGY model—a new model for the 1990's. *J Pall Care* 1993:26–32.

22. Lindop E, Beach R, Read S. A composite model of palliative care for the UK. *Int J Pall Nurs* 1997; 3(5):287–292.

23. Stjernsward J, Colleau SM, Ventafridda V. The World Health Organization cancer pain and palliative care program past, present and future. *J Pain Symptom Manage* 1996; 12(2):65–72.

24. Broadfield L. Evaluation of palliative care: current status and future directions. *J Pall Care* 1988; 4(3):21–28.

25. Maltoni M, Travaglini C, Santi M. Evaluation of the cost of home care for terminally ill cancer patients. *Supp Care Canc* 1997; 5:396–401.

26. Scott JF. Palliative care 2000: what's stopping us? *J Pall Care* 1992; 8(1):5–8.

27. Munn B, Worobec F. Data collection as the first step in program development: the experience of a chronic care palliative unit. *J Pall Care* 1997; 13(2):39–42.

28. Cummings Ajemian I. Palliative Care in Canada: 1990. *J Pall Care* 1990; 6(4):47–58.

29. Jarvis H, Burge FI, Scott CA. Evaluating a palliative care program: methodology and limitations. *J Pall Care* 1996; 12(2):23–33.

30. Degner LF, Henteleff PD, Ringer C. The relationship between theory and Measurement in evaluations of palliative care services. *J Pall Care* 1987; 3(2):8–13.

31. Ferris FD, Adams D, Balfour HM, et al. How close are we to consensus? A report on the first cycle of the national consensus-building process to develop national standards of practice for palliative care in Canada. Ottawa, Ontario: *Canadian Palliative Care Association* 1999.

32. Canada Health Act. 1984., c. 6, s. 1. pp. 1–12.

33. O'Donnell NM. A regional approach to palliative care services. *J Pall Care* 1992; 8(1):43–46.

34. Bruera E, Neumann C, Gagnon B, et al. Edmonton Regional Palliative Care Program: impact on patterns of terminal Cancer Care. *Can Med Assoc J* 1999; 161:290–293.

35. *Guidelines for Developing an Integrated Palliative Care Service*. Saskatchewan Health. April 1994.

36. Quality End-of-Life care: The right of every Canadian. Subcommittee to update "of life and death" of the Standing Senate Committee on Social Affairs, Science and Technology. *Senate of Canada* June, 2000
http://www.parl.gc.ca/36/2/parlbus . . . m-e/upda-e/rep-e/repfinjun00-e.htm.

37. *Palliative Care: A Policy Framework*. Alberta Health. December 1993.

38. Bruera E, Kuehn N, Miller MJ, et al. The Edmonton symptom assessment system (ESAS): a simple method for the assessment of palliative care patients. *J Palliat Care* 1991; 7(2):6–9.

39. Folstein MF, Fetting J, Labo A, et al. Cognitive assessment of cancer patients. *Cancer* 1984; 53(suppl 10):2250–2257.

40. Bruera E, Miller MJ, McCallion J, et al. Cognitive failure (CF) in patients with terminal cancer: a prospective study. *J Pain Symptom Manage* 1992; 7:192–195.

41. Bruera E, Moyano J, Seifert L, et al. The frequency of alcoholism among patients with pain due to terminal cancer. *J Pain Symptom Manage* 1995; 10(8):599–603.

42. Moore R, Bone L, Geller G, et al. Prevalence, detection and treatment of alcoholism in hospitalized patients. *JAMA* 1989; 261:403–407.

43. Bruera E, Macmillan K, Hanson J, MacDonald RN. The Edmonton staging system for cancer pain. Preliminary report. *Pain* 1989; 37:203–209.

44. Pereira J, Bruera E. The Edmonton Aid to Palliative Care. Edmonton: *Regional Palliative Care Program*, 1998.

45. Pereira J, Otfinowski P, et al. eds. Alberta Palliative Care Resource, Edmonton, *Alberta Cancer Board*, 1999.

46. Brenneis C, Perry B, Read-Paul L, et al. 99 common questions (and answers) about palliative care: a nurses' handbook. Edmonton: *Regional Palliative Care Program*, 1998.

47. MacMillan K, Peden J, Hycha D, et al. eds. A Caregiver's guide A handbook about end of life care. *Palliative Care Association of Alberta*, 2000.

48. Fainsinger RL, Bruera E, Macmillan K. Innovative palliative care in Edmonton. *Can Fam Physician* 1997; 43:1983–1992.

49. Brenneis C, Bruera E. The interaction between family physicians and palliative care consultants in the delivery of palliative care: clinical and educational issues. *J Palliat Care* 1998; 14(3):58–61.

50. Bruera E, Selmser P, Pereira J, Brenneis C. Bus rounds for palliative care education in the community. *Can Med Assoc J* 1997; 157(6):729–732.

51. Kanji T, Hanson J, Bruera E. Community liaison for terminally ill patients discharged from a cancer center. *Support Care Cancer* 1996; 4(3):240.

52. Regional Palliative Care Program. Annual Report April 1, 1996 to March 31, 1997. *Capital Health Authority*. Edmonton, Alberta. 1997.

53. Alberta Management Group. An evaluation of the Regional Palliative Care Program—Final Report. Prepared for the Capital Health Authority. Edmonton: Alberta Management Group, 1996.

54. O'Neill WM, O'Connor P, Latimer EJ. Hospital palliative care services: three models in three countries. *J Pain Symptom Manage* 1992; 7(7):406–413.

55. Dudgeon DJ, Raubertas RF, Doerner K, et al. When does palliative care begin? A needs assessment of cancer patients with recurrent disease. *J Pall Care* 1995; 11(1):5–9.

2

Models for the Delivery of Palliative Care:
The Spanish Model

CARLOS CENTENO AND
MARCOS GÓMEZ-SANCHO

Before describing the model of palliative care in Spain, it is necessary to give a brief description of the country's current health care model. Our country has approximately 40 million inhabitants. The public health system offers universal access and is publicly financed. In accordance with the constitutional principle of territorial decentralization in the healthcare field, public health services and functions have been transferred from central government to 7 of the 17 Autonomous Regions, affecting some 62% of the country's population.[1] The Instituto Nacional de Salud (INSALUD), the central government's public body directly responsible for providing health care services, covers more than 14 million citizens. In the rest of the country, health care is in the hands of the so-called Regional Health Systems, rather than the INSALUD. In these regions, care is provided within the same public framework and is free of charge.

When analyzing health problems in Spain there is not just one health care scenario. We are experiencing a decentralizing process now and the public health situation is diverse.

We should be quite clear that the Spanish public health system enjoys a high technical and human level, and is at least at the same level as that of the other European countries. It is also true, however, that all European countries that have incorporated what we know as the "Welfare State" into their social policy are experiencing financial and management problems that affect health care policy overall. This explains some difficulties in incorporating new solutions and approaches to health care problems. It is because of these problems, of decentralization and of management, that palliative medicine in Spain has found it difficult to move forward in its proposals for new kinds of care for advanced-stage cancer patients and those with other terminal illnesses.

Nevertheless, our traditions and culture have helped us overcome these structural difficulties. Palliative medicine in Spain, as is reflected in numerous works of art,[2] from Velazquez to Picasso, has continued a long history of humanistic doctors. One can also appreciate the influence of Catholic-inspired organizations that have always worked with the sick and the dying. The deeply rooted family structure in our society, the Mediterranean culture with people of open, communicative character, are factors that have influenced the rapid development of palliative medicine in Spain.

The Beginnings of Palliative Medicine in Spain

Doctors and nurses have always been involved with palliative medicine in Spain. It was in the 1980s that some professionals became aware that there existed an alternative way of tending to terminal phase patients using specifically trained and dedicated teams. As true pioneers, individuals sought training and emerged knowing more of the true situation. With the risk of overlooking a fair number of them, we cite Jaime Sanz Ortiz, Marcos Gómez Sancho, Juan Manuel Núñez Olarte, Xavier Gómez Batiste, Antonio Pascual, Pilar Torrubia, Josep Porta, and others.

Professor Sanz Ortiz, an oncologist, undertook a trip to London in 1984 to see the work of some of the London hospices. On his return, he incorporated the palliative care philosophy into the Oncology Department where he was working in Santander. In 1984, Sanz Ortiz published the first study in the Spanish language on the topic of the terminal patient.[3] Professor Sanz has worked ceaselessly all over Spain, transmitting his enthusiasm for this for way of working.

In 1986 and 1987, J. Porta, a specialist in internal medicine, and X. Gómez, an oncologist, both spent time at St. Christopher's Hospice in London. In December of 1987, Gómez and J. Roca set up the Palliative Care Unit at the Santa Creu Hospital, in Vic (Barcelona). In 1989, Porta established a Palliative Care Unit at the Cruz Roja Hospital in Lleida.

In 1989, M. Gómez, an anesthetist, founded the Palliative Medicine Unit in Las Palmas de Gran Canaria, after a time spent in Milan with Professor Ventafridda. The El Sabinal Hospital of Las Palmas in the Canary Islands, as we shall see further on, has generously hosted many of those professionals who today work in palliative care. It has also been like a beacon in the field of palliative care, enlightening the work in the rest of the country.

In 1990, Dr. Nuñez Olarte, an internist, traveled to the Royal Victoria Hospital in Montreal, and had the opportunity of working with B. Mount. In 1991, he worked toward the founding of Spain's largest and busiest Palliative Care Unit at the Gregorio Marañón Hospital in Madrid. The service maintains important links with diverse Latin American countries.

These more personal individual initiatives gave rise to actions organized by the health authorities. The most important of these was that of X. Gómez, in

Catalonia, a region in North East Spain. This was the Catalonian Palliative Care Planning and Implementation Pilot Program, 1990–1995.[4] This program has been vital to the development of palliative medicine not only in Catalonia, but also in the rest of Spain and in Europe. It is a World Health Organization (WHO) pilot that gave successful, wide range solutions to the incorporation of palliative care into the public health system, both in home care and in the hospitals of the public network. With the Catalonian programs, many other teams have had a model to follow, or more accurately, a model to adapt to their own regional characteristics. More recently, in 1998, a Regional Program of Palliative Medicine was approved in Castilla y León. It is in this very region, the largest in Europe, that modern techniques of telemedicine are being applied to training, information, and clinical support for the teams who work with terminal patients. In Valencia, on the Mediterranean Coast, a number of planning measures have been adopted and in the Canary Islands, a strategy was designed in 1998 in an attempt to spread the work of the El Sabinal center from Gran Canaria to the rest of the Islands. The INSALUD, the central administration, has, up to now, adopted only discrete local measures in some health districts in Madrid, Spain's capital city. It has tolerated, and not without difficulties, the development of other new programs in the rest of the nation.

Two institutions, the Spanish Association Against Cancer (Asociación Española Contra El Cáncer [AECC]) and The Orden de los Hermanos Hospitalarios de San Juan de Dios (Saint John's Religious Order of Hospital Brothers), have also done much to earn the title of pioneers in the field of palliative medicine in Spain. In 1991, the AECC, a nongovernmental organization, launched its first Home Care Mobile Unit for terminal patients. This model has spread to the rest of Spain and the work of the AECC must be recognized for its merits in helping the early stages of palliative medicine in many provinces of Spain. The AECC provided resources and personnel to work with terminal patients. Many more complete programs in a number of areas, working within the public health network has come from this.

The Order of St. John holds as its philosophy the treatment of all kinds of patients in its hospitals, with special interest in those with chronic degenerative illnesses and other processes that mark the patient, such as the terminal phase. In 1991, J. Viguría established the first Palliative Care Unit at St. John's Hospital in the city of Pamplona near to the Pyrennees. The work is carried out through agreements with the public health authorities.

In 1997 and 1998, a number of private palliative care programs were launched in cities such as Seville, Barcelona, and Madrid. In these cases, it is the patient, or his or her insurance company, who pays for care in the terminal phase. It is still too early to know whether this type of initiative will prosper. Nevertheless, current data show that even for countries such as Spain with a public health care system, there is still room for private programs offering high quality attention, excellent scientific quality, and the flexibility to adapt to the needs of the patient and his or her family whether in the hospital or at home.

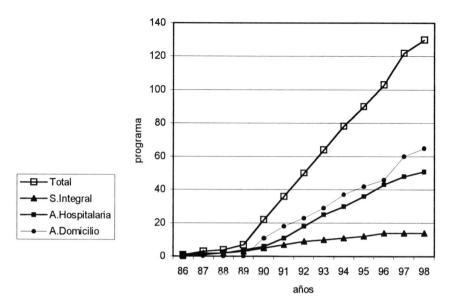

Figure 2.1. Palliative Care Programs, Spain 1986–1998 (data from 130/143 programs).

It is not possible here to give a complete picture of palliative medicine in Spain. Others offer more data and have dealt with the history and initial development of palliative medicine in Spain.[5–9] To summarize, it is enough to state that palliative medicine has been the result of personal efforts in the majority of cases, and has enjoyed neither planning nor financing of public health institutions. Great advances are to be expected once the health administration starts to move and contributes to what now seems inevitable.

Palliative Care Programs in Spain

Two national studies have evaluated the care for terminal patients as part of palliative care programs. The latest was published in May 1998 and gathers activity data for those programs running in January 1998.[10,11] From the data presented in the 1998 Directory, it can deduced that at least 25,000 patients are attended by specific palliative care teams each year in Spain. To obtain a clearer perspective of the real meaning of this figure, we should point out that each year some 80,000 people die of cancer in Spain and approximately 20,000 patients, or 25%, are cared for in their final months through some sort of palliative care program.

In 1998, there were 143 teams working in palliative care in Spain. Figure 2.1 shows the evolution of palliative care programs, showing constant growth since 1986.[12] There are three main types of programs: integral systems, programs for hospitalized patients, and home care programs. Table 2.1 shows the number of

Table 2.1. Palliative care programs in Spain in 1998 and activity in the last year

Programs	Identified N	Responses N	%	Activity communicated N	%	Cancer patients attended in 1997° N	%	Total patients attended en 1997° N
Integral systems[+]	15	14	93	14	93	5,281	85	6,214
Hospitalized patients	53	52	98	41	77	8,378	90	9,298
Home-based Patients	75	62	83	50	67	6,307	69	9,182
Total	143	128	89	106	74	19,996	81	24,694

° Non exclusive data.

[+] An integral system is one that involves patient attention at different levels—acute care hospitals, medium, or long-term stays and home-based—within the same coordinated program.

Source: SECPAL Directory of Palliative Care Programs, 1988.

teams and gives an idea of their relative activity. Integral care systems are programs that address the full range of patient needs. They are based usually in an acute care center, which acts as coordinator and houses the support teams that attend the patient once he or she is discharged and sent home. When the patient has additional social problems or when a longer stay with less technical assistance is required, the integral system should offer the possibility of admittance to a medium or long-term stay center. To name but a few, this method is followed by the teams of the Catalonian Oncology Institute, from the Duran i Reynals Hospital, the El Sabinal Hospital program, coordinated with home care offered by the AECC and the regional health system, and the program of the Virgen de la Poveda Hospital, which offers a support center for medium-term stays, the acute care center with AECC teams, and coordination of a health center. We might say that this would be the ideal most local solution. In Spain there is a great administrative separation between specialized attention, generally based in hospital centers, and primary health care teams. Although there may be a number of advantages in other aspects, for advanced stage patients the conflicts and confusion produced by this separation and the resulting lack of coordination between the two areas represent a serious inconvenience. At times, the patient may find him or herself in no-man's land, where it is not clear as to who is responsible for providing him or her with health care.

The integral systems have the advantage of providing flexibility in care and resource integration. At the present time, the lack of planning means that we only have integral systems in Catalonia and in certain other areas.

In Spain, a wide network of hospitals is oriented toward high technology care for diagnosis or treatment. In these centers, designed for acute patients, there are hospital support teams similar to those that have existed in other countries,

Table 2.2. Activity of palliative care programs for hospitalized patients, Spain 1998

Type of center	Hospitals for acute patients		Medium- or long-term stay centers		Total hospitalized units	
	N	Units evaluated (%)	N	Units evaluated (%)	N	Units evaluated (%)
Programs Identified	32	32 (100)	36	34 (94)	68	66 (97)
No. of cases	9,523	27 (84)	5,989	29 (81)	15,512	55 (81)
No. of cases with cancer	9,173	27 (84)	4,497	29 (81)	13,671	56 (82)
% of cancer	96	27 (84)	75	29 (81)	88	55 (81)
Total number of beds	283	25 (71)	529	30 (83)	812	55 (81)
Average stay	10.7	25 (78)	26.3	26 (72)	16.9	51 (75)
Average survival	37.5	20 (62)	30.4	22 (61)	33.6	42 (62)

Source: Data from the SECPAL Directory 1998: Not all the programs gave figures in all the sections.

such as Canada or England, for a number of years. These are programs based on advisory teams that do not have their own beds assigned, but rather, monitor situations where and when needed and that then continue in an advisory role, coordinating patient care on discharge. They may be autonomous, or they may be based in other departments, generally oncology, internal medicine, or in a palliative care unit. This is an ideal solution for large hospitals and has been shown to be efficient in other countries. The model has been applied successfully in Catalonia. The greatest difficulty in expanding this model is that the tradition simply does not exist in our health care system.

Up to now, in the large centers, working specifically with terminal stage patients has been based on the creation of a physical structure with its own beds and space. Some characteristics of the hospital programs are detailed in Table 2.2. There are 32 acute care hospitals with palliative programs under way. In the 300 beds belonging to these units, the majority of the patients have advanced cancer and the average stay is short, generally around 10 days.

The support hospitals for medium-term stays, centers for chronic patients or socio-sanitary centers, would be the equivalent of the hospices in Great Britain. These centers are still in the early stages of development and represents an area to be rectified in the Spanish health care system. The INSALUD hardly has any centers of this type and those that do exist are generally in areas where health care has been transferred to the regional authorities.

Dedicated centers for terminal stage patients do not exist in Sapin and this may be because they are not well-accepted culturally. There is a privately managed project for the construction of a hospice on the Costa del Sol, an area where people from other European countries often retire.

The shortage of public centers of this type has led to a situation where agreements are frequently made with privately run hospitals to find beds for terminal patients. In Spain, general practitioners are not responsible for the hospitalization of this kind of patient and hospital centers must offer complete multidisciplinary teams. There are at least 36 hospitals for chronic patients that offer these palliative programs. These provide more than 500 beds for terminal patients. The average stay in these is longer, approximately 26 days. The Hospitals of the Order of St. John, which we mentioned previously, are this type of center when they offer palliative care units.

We can identify three different types of hospital care programs: (1) those developed in Catalonia and known as PADES (Programa de Atención Domiciliaria y Equipos de Soporte [Program for Home Care and Support Teams]), (2) the AECC teams, and (3) a number of others, mainly from the INSALUD. A comparison of their characteristics and activities is shown in Table 2.3. The AECC works in a similar way to charities found in Anglo-Saxon countries. Using its own financial resources, it forms teams for care at the terminal cancer patients' homes. These are mobile units that are located in, or at least backed up by, a hospital. Agreements exist for patients to be admitted to those centers when required. The hospital also supplies medication and normally provides an office or room from which the unit's work is coordinated. There are approximately 40 teams of this type and they have developed principally in the area covered by the INSALUD at moments when the INSALUD itself has not taken firm action to establish a solid model for care.

At the same time that these teams were being formed by the specialized care services, something of a paradox arose, as the INSALUD tried out other, conflicting pilot schemes from primary health care services. These were based in health centers and were not specifically for cancer patients and not only for terminal cases, but for any patient requiring health care. The future is not clear for either of these kinds of team. For now it seems that development is focused on the teams that began first.

PADES teams were created in the 1990s as part of the pilot scheme in Catalonia. They represent an important step forward as they have now been established all over that region, meaning that cover is provided, in theory at least, for 100% of all terminal cancer patients in Catalonia. At first they were located indistinctly, in health centers, acute care hospitals or in socio-sanitary centers. At this moment, experience points to the acute care centers as preferable. The specific nature of the programs has not produced uniform results, given that some teams are oriented totally toward terminal stage patients and others, toward all kinds of home-based patents. In any case this may be considered an advance.

None of these three models of home care solves the problem of the duplication of resources for similar functions within the same health care system. In theory, all the palliative teams should work as support teams. Those with the real responsibility are still the primary health care teams with their respective general

Table 2.3. Activity of palliative care programs for home-based patients, Spain 1998

Type of team	AECC		PADES		Other		Total	
	N	Teams evaluated (%)	N	Teams evaluated (%)	N	Teams evaluated (%)	N	Teams evaluated (%)
Programs identified	27	24 (89)	41	31 (76)	7	7 (100)	75	62 (83)
Number of cases	2,249	20 (74)	5,504	24 (59)	1,424	6 (86)	9,182	50 (67)
Number of cases	2,246	20 (74)	2,769	24 (59)	1,291	6 (86)	6,306	50 (67)
Percent of cases with cancer	100	22 (81)	50	31 (76)	90	6 (86)	69	59 (79)
Average visits per patient	8.6	11 (41)	10.0	26 (63)	12	3 (43)	9.7	40 (53)
Average survival	45	17 (63)	58	12 (29)	53	4 (57)	50	33 (44)
Doctors per team (average)	1.5	24 (89)	1.1	31 (76)	2.7	7 (100)	1.39	62 (83)
Nurses per team (average)	1.1	24 (89)	2.3	31 (76)	3.3	7 (100)	1.8	62 (83)
Psychologists (total)	22	24 (89)	5	31 (76)	3	7 (100)	30	62 (83)

AECC, Spanish Association Against Cancer; PADES, Program for Home Care and Support Teams.
Source: Data from the SECPAL Directory 1998: Not all the programs gave figures in all the sections.

practitioners. What we find in reality is quite different and there is a tendency in all cases toward exclusivity in the care. This means that the so-called support teams become care teams, saturated with work because of their reduced size compared to what is considered necessary for exclusive attention. Again, the lack of tradition with advisory teams and the novelties of the palliative programs give rise to problems, which have not, to date, been solved.

Use of Opioids for Cancer Pain in Spain

In 1992, Spain was first in the world ranking for the increase in the consumption of morphine for pain control. These levels have stabilized at present and we are still far from what the WHO considers the optimum level to meet the needs of terminal patients. According to the latest figures,[13] Spain occupies the 11th place in Europe as far as morphine consumption is concerned, with 9 mg per inhabitant per year. It is preceded by Denmark, Sweden, the United Kingdom, France, Iceland, Ireland, Norway Austria, Switzerland, Holland, and Germany, nearly all with over 20 mg per capita annually, and it is followed by Belgium, Finland, and Luxembourg. Spain remains below the level determined by the WHO as optimum for the treatment of pain in cancer.

Over the last 10 years, Spain has witnessed an increase in the use of slow-release, orally administered morphine preparations. Quite different from other countries, the slow-release formulation was introduced in 1988, and the commercialization of immediate-release morphine tablets occurred only in 1995. The use of immediate-release morphine is still far from common. In June 1998, the use of transdermal fentanyl was approved. Other opioids, such as hydromorphone and oxycodone, are not available in Spain and neither are other forms of morphine. Methadone is an exclusively hospital prescription and is not available from pharmacies. A commercial morphine-based syrup will soon be available in Spain but the introduction of other presentations or forms is not likely. The development of palliative care has made a decisive contribution to the greater use of opioid medication.

The Spanish Society of Palliative Care

The Spanish Society of Palliative Care (SECPAL) was founded in January 1992 (see Fig. 2.2). It has spread the palliative care philosophy throughout the country through the tireless efforts of some of its members in numerous activities such as courses, symposia, and conferences. In order to meet the objectives that led to its foundation, the Society has incorporated over 600 members from different professions and specialties. Since 1992, its activities have included the following:[14]

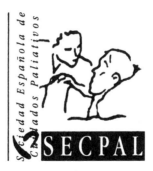

Figure 2.2. Logo of the Spanish Society of Palliative Care.

- Organization of two national congresses, Barcelona-95 and Santander-98, with the participation of more than 1000 professionals in each.
- Many regional congresses and scientific meetings in different regions.
- The Society sponsored numerous training activities at basic, intermediate, and advanced levels in many parts of Spain.
- The multidisciplinary journal, *Medicina Paliativa*, now in its fifth year, is published four times each year and is the Society's official publication. It is the first periodical publication on palliative care in Spanish. Its editor is Josep Porta.
- The dedicated publication *SECPAL Recommendations for Palliative Care* has been distributed to more than 20,000 health care professionals.
- The participation of SECPAL members has been noteworthy in numerous editorial projects, in guidelines and manuals, which have been widely spread in Spain and in Latin America.
- In 1997 and 1998, the SECPAL Directory of Palliative Care Programs was published with information and data on the organization, structure, and activities of the teams at work in Spain. In the most recent Directory, there is a list of over 1200 professionals involved in offering care to terminal stage patients in our country.
- A joint pilot scheme, with the WHO and the Spanish Pain Society, was carried out in 11 Spanish hospitals, under the title "Towards a Painless Hospital." It reached the objectives previously established.
- Through its many meetings with the Ministry of Health, the Society contributed to the development of a new set of rules for the prescription of opioids, which was applied in 1994 and which allows access to morphine.
- SECPAL has incorporated a number of regional organizations into its structure and is an active part of the European Society of Palliative Care, in which it participates as a collective member. At an international level, it has formed a part of numerous research, teaching, and legislative commissions.

With the aim of continuing the improvement in the care of patients and their families, SECPAL proposes the following projects in the short-term:

- From May 3 to May 6, 2000 the Society's 3rd National Congress will be held in the Valencia Palace of Congresses. For that occasion, certain new innovative events are planned, such as Debate Forums and Consensus Sessions with other Scientific Societies.
- A Web site has been created and maintained for SECPAL. This Internet presence (www.secpal.com) aims to provide continuous information on the Society's different facets. It will also make scientific information available to Spanish-speaking professionals, regarding the specialty's most important journals and books, through a virtual library.
- A new, revised format of the magazine *Medicina Paliativa*, in its second phase, has been launched. With this initiative, the idea is to increase its diffusion in all the countries of Latin America. This is in response to requests that we have received repeatedly.
- At present, work is continuing on training standards and program organization. Basic Recommendations of the SECPAL will be published for the health care authorities, advising on the training and organization of teams.
- The campaign "Towards a Painless Hospital" will be extended to Basic Health Teams and hospitals in all regions, as well as an evaluation and diffusion of the final results.
- The permanent objective of this Society is to maintain its multidisciplinary nature and its contacts with all kinds of institutions, societies, and organizations involved in caring for terminal patients and their families.

Teaching and Research in Palliative Medicine

From the beginning, those teams with sufficient experience have been essential components in training new teams. They have given their support to a great number of basic palliative care courses. The demand for this initial training in palliative care over these years has been quite striking. To help with this task of educating, a number of guides and manuals of unmistakable quality have been published in Spanish in recent years.[15-19] A singular phenomena has been the distance training course organized by the El Sabinal in Las Palmas. Those who applied received a book, a video, and a questionnaire with which to answer the 432 questions contained in the test. The course was a success in the whole of Spain and was completed by 11,107 students, of which 92% passed the final test.[20] The second edition of this course is underway and a number of Latin American professors are now taking part.

Finally, to bring this quick summary of the current state of palliative medicine in Spain to an end, we should mention the universities. Some faculties have already included palliative medicine as an optional subject in their new degree syllabi, thus putting the topic within reach of all the future graduates concerned with the treatment of terminal patients. In the consensus meeting on university training at the National Congress in Santander on May 6, 1998, a group of Spanish medical faculty deans met together with several palliative medicine professors and other professionals. This resulted in the publication of a document recognizing the need to include palliative medicine as part of the undergraduate curriculum in medical faculties and the recommendation that this directive be implanted in all universities and nursing schools.

Little by little, having satisfied the most urgent need to change attitudes and induce a new way of thinking about care, there arose demands to form teams with advanced training. Training has become a little more structured and in 2000 in Spain there are important postgraduate university programs. Specialist university programs and Masters degrees for nurses and doctors are offered at the Universities of Valladolid, Barcelona, Madrid, Salamanca, Deusto, Granada, and Extremadura. Some of these postgraduate programs are decisive for the consolidation of new ideas. The Spanish Society of Palliative Care is involved in setting the minimum standards required in advanced training.

Regarding research, the studies carried out up to now have been focused on describing organizational aspects and evaluating the results, the problems of communication, and diagnostic information in our environment, and clarifying psychosocial aspects. Hardly any clinical tests or comparative studies have been published on the difficult subject of symptom control in the terminal phase. Research in palliative medicine can be thought of as one of the great tasks left to fulfill in Spain and special attention will have to be given to this area in the coming years.

It is with satisfaction that we are able to view the development or culmination of certain doctoral projects directly related to palliative medicine. Doctoral theses have been defended in Valladolid, Madrid, Granada, Lerida, Valencia, and the Canary Islands. These studies have been encouraged by university professors who have become aware of the problem and have thus made palliative medicine the focus of their lines of investigation. Perhaps the moment is coming when some of these professors, or others returning from the clinical field, will start to show some preference for, or dedication to, research in the field of palliative medicine. This would mean that the discipline had reached maturity and would contribute to the definitive acceptance of palliative medicine at the scientific level that it deserves. It should coexist in a fruitful relationship with medical oncology, internal medicine, radiotherapy, oncology and, surgical oncology.

We are of the opinion that, in Spain, we should train new doctors and nurses in palliative medicine, from the faculties and university schools. There will be those, due to their chosen specialty, who will require a higher level of preparation in order to treat terminal patients. Nevertheless, all should be acquainted with the fundaments of palliative treatment and the control of symptoms, and integrate these into their own fields. That way we can assure the welfare of the highest possible number of future terminal-cancer sufferers. Furthermore, we believe that university training in the philosophy of palliative care will influence, to a great extent, the much needed regeneration in the field of medicine in the future.

References

1. INSALUD, What is INSALUD?. http://www.msc.es/insalud/introduction/english.htm.
2. Fernàndez-Shaw Toda M. Ars moriendi images of death in Spanish art. *Eur J Pall Care* 1997; 4(5):164–168.
3. Sanz J, Bild RE. El paciente en enfermedad terminal. Los intocables de la medicina. Editorial. *Med Clin* 1985; 84:691–693.
4. Gómez-Batiste X, Fontanals M, Roca J, et al. Catalonia WHO Demonstration Project on Palliative Care Implementation 1990–1995. Results in 1995. *J Pain Symptom Manage* 1996; 12(2):73–78.
5. Bondjale O, Marrero M, Sosa R, Mendoza NM. Cuidados paliativos y medicina paliativa en España. In: Gómez M, ed. *Cuidados Paliativos e Intervenzción Psicosocial en enfermos terminales*. Las Palmas: ICEPSS, 1994;146–149.
6. Centeno C. Panorama actual de la medicina paliativa en España. Oncología 1995; 18(4):173–183.
7. Nabal M, Porta J, Ramírez M. Unidades de cuidados paliativos en España: situación actual y tendencias. *Medicina Paliativa* 1996; 3:9–10
8. Centeno C, Gómez M. Programas de cuidados paliativos en España: una realidad en auge. Datos del directorio SECPAL de cuidados paliativos 1997. *Medicina Paliativa* 1997; 4(3):125–134
9. Porta J, Albó A. Cuidados paliativos: una historia reciente. *Medicina Paliativa* 1998; 5(4):33–41
10. Centeno C. *Directorio de Programas de Cuidados Paliativos, España 1997*. Madrid: Sociedad Española de Cuidados Paliativos, 1997.
11. Centeno C, Arnillas P, López-Lara F. *Directorio de Programas de Cuidados Paliativos, España 1998*. Valladolid: Sociedad Española de Cuidados Paliativos, 1998.
12. C. Centeno, F. López-Lara, M. Gómez Sancho. Palliative Care Programmmes In Spain, A Rising Reality. Communication to: Fifth Congress of the European Association for Palliative Care, 10–13 September 1997, London Book of Abstracts, P-221, (S78).
13. International Narcotics Control Board. University of Wisconsin: Pain & Policy Studies Group / WHO Collaborating Center, 1997
14. Sociedad Española de Cuidados Paliativos. Acta de la Reunión del Comité Ejecutivo, El Escorial, 29 de enero de 1999 (pro manuscrito).
15. Gómez Sancho M. Cuidados paliativos e intervención psicosocial en enfermos terminales. ICEPS, Instituto Canario de Estudios y Promoción Social y Sanitaria, Las Palmas, 1994.
16. Gómez-Batiste X, Planas Domingo J, Roca Casas J, Viladiú P. Cuidados paliativos en oncología [editorial]. Barcelona: *JIMS*, 1996.
17. González Barón M, Ordõez A, Feliú J, Zamora P, (eds). Tratado de Medicina Paliativa y tratamiento de Soporte en el enfermo con cáncer. Madrid: Ed. Médica Panamericana, 1996.

18. Astudillo W, Mendinueta C, Astudillo E, (eds). Cuidados del enfermo en fase terminal y atención a su familia. Pamplona: EUNSA, 1995.
19. López Imedio E. *Enfermería en Cuidados Paliativos*. Madrid: Editorial Panamericana, 1998
20. Gómez M, Ojeda M, García E, Navarro MA, Marrero MS. Curso de formación a distancia en medicina paliativa. Comunicación al II Congreso Nacional de Cuidados Paliativos, Santander, May 5–9, 1998 [Abstract 0019].

3

Models for the Delivery of Palliative Care in Developing Countries: The Argentine Model

ROBERTO WENK AND MARIELA BERTOLINO

Half of Argentina's 35 million inhabitants live in the urban areas scattered throughout the country's 23 provinces, while the other half live in rural districts.[1] Health care development varies considerably, with areas of excellent medical facilities and others with insufficient basic primary care. This chapter describes the development and current status of palliative care in Argentina, noting that the information could be incomplete because of lack of up-to-date national data. The description that follows could be applied to the rest of Latin America because many of these countries face the same challenges.[1–10]

Health Aspects

To understand fully palliative care's status in Argentina and the diverse forms of delivering it, a brief description of the country's health system is required.[1]

The health services comprise three sectors:

- Public services: free or with a minimum payment. These services rely on federal, provincial, or municipal governments; there are 81,000 hospital beds and 6880 facilities.
- Mutuals or social plans: approximately 300 in number, financed by employer and employee contributions, and generally administered by trade unions.
- The private sector, prepaid care institutions, or non-profit entities. There are some 200 of these institutions. Affiliation is on a voluntary basis.[1]

According to 1995 data, 62% of the population has some type of health coverage through prepaid or social plans.[1] The public health expenditure in 1995 was 1.75 of PBI or US$388 per capita.[1]

Life expectancy is 75.6 years and the mortality rate is 7.7 per 1000 inhabitants. The three most common causes of death are cardiovascular disease, cancer, and cerebrovascular disease.[1] The global mortality rate for cancer in 1995 was 141.6 per 100,000 inhabitants. The three most frequent types of cancer in men are lung, prostate, and stomach, and in women, breast, colon, and lung cancer.[1] The incidence of human immunodeficiency virus (HIV) and acquired immunodeficiency syndrome (AIDS) is growing every year. Since the first cases were reported in 1982, the number of AIDS cases rose to a reported 14,289 in 1998. It is estimated that only 40% of cases are actually reported.[11]

The health care system is complex and is undergoing major changes. The economic resources assigned for public health do not effectively solve the problems. Poor administration combined with bureaucracy at the professional and administrative levels aggravate the problem. All of these factors result in an elevated percentage of the population having difficulties in obtaining qualified and efficient medical attention, and this is more so in the lower socioeconomic classes.

Educational Aspects

The university system, with 16 schools of medicine, graduates approximately 3500 doctors every year, but palliative care still is not part of the undergraduate curriculum.[1] A health professional acquires his/her palliative care knowledge and skills after graduation, generally through a combination of courses, seminars, and conferences. A survey conducted in 1995 among 226 MDs in the Buenos Aires province (general practitioners, oncologists, anesthetists, and pulmonologists), who provide symptom control to an average of 25.8 terminal patients per year, indicated that 70% of them learned only the pharmacological aspects of analgesics and opioids as undergraduates.[12] Postgraduate education relied mostly on reading material, and only 5% had some sort of actual palliative care clinical training.

The data from another palliative care survey, conducted in 1996 among 71 health professionals (MDs, nurses, students, and nurses' aides) who attended classes or clinical rotations in the Palliative Care Unit of Hospital Tornú— FEMEBA (Federacion Medica de la Provincia de Buenos Aires) Foundation, showed that less than 30% had any knowledge of immediate-release morphine conversion to a slow release form, oral/intramuscular equianalgesic dosages, and the concept of the rescue dose. The same percentage of surveyed professionals were unable to name the morphine when prescribing it, were unaware of the frequency of delirium in the final stages of life, and did not know what type of drugs could be administered by the subcutaneous route.[13] This lack of professional training could expose patients to inefficient or unsuitable treatments for their specific needs.

These survey results highlight the strong need to promote clinical training in the different health professions, and several training systems actually have been implemented: university or nonuniversity courses, a distance education system, or through a heavy hourly practice. These diverse types of learning methods allow professionals or volunteers to acquire or complete their education, or both.

A rising interest in palliative care is seen in other medical specialities, especially oncology, internal medicine, geriatrics, pediatrics, and infectious diseases. The curriculum for oncology at the Catholic University of Buenos Aires and El Salvador University includes specific palliative care modules.

Socioeconomic Aspects

The monthly average income per capita is US$400. The poverty rate fluctuates between 8.5% and 35.5% of the population, depending on the region.[1] The great concentration of poor people reside in the outskirts of the cities, where there is poor water, energy, transportation, and community/health services.

Sociocultural Aspects

Argentina is a country with a strong Latin culture, the product of a large Spanish and Italian immigration. Some of these sociocultural characteristics influence trends related to palliative care.

Diagnosis and prognosis disclosure

A great majority of the members of the health care community, in keeping with the cultural paternalistic doctrine, consider it important to keep patients uninformed about a diagnosis of cancer or another life-threatening disease. Health care professionals argue that, in this way, they shield the patient from anxiety and suffering. Frequently, family members filter and influence information for the same purpose. Therefore, many patients with cancer and other incurable diseases are not aware of their illness and lack the information necessary to make informed decisions about their care.

Patients' misinformation varies with the type and location of the facilities. In a group of 76 cancer patients at the end of life, cared for consecutively by a community volunteer palliative care group in San Nicolás, only 25% knew of their diagnosis at the first consultation.[12] In another group of 100 cancer patients receiving palliative care and active oncological treatment at a university hospital, 55% fully knew their diagnosis and 14% had partial knowledge of it at the first consultation with the palliative care team.[14] This data let us presume that early palliative care intervention, with concomitant therapies, favors the disclosure of diagnosis and prognosis.

Recently, a more open discussion of incurable diseases like cancer, AIDS, and others is taking place at the individual level between doctor–patient or family–patient, and in the media.[15]

Misconceptions about use of morphine and other strong opioids

The association of morphine and its derivatives with drug addiction and imminent death is still strong.[16] There is little actual knowledge in the public domain, but the acceptance of the use of opioids is easily achieved when detailed information is made available to patients and families.

A study on prognostic and limiting factors in pain control from day 1 to day 21 of treatment shows a certain reluctance to increase the dosage during treatment.[17] On day 1, the most prevalent limiting factors in pain control were incorrect prescriptions (drugs, doses, intervals), but on day 21, the factors related to patient attitude (reluctance to increase opioid dosage, nonutilization of rescue doses, or noncompliance with prescribed indications).[17]

Decisions at the end of life

Discussions about resuscitation or admission to the intensive care unit, when the chances for improvement are little or nonexistent, are not conducted in a systematic manner. Few patients speak easily of these decisions and few palliative care teams try to broach the subject. The use of living wills or advance directives is not common and they do not carry much legal weight.

Palliative care seems, without confirmation at the moment, to be influencing great changes in this regard, making it more acceptable and easier to discuss diagnosis and prognosis, and recognizing the ethical necessity of informed consent regarding treatment and other important decisions. During the last 5 years, an increased interest in ethics at the end of life has been noted, questioning some of the points mentioned above, and attitude changes have been detected.

Nevertheless, a survey conducted by Przygoda et al.[18] among young MDs (those with less than 10 years' experience) about practices related to the end of life shows an important need for discussion on the subject. This study asked questions about nontreatment, assisted suicide, and active euthanasia without the patient's consent. Seventy-one percent agreed with the decision of nontreatment, 24% favored assisted suicide, and 61% agreed with active euthanasia without the patient's consent. In this last group, 63% (39.8% of the overall survey) admitted ending the life of terminal patients without explicit consent.[18] It is frightening that such a high percentage of doctors make these kinds of illegal decisions without patient consent and it shows the need for an open debate and continuing education about palliative care.

Palliative Care Development in Argentina

Under the influence of the Hospice Movement and the World Health Organization's Cancer Pain Program, modern palliative care concepts began to be offered in an organized manner in 1982, both in the Federal District and in the provinces.[19–22] Palliative care development was unlike that in Europe or the United States because cultural and economic characteristics made it difficult to follow those models. The development basically followed three paths in consecutive and interrelated stages. We describe them as horizontal, ascendant, and descendent models (Fig. 3.1).

Horizontal
This is the initial model that has a sustained development and reflects the need and increased interest in palliative care. It works and expands on the surface at the same level of motivation and dedication within the community and non-

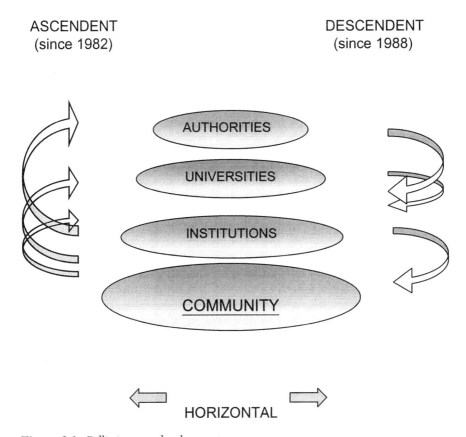

Figure 3.1. Palliative care development.

governmental entities. In numerous cities, volunteers and professionals from different health disciplines assist patients in various ways: individually or in a team, using a single or interdisciplinary approach, in institutions or at home, and as paid or unpaid professionals. They not only bring medical and psychological assistance to the patient–family unit, but also do social work—determining need, providing resources, and establishing links with the health care community.

Actually, the complexity of the attention provided depends on the local culture and rational use of available resources. Two examples of this model, among others, are the Centro de Cuidados Paliativos de LALCEC San Nicolas and the Praguer-Bild Foundation in Buenos Aires, both established in 1985.

Ascendant

This model is the result of promoting and achieving more awareness of the needs of patients with incurable illnesses and the benefits of palliative care at the higher levels of organization in the community (i.e., municipalities and hospitals) through motivated professionals in diverse executive positions.

The results obtained through the policy and organization of voluntary work in the private sector or nongovernmental organizations strives to capture the interest of political and health authorities. The practical aspect is that it provides hospitals and universities with the two most important activities of the teams initiated and developed in the community: clinical assistance and teaching.

Examples of this model are the teams in several hospitals: Jose de San Martín, Garraham, Elizalde, Tornú, Udaondo y Roffo in Buenos Aires; San Roque in Córdoba, Británico, Centenario or Baigorria in Rosario, and Humberto Noti in Mendoza.

This model also provides the basis for pre- and postgraduate teaching of palliative care in the public universities (Universidad Nacional de La Plata, de Buenos Aires, and Rosario) and private universities (Universidad Católica Argentina and Universidad del Salvador). At the same time, it contributes to the training of volunteers in philanthropic or charitable institutions.

Descendent

This model promotes official palliative care programs from inception to management in different institutions. It represents the concepts, with varied results, of shared responsibilities in collaborative work with health authorities, professional organizations, and the community in developing these clinical and educational programs. Some of these programs are:

- 1988. *Programa de Medicina Paliativa del Ministerio de Salud Publica de la Provincia de Buenos Aires*, to provide palliative care in its institutions in Zone IV. Deactivated in 1992 for lack of distribution of the necessary existing resources.
- 1991. *Programa de Dolor y Cuidados Palliativos del Programa Nacional de Control de Cancer*, to promote palliative care in institutions of the

national health net. Due to a change in administrative health authorities, the program never went into effect.

- 1994. *Federacion Medica de la Provincia de Buenos Aires (FEMEBA)*, a corporation of 14,000 MDs and the *Programa Argentino de Medicina Paliativa* began a medical education program that provides theoretic/practical training in palliative care.
- 1995. *Ministerio de Salud del Gobierno de Mendoza* created a provincial agency for the provincial palliative care program. Two hospital units are active in palliative care and pain control.
- 1996 and 1998. In the *Camara de Diputados de la Nation* (Federal House of Representatives), two bills were introduced for the implementation of a National Palliative Care Program. The slow political process has hindered its progress.
- 1998. *Camara de Diputados de la Provincia de Buenos Aires* (Bs.As. Province Legislature). One bill was introduced for the creation of a Palliative Care Provincial Agency to provide assistance teams in provincial hospitals. It is in the development stage.
- 1999. *Ministerio de la Salud de la Nación* (National Health Department) approved the Integral Continuing Assistance Program (PACI). This is a multidisciplinary program that combines education, prevention, diagnosis and treatment of HIV, and palliative care for cancer patients in the Hospital Nacional Baldomero Sommer. The PACI will be active by the end of October 2000.
- 1999. *Legislatura de la Provincia de Jujuy* (Jujuy Legislative Branch) created a Program of Integral Attention for Oncologic Patients and a Provincial Executory Unit. This unit is in the development stage and will provide palliative care to cancer patients throughout the Jujuy Province.
- 1999. *Programa de Garantía de Calidad de la Atención Medica del Ministerio de Salud y Acción Social* (Program for the Guarantee of Quality of Medical Care), began the drafting of organizational, functional, procedural, diagnostic, and treatment standards for palliative care programs. The standards are in the approval stage.

Contemporary Models for Providing Palliative Care

The great diversity of health care system resources in different regions has led to different ways to provide palliative care at this time.[23-26]

Palliative work approach

Individual care provided by professionals of various specialties with training in palliative care. They work to establish a functioning team for the assistance of certain patients and their families. When this occurs, professionals from multiple disciplines specify a care and treatment plan to address the patient's particular needs.

Palliative care teams

There are approximately 25–30 active teams throughout the country, with different configurations depending on the characteristics of each institution and other factors.

Disciplines involved

Palliative care has a predominance of MDs over nurses and psycho-social professionals. This also occurs in other specialized fields—few general practitioners compared to the number of specialists, and a reduced number of nurses compared to the overall number of doctors. Teams can include two or more disciplines, depending on the availability of professionals in each area. All teams have a minimum of one MD and nurses, psychologists, social workers, pharmacists, volunteers, chaplains, et al. are added.

Dedication

Most teams comprise part-time palliative care professionals. Very few can dedicate themselves full-time because the remuneration does not encourage it.

Dedicated institutions

Non-Government Organizations NGO (Palliative Care Centers of the Argentine Cancer League Against Cancer: San Nicolás, Bolivar, Caseros, etc.), public hospitals, university hospitals, and a handful of private clinics and social organizations.

Members' earnings

Some are paid and some work ad honorem; some groups have mixed personnel. Few health systems pay fees for palliative care services, and those teams that do receive remuneration are not highly paid. In the public system teams, a high percentage of professionals work ad honorem.

Development stage

Some teams are just in the preliminary project stage, others are developing, and still others are fully implemented. There has been an increase in the number of teams in development and those fully implemented, as well as an increase in the number of professionals interested in creating new teams.

Teaching and research

All teams perform internal teaching duties in their institution and frequently lend a hand in outside teaching. Research is in the initial stage; several teams have recognized the necessity and importance of producing local data to achieve advances in the field. Multicenter studies involving other Latin American countries, the Edmonton Group (Canada), and several local teams are in progress.

Patients

Most of the team's work is geared to cancer patients, but lately patients with AIDS and other chronic or degenerative diseases have been included. A greater number of teams treat adult patients than pediatric patients. There are two pedriatic teams in the city of Buenos Aires, and one each in the cities of Rosario, Mendoza, and Neuquén cities. Other teams are in the preliminary stages of development. Generally, these teams take care of patients with congenital/degenerative pathologies.

Work place

Outpatient consultations are available in all programs. Admission to hospital is done in another specialty's ward. At the present time, there is only one specific palliative care ward available for inpatients. Day hospital services are provided in few institutions; this area is still in the development stages. Home care is practically nonexistent in the public system, with some exceptions in the cities of Rosario and Buenos Aires, but has been widely developed in the private sector and social organizations. The scarcity of specific home care teams and the great distances between institutions and homes hinder the small proportion of the population that has access to palliative care. The common belief that only health institutions are capable of providing all resources and services is also a factor in the general preference for inpatient treatment.

Obstacles to the Implementation of Palliative Care

Distribution of resources

Patients suffering incurable diseases face a series of problems that hinder their primary care and the availability of palliative care:

- Palliative care as a medical practice is not recognized and is not included in health plans.
- A 1996 survey showed that fewer than 10% of both prepaid and social health plans paid for palliative care.[12]
- A 1998 poll revealed that only 6 of 36 public hospitals in Buenos Aires have active palliative care teams.[27]

As a general rule, most of the human and material resources are dedicated to curative treatments and few or none to palliative care.

Opioid analgesics: availability and access

Since 1999, 12 different opioid analgesics have been available (Table 3.1), and according to the International Narcotic Control Board, the annual consumption of morphine is increasing.[5] However, high prices place a restriction to their use (Table 3.2). Given that the average monthly income is US$400, opioids are very

Table 3.1. Opioid availability in Argentina in 1999

Buprenorphine	Pethidine
Codeine	Morphine
Dextropropoxyphene	Methadone
Hydrocodone	Nalbuphine
Hydromorphone	Oxycodone
Fentanyl	Tramadol

Table 3.2. Costs of "strong" opioids in Argentina (Daily dose: 180 mg. equivalent of oral morphine.)

	Cost Per Month
Morphine	
Compounded: aqueous solution morphine HCl	
—Prepared in hospital pharmacy (1 g: $4.8)	$26.
—Prepared in community pharmacy (1 g: $10)°	$52.
Compounded: tablets of immediate-release morphine HCl	
—Prepared in community pharmacy (30 mg tablets: $0.4)°	$72.
Commercial: tablets of immediate-release morphine HCl	
—30 mg tablets: $0.7	$133.
Commercial: slow-release morphine sulfate tablets	
—10 mg tablets: $2.2; 30 mg tablets: $3.7	$582.
Oxycodone	
Compounded: aqueous solution of oxycodone HCl	
—Prepared in hospital pharmacy (1 g: $8.5)	$32.
—Prepared in community pharmacy (1 g: $17)°	$64.
Commercial: slow-release oxycodone HCl tablets	
—20 mg tablets: $4.7; 40 mg tablets: $7	$702.
Fentanyl	
Commercial	$400.
25 μg/h patch: $40; 50 μg/h patch: $78; 75 μg/h patch: $109,	
100 μg/h patch: $137	
Methadone	
Commercial. methadone HCl tablets	
5 mg tablets: $1.0; 10 mg tablets: $1.6; 40 mg: $3.7	$89.

° According to the minimum tariffs suggested by the Colegio de Farmacéuticos de la Provincia de Buenos Aires.
1$ = 1 US$. Every price includes taxes.
Very few health system sectors (publics or privates) pay for compounded preparations.
Source: From the *Manual Farmacéutico* 465, Feb. 1999.[28] The least expensive prices for commercial products were used.

expensive, despite the fact that some health systems partially cover the cost of commercial preparations. Only a small number of patients can afford the treatment.

Most public hospitals in the city of Buenos Aires City do not have oral morphine or other strong opioids, which makes opioid rotation impossible.[27] Another problem has arisen: because commercial products are expensive, it has been necessary to prescribe the less expensive compounded medications. However, in some cases, compounded medicines have became more expensive than the commercial ones.

Insufficient professional training and insufficient public information

Information that refers to the end of life and the options available are rarely mentioned, both in the professional teaching setting and in the media.

The Argentine Association of Medicine and Palliative Care

The Argentine Association of Medicine and Palliative Care (AAMyCP), created in 1991, is an interdisciplinary scientific association with approximately 500 members. The Association's goals include:

- Conduct a national census of teams and professionals to facilitate networking
- Increase the technical capacity of its members with annual meetings, monthly clinical seminars, bimonthly technical meetings, development of standards and clinical models, and the creation of a Web page and a quarterly publication[28]
- License professionals and teams for clinical work
- Interact with the responsible authorities to achieve the recognition of palliative care as a specialty with corresponding remuneration

Conclusion

The development of palliative care in Argentina described here spans 15 years. Its increased development and activity has resulted in better care for a great number of patients and, at the same time, a greater awareness and interest from the community and health professionals. Difficulties have been identified, but there is also a willingness to solve the problems. Changes have encouraged a permanent collaboration that will enable us to succeed in:

Care issues

- Recognition of palliative care teams in the structure of public and private institutions

- Increase access to palliative care in public, private, and social institutions throughout the country, with a broader percentage of coverage
- Establish guidelines for referral/admission of intermediate and high complexity palliative care teams
- Develop a list of drugs (vademecum; mostly potent opioid analgesics) that should be distributed free to patients lacking health coverage

Education issues

- Ensure the systematic inclusion of palliative care in pre- and postgraduate curricula
- Establish a system of accreditation for palliative care caregivers

Research issues

- Obtain reliable epidemiological data
- Compile information for future development and monitor the existing clinical programs

Perseverance of our goals and continued improvement of our models will allow the introduction of palliative care on a greater scale to assist Argentinean patients with incurable diseases.

References

1. Argentina, In: *La Salud en Las Américas. Eds Oficina Sanitaria Panamericana.* Oficina Regional Organización Mundial de la Salud. Washinton DC: EUA; 1998; Vol II:24–48.
2. Bruera E. Palliative care programs in Latin America. *Palliat Med* 1992; 6:182–184.
3. Wenk R. Cancer pain management problems in developing countries. In: Patt R, ed. *Cancer Pain.* Philadelphia: J.B. Lippincott Co., 1993:501–508.
4. De Lima L, Bruera E, Stjernsward J, et al. Opioid availability in Latin America: the Santo Domingo Report. Progress since the Declaration of Florianopolis. Working draft and personal communication.
5. Joranson DE, Gilson AM, Nelson JM, Colleau SM. Disponibilidad de opioides para el alivio del dolor en cancer: puntos relevantes en America Latina (monografía). Division of Policy Studies; University of Wisconsin Pain Research Group/WHO Collaborating Center, Madison, Wisconsin. 1999.
6. Stjernsward J, Bruera E, Joranson D, et al. Opioid availability in Latin America: The declaration of Florianopolis. *J Pain Symptom Manage* 1995; 10(3)3:233–236.
7. Bruera E. Palliative care in Latin America. *J Pain Symptom Manage* 1993; 8(6):365–368.
8. Quesada L. Costa Rica: Status of cancer pain and palliative care. *J Pain Symptom Manage* 1993; 8(6):407–408.

9. De Lima L. Status of cancer pain and palliative care. *J Pain Symptom Manage* 1993; 8(6):404–406.
10. Rico MA. Les soins Palliatifs au Chili. European *J Palliat Care* 1997; 4(4):138–139.
11. *Boletín sobre el SIDA en Argentina*. Ministerio de Salud y Acción Social, VII, N° 16. Marzo 1999:9–20.
12. Wenk R, Marti G. Palliative care in Argentina: deep changes are necessary for its effective implementation. *Palliat Med* 1996; 10:263–264.
13. Bertolino M, Wenk R, Pussetto J, Ochoa J. Surveys on knowledge of the participants of courses or rotations in a palliative care unit. Fifth Congress of the European Association for *Palliat Care* 1996; P-347:S107.
14. Bertolino M, Wenk R, Aresca L, Bagnes C, Rogel M, Vicente H. Awareness of cancer diagnosis in patients at the first consultation with a palliative care team in Argentina. Proceedings of the Fifth Congress of the European Association for Palliative Care 1996; 133:S57.
15. Bertolino M, Felippo R, Leone F, et al. Condiciones del final de vida en pacientes con cáncer tratados por una Unidad de Cuidados Paliativos. VII Congreso Nacional de Medicina 1999; S-04-01:316.
16. El miedo a la adicción: Obstáculo al alivio del dolor de cáncer. *Cancer Pain Release* 1998; 11(3):1–8.
17. Bertolino M, Lassauniere JM, Marchand H, Leone F, Wenk R, Zittoun R. Prognosis factors in the relief of cancer pain. A French-Argentinian Study. Proceedings of the Fifth Congress of the European Association for Palliative Care 1996; 003:S29.
18. Przygoda P, Saimovici J, Pollán J, Figar S, Cámera MI. Posición de los jóvenes médicos sobre las prácticas relacionadas con el fin de vida. *Revista Argentina de Medicina* 1999; 1(3):135–139.
19. World Health Organization. *Cancer Pain Relief and Palliative Care*. Geneva: World Health Organization, 1990.
20. Stjernswärd J, Colleau S, Ventafridda VJ. The WHO cancer pain and palliative care program. Past, present and future. *J Pain Symptom Manage* 1996; 12(2):65–72.
21. Saunders C. Foreword. In: Doyle D, Hanks G, MacDonald N, eds. *Oxford Textbook of Palliative Medicine*. First Edition. Oxford: Oxford University Press, 1993:v–viii.
22. Stjernsward J, Koroltchouk V, Teoh N. National policies for cáncer pain relief and palliative care. *Palliat Med* 1992; 6:293–298.
23. Wenk R, Diaz C, Echeverría M, et al. Argentina's WHO Cancer pain relief program: a patient care model. *J Pain Symptom Manage* 1991; 6:40–43.
24. Wenk R. Los Cuidados Paliativos en la República Argentina: la necesidad de centros de asistencia y entrenamiento. *Rev Arg Anest* 1993; 51(2), 2:107–111.
25. Wenk R. Argentina: status of cancer pain and palliative care. *J Pain Symptom Manage* 1993; 8:385–387.
26. Wenk R, Pussetto J. Resultados de la actividad de una hot-line de cuidados paliativos. Proceedings of the Fifth Congress of the European Association for Palliative Care. Barcelona, 1995.
27. Bertolino M, Laje E, Contissa D, Vugalter B, Ponczeck B, Wenk R. Disponibilidad de opioides en los hospitales públicos de la Ciudad de Buenos Aires. *II Jornada de la Unidad de Cuidados Paliativos Hospital Tornú-Fundación FEMEBA*. November 1998.
28. *Boletín Científico de la Asociación Argentina de Medicina y Cuidados Paliativos 1999*, año V, N° 10.

II

PALLIATIVE CARE IN GERIATRICS

4

Exploring the Need for a Special Model of Geriatric Care

R. SEAN MORRISON AND DIANE E. MEIER

Popular images of death and dying are a jumble of gun violence; young and middle-aged adults on television fighting for life with the help of tubes, intensive care units (ICU^L_F), and other modern machinery; and nineteenth century images of feverish mothers or children attended at home by their grieving families and helpless physicians. In reality, these media visions bear little relationship to the actual human experience of dying in the United States. In our society, the overwhelming majority of people who die are elderly. They typically die slowly of chronic diseases, over long periods of time, with multiple coexisting problems, progressive dependency on others, and heavy care needs met mostly by family members. They spend the majority of their final months and years at home but, in most parts of the country, die in the hospital or nursing home surrounded by strangers. Many of these deaths become protracted and negotiated processes, with health care providers and family members making difficult, often wrenching, decisions about the use or discontinuation of life-prolonging technologies, such as feeding tubes, ventilators, and intravenous fluids. There is abundant evidence that the quality of life during the dying process is often poor, characterized by inadequately treated physical distress, fragmented care systems, poor to absent communication between doctors and patients and families, and enormous strains on family caregiver and support systems.

Demography of Dying and Death in the United States

The median age at death in the United States is now 77 years, associated with a steady and linear decline in age-adjusted death rates since 1940. Whereas in 1900, life expectancy at birth was less than 50 years, a girl born today may expect to live to age 79 and a boy to age 73. Those of us reaching 75 years can expect to live another 10 (men) to 12 (women) years on average. This dramatic and unprecedented increase in life expectancy (equivalent to that occurring between the Stone Age and the year 1900) is due primarily to decreases in maternal and infant mortality, resulting from improved sanitation, nutrition, and effective control of infectious diseases. The result of these changes in demography has been an enormous growth in the number and health of the elderly, so that by the year 2030, 20% of the United States' population will be over age 65, as compared to fewer than 5% at the turn of the twentieth century.

Death at the turn of the twentieth century was largely attributable to infectious diseases, whereas today the leading causes of death are heart disease, cancer, and stroke. Advances in treatment of atherosclerotic vascular disease and cancer have turned these previously uniformly fatal diseases into chronic illnesses, which people often live with for many years before death. In parallel, deaths that occurred at home in the early part of the twentieth century now occur primarily in institutions (57% in hospitals and 17% in nursing homes).[1] The reasons for this shift in location of death are complex, but are related to Medicare reimbursement for hospital-based care, with the subsequent rise in the availability of hospitals and hospital beds, and the care burdens of chronicity and functional dependency typically accompanying life threatening disease in the elderly. The older the patient, the higher the likelihood of death in a nursing home or hospital, with an estimated 58% of persons over 85 spending at least some time in a nursing home in the last year of their life.[2]

These statistics, however, should not hide the fact that the majority of an older person's last months and years is still spent at home in the care of family members, with hospitalization or nursing home placement, or both occurring only near the very end of life. Additionally, national figures such as these hide the substantial regional variation in location of death. In Portland, Oregon, for example, only 22% of adult deaths occur in hospitals[3] as compared to more than 68% in New York City.[1] This disparity is associated, at least in part, with differences in regional hospital bed supply and availability of adequate community supports for the dying. Finally, national statistics also obscure the variability in the experience of dying that characterizes our highly diverse nation. For example, need for institutionalization or paid formal caregivers in the last months of life is much higher among the poor and among women. Similarly, persons suffering from cognitive impairment and dementia are much more likely to spend their last days in a nursing home compared to cognitively intact elderly persons dying from non-dementing illnesses.

The incentives promoting an institutional death—as opposed to death at home—persist despite evidence that patients prefer to die at home and despite the existence of the Medicare Hospice Benefit. The hospice benefit was designed to provide substantial professional and material support (medications, equipment) to families caring for the dying at home during their last 6 months of life.

Reasons for the low rate of utilization of the Medicare Hospice Benefit (serving only 17% of adult deaths) vary by community but include the inhibiting requirements that patients acknowledge that they are dying in order to access the services, that physicians certify a prognosis of 6 months or less, and that very few hours (usually 4 or less) of personal care home attendants are covered under the benefit. In addition, the fiscal structure of the Medicare Hospice Benefit lends itself well to the predictable trajectory of late-stage cancers or AIDS, but not so well to the unpredictable chronic course of other common causes of death in the elderly, like congestive heart failure, chronic lung disease, stroke, and dementing illnesses.

The Dying Experience

Although death occurs far more commonly in the elderly than in any other age group, most research on the experience of dying has been done in younger populations. Remarkably little is known about how death occurs in the oldest-old, those over age 75. To date, most studies have focused on patient's preferences for care as opposed to actual care received.[4] The largest and most detailed study of dying persons in the United States (The Study to Understand Prognoses and Preferences for Outcomes and Risks of Treatments [SUPPORT]) studied hospital deaths and enrolled subjects with a median age of 66 (while the median age of death in the United States is 77) and many of the old-old spend most of their last days in nursing homes or at home.

State and Medicare discharge data suggest that costly aggressive and potentially burdensome life prolonging interventions are less frequently used among the oldest patients, independent of functional status.[5,6] This may represent a form of implicit rationing based on age. These data are disturbing given the suggestion that 50% of the highest-cost Medicare enrollees survive at least 1 year after the medical costs are incurred.[7]

Studies focusing specifically on the prevalence of pain have shown consistently high levels of untreated or undertreated pain in the elderly. In one study of elderly cancer patients in nursing homes, 26% of patients with daily pain received no analgesic at all and 16% received only acetaminophen.[8] Another study comparing pain management in cognitively intact versus demented elderly with acute hip fracture also found a high rate of undertreatment of pain in both groups, a phenomenon that worsened with increasing age and cognitive impairment.[9,10] A large study of outpatients with cancer found that age and female sex were predictors of undertreatment, a disturbing observation given the dramatic rise in cancer prevalence with increasing age.[11,12] Finally, chronic pain due to arthritis, other bone and joint disorders, and low back syndrome, which is probably the most common cause of distress and disability in the elderly (affecting 25%–50% of community-dwelling older adults) is, similar to cancer pain, consistently undertreated.[13] These data suggest that the time before death among elderly persons is often characterized by significant physical distress, which is neither identified nor properly treated.

Despite the high prevalence of pain and other symptoms in the elderly, most studies focusing on the assessment and treatment of pain and other symptoms have enrolled young cancer patients. It is unclear whether these results are generalizable to a geriatric population. For example, elderly patients may have difficulty using widely recommended assessment instruments (e.g., visual analogue scales) because of cognitive or sensory impairment.

The World Health Organization (WHO) analgesic ladder may not be appropriate for the elderly because of the increased risk of side effects (renal failure, gastrointestinal bleeding) observed with nonsteroidal anti-inflammatory drugs. Indeed, the American Geriatrics Society has recently recommended that opioids be considered as a first step treatment rather than nonsteroidal anti-inflammatory drugs (NSAIDS).[13] Unfortunately, these recommendations were made based upon expert opinion rather than empirical data, as empirical data are simply not available. The use of opioids themselves present problems because of the increased prevalence of difficult to manage side effects in the elderly (e.g., sedation, delirium, constipation).

Finally, the constellation of symptoms seen in dying elderly patients is different from that of young adults. For example, delirium, sensory impairment, incontinence, dizziness, and cough are more prevalent in the elderly.[14] The elderly, on average have a mean of 1.5 more symptoms than younger persons in the year prior to death and 69% of the symptoms reported for people aged 85 or more lasted more than a year, as compared to 39% of those for younger adults.[14]

Aside from pain and other sources of physical distress, the key characteristic that distinguishes the dying process in the elderly from that experienced by younger groups is the nearly universal occurrence of long periods of functional dependency and need for family caregivers in the last months to years of life. SUPPORT, focusing on a younger age cohort, found that 55% of patients had persistent and serious family caregiving needs during the course of a terminal illness,[15] a figure that rises exponentially with increasing age. Although the vast majority of caregiving is done by unpaid family members (transportation, homemaker services, personal care, and more skilled nursing care), paid care supplements provide the sole source of care in 15%–20% of patients, especially among poor elderly women living alone. Most family caregiving is provided by women (spouses and adult daughters and daughters-in-law), placing significant strains on the physical, emotional, and socioeconomic status of the caregivers. Those ill and dependent patients without family caregivers, or those whose caregivers can no longer provide nor afford needed services, are placed in nursing homes, where 20% of the over-age-85 population resides.[16] Thus, the dying process in the oldest-old is characterized by a high prevalence of untreated pain and other symptoms due to chronic conditions associated with progressive functional dependency, unpredictable disease course, and high family caregiver needs.

Mismatch Between Our Health Care System and the Needs of the Dying Elderly

The current payment system is poorly matched to the needs of the chronically ill and dying elderly. Medicare fee-for-service promotes use of procedure-based payments, hospitalization, and associated specialization and discontinuity of care. Capitated managed care systems attempt to avoid seriously ill or dying patients with high intensity service needs, focusing instead on healthier, lower cost patient populations. The Medicare hospice benefit was designed for patients with cancer and predictably short life spans, who are willing to give up efforts to prolong life and whose families can provide for the majority of their care needs at home. None of these payment systems address the long-term care needs—whether at home or in a nursing home—of chronically ill and functionally dependent individuals whose prognoses are uncertain and whose medical care usually requires simultaneous efforts to prolong life, palliate symptoms, and provide support for functional dependency. Neither paid personal care services at home nor nursing home costs for the functionally dependent elderly are covered by Medicare, but instead are paid for approximately equally from out-of-pocket, and from Medicaid budgetary sources originally intended to provide care for the indigent.

Even in nursing homes, standards of care focus on improvement of function, and maintenance of weight and nutritional status, and evidence of the decline that accompanies the dying process is regarded typically as a measure of sub-standard care.[17] Thus, a death in a nursing home is often viewed as evidence, particularly by state regulators, of poor care rather than an expected outcome for a frail chronically ill older person. Similarly, quality indicators required in long-term care settings fail to either assess or reward appropriate attention to palliative measures, including relief of symptoms, spiritual care, and promotion of continuity with concomitant avoidance of brink of death emergency room and hospital transfers.[18]

Improving End of Life Care for the Elderly

Because of unprecedented improvements in maternal and infant mortality and successes in the control, if not cure, of common chronic diseases, most people who die in the United States are old and frail. They die of chronic, progressive illnesses (such as end-stage heart and lung disease, cancer, stroke, and dementia), with unpredictable clinical courses and prognoses. Current hospice and palliative care programs are not well adapted to the trajectory of illness or the clinical needs of this group of patients.[19] Furthermore, these patients have unrecognized and untreated symptoms and an extremely high prevalence of functional dependency and associated family caregiver burden. Current reimbursement systems outside of hospice are unresponsive to this patient population and their families, failing to provide primary care with continuity, support for family caregivers, and home care services, and instead promoting fragmented specialized care tied to procedures and hospitals for lack of any other coherent alternative financing mechanism. This phenomenon has prompted widespread calls for change and reorganization that would ensure accountability for outcomes, processes, and costs of care for the growing population of frail, functionally dependent, and chronically ill elderly in their last phase of life.

Because care for a dying person typically includes preventive, life-prolonging, rehabilitation, and palliative measures in varying proportion and intensity based upon the individual patient's needs and preferences, any new model of care will have to be responsive to this range of service requirements. For example, an 88-year-old woman with congestive heart failure and deconditioning after hospitalization for pneumonia requires life-prolonging measures (treatment of heart failure with diuretics, angiotensin-converting enzyme inhibitors, digoxin, oxygen, and antibiotics), preventive measures (annual influenza vaccination), rehabilitation (home physical therapy to restore independent bed-to-chair mobility), and palliative care (advance care planning, appointment of a health care proxy, treatment of depression, diuretics, oxygen, and low-dose opioids for dyspnea). If her daughter works during the day, she also needs a 12-hour-a-day home-health aide as she is unable to care for herself independently. Thus, the model of care needed provides simultaneous life-prolonging, palliative, and personal care (in this patient they are nearly one and the same), and, given the difficulty of prognosticating time of death in heart failure, will have to continue to do so for the remainder of the patient's life—which may be up to several years prior to a sudden and unpredictable death from an arrhythmia.

Several mixed-management models of care have been recently proposed to address the needs of the frail elderly. The PACE (Program of All-Inclusive Care for the Elderly) Demonstration Program[20] is a capitated Medicare and Medicaid waiver program of full service primary care for the elderly focusing on continuity, avoidance of hospitalization, and bringing needed services to the patient. Each PACE site is staffed by an interdisciplinary team that coordinates care across home, clinic, hospital, and the day health centers. The PACE sites serve approximately 120 to 150 enrollees and the average patient is 80 years old, has 7.8 medical conditions, and is dependent in 2.7 activities of daily living.[20] Preliminary results from the PACE project suggest that this high-risk population utilized fewer hospital days than the general Medicare population (2399 hospital days/1000 persons/annum compared to 2448 days/1000 persons/per annum) and had shorter hospital lengths of stay (4.9 days as compared to the Medicare length of stay of 7.6 days/admission for all Medicare recipients), with no increase in mortality rates.[20] It is estimated that PACE yields actual savings to Medicare of 14% to 39% compared with fee for service care.[20] Whether the PACE program is generalizable to non-urban settings and whether the model can work on a larger scale has yet to be determined.

Another promising model developed by Lynn and colleagues[19] is about to undergo extensive pilot evaluation in a chronically ill veterans population with lung and heart disease. The *MediCaring* model will (1) define eligibility in terms of chronic disease severity (e.g., congestive heart failure with an ejection fraction of less than 30% and 2 hospitalizations in the last year), *not* by predicted time of death, (2) provide services that span the range of patient and family needs described above through use of interdisciplinary teams, consistent primary care providers across all care settings, and delivery of as much care as possible in the home setting, whether the focus be on life prolongation, palliation, rehabilitation, or, as is typical, all three; and (3) organize payment through a Medicare waiver combination of capitation (for team services, equipment) and fee for service or salary for participating physicians.[19,21]

Substantial change using approaches such as PACE and *MediCaring* will be necessary if the health care system is to bear any relationship to the needs of the patients seeking care, patients who are predominantly old and chronically ill and in urgent need of help truly fitted to their needs. Though the problem is daunting, the increase in attention to medical education, research, and clinical service delivery for patients near the end of life are indicators that the recognition necessary to begin the process of change has occurred. The next steps, testing new models and seeing what works, will define the new structure of health care services for future generations.

Whereas a century ago, when virtually everyone died at home, surrounded by family and cared for by physicians whose primary role was the relief of suffering, today the vast majority of Americans die in institutions, surrounded by medical technology and physicians who believe there is nothing else that they can do. Although the past 100 years have seen tremendous advances in the treatment of disease, such that previously fatal illnesses (e.g., diabetes, congestive heart failure) have become chronic conditions, this progress has come at a substantial cost. We have transformed the culture of death from an accepted part of life's experience to an unfamiliar and much feared event. The majority of Americans have never witnessed a loved one die (a common experience at the turn of the century) and physicians are ill-trained, ill-equipped, and uncomfortable taking responsibility for the care of dying patients. It is clear that the time has come to restore the balance so that "relief of suffering and cure of disease [are] seen as twin obligations of a medical profession that is truly dedicated to the care of the sick."[22]

References

1. National Center for Health Statistics. Vital Statistics for the United States, 11, Mortality, Hyattsville, Maryland, 1993.
2. National Center for Health Statistics. National mortality followback survey: 1986. Summary, United States, Series 20. Hyattsville, Maryland: Vital and Health Statistics, 1992.

3. Tolle SW, Rosenfeld AG, Tilden VP, Park Y. Oregon's low in-hospital death rates: What determines where people die and satisfaction with decisions on place of death? *Ann Intern Med* 1999; 130:681–685.

4. Tsevat J, Dawson NV, Wu AW, et al. Health values of hospitalized patients 80 years or older. HELP Investigators. Hospitalized Elderly Longitudinal Project [see comments]. *JAMA* 1998; 279:371–375.

5. Hamel M, Phillips R, Teno J, et al. Seriously ill hospitalized adults: Do we spend less on older patients? *J Am Geriatr Soc* 1996; 44:1043–1048.

6. Peris T, Wood E. Acute care costs of the oldest-old: They cost less, their care intensity is less, and they go to nonteaching hospitals. *Arch Int Med* 1996; 156:754–760.

7. Lubitz JD, Riley FF. Trends in Medicare payments in the last year of life. *N Engl J Med* 1993; 328:1092–1096.

8. Bernabei R, Gambassi G, Lapane K, et al. For the SAGE Study Group. Management of pain in elderly patients with cancer. *JAMA* 1998; 279:1877–1882.

9. Feldt KS, Ryden MB, Miles S. Treatment of pain in cognitively impaired compared with cognitively intact older patients with hip-fracture. *J Am Geriatr Soc* 1998; 46:1079–1085.

10. Morrison RS, Siu AL. A comparison of pain and its treatment in advanced dementia and cognitively intact patients with hip fracture. *J Pain Symptom Manage* 1995; 10:591–598.

11. Cleeland CS, Gonin R, Hatfield AK, et al. Pain and its treatment in outpatients with metastatic cancer. *N Engl J Med* 1994; 330:592–596.

12. Stein W. Cancer pain in the elderly. In: Ferrell BR, Ferrell BA, eds. *Pain in the Elderly*. Seattle: IASP Press, 1996:69–80.

13. AGS Panel on Chronic Pain in Older Persons. The management of chronic pain older persons. *J Am Geriatr Soc* 1998; 46:635–651.

14. Seale C, Cartwright A. *The Year Before Death*. Brookfield, VT: Ashgale Publishing Co., 1994.

15. Covinsky K, Goldman L, Cook E, et al. The impact of serious illness on patients' families. *JAMA* 1994; 272:1839–1844.

16. Ferrell B. Overview of aging and pain. In: Ferrell BR, Ferrell BA, eds. *Pain in the Elderly*. Seattle: IASP Press, 1996.

17. Keay TJ, Fredman L, Taler GA, Datta S, Levenson SA. Indicators of quality medical care for the terminally ill in nursing homes. *J Am Geriatr Soc* 1994; 42:853–860.

18. Engle VF. Care of the living, care of the dying: reconceptualizing nursing home care. *J Am Geriatr Soc* 1998; 46:1172–1174.

19. Lynn J. Caring at the end of our lives [editorial; comment]. *N Engl J Med* 1996; 335:201–202.

20. Eng C, Pedulla J, Eleazer GP, McCann R, Fox N. Program of All-Inclusive Care for the Elderly (PACE): an innovative model of integrated geriatric care and financing [see comments]. *J Am Geriatr Soc* 1997; 45:223–232.

21. Field MJ, Cassel CK. (eds) Approaching death: improving care at the end of life. *Institute of Medicine*. Washington DC: National Academy Press, 1997.

22. Cassell EJ. The nature of suffering and the goals of medicine. *N Engl J Med* 1982; 306:639–645.

5

Care of the Elderly with Advanced Diseases: Caregiver Issues

TAMI BORNEMAN AND BETTY FERRELL

In many ways, family members caring for the elderly with an advanced disease experience a solitary journey. While some have been down this road before, many are not prepared for the journey. Throughout history, family members have assumed responsibility for caring for their own sick with more deaths occurring in the home rather than in the hospital setting. In the 1940s, a shift occurred with more deaths occurring in hospitals.[1-2] Over the last 2 decades, there has been a shift in care back to the home setting along with an increase in deaths. This is largely due to increased home care technology, earlier patient discharge, increased numbers in the elderly population, and increased incidence of chronic diseases.[3-5]

Not only are family caregivers struggling with the emotional impact of their loved one's condition and their own impending sense of loss, but they also are sharing the pain and suffering felt by the patient. Given this shared suffering, Lederberg[6] has referred to family caregivers as *second order patients*. They are critical in either helping or actually providing care to the patient, and in essence, become part of the health care team. However, although the family functions as part of the health care team, they need as much support and care from the professionals as does the patient.

It is important to remember that while the patient and the family caregiver have individual needs, they are not independent of each other. Both must also be assessed as part of the family unit. How the family has worked through or coped with prior illness experiences provides insight into present behavior and provides a springboard for planning effective interventions. Seeking to better understand and learn from the family as a unit, and not just as a group of isolated individuals, creates and promotes a sense of being valued. As a by-product of feeling valued and of being heard, there is a much higher likelihood of overall adherence from the patient and family. Also important to understanding the family as a whole, is knowing their developmental stage, because this effects the types of concerns and problems they have, their responses, their relationships and roles, the availability of those working to provide care, and the availability of secondary caregiving support.[7–9]

This chapter provides an overview of recent literature on issues faced by family members caring for the elderly with advanced diseases, findings from a current qualitative study as it relates to family caregiver issues, and finally, suggestions are provided for interdisciplinary interventions.

Review of the Literature

Family caregiver literature is replete with information on how caring for a loved one with an advanced disease is difficult. Caregiving is difficult, not only emotionally, but physically, socially, and spiritually as well. This review describes major consistent findings in family caregiver literature. To advance this area of research and clinical care, it is important to acknowledge prior studies and the wealth of information they have provided. Not only have these previous studies provided a foundation of knowledge in this area, but the research has given clear direction for future work as well.

Viewing family caregiver issues from a quality of life perspective allows us to focus attention on needs of the caregiver as well as on the demands of caregiving. The quality of life needs of caregivers fall into four categories: physical, psychological, social, and spiritual well-being. The existing literature is discussed according to these categories.

Physical well-being

The primary focus of physical well-being and family caregivers has been in relation to the physical demands of caring. Investigators have portrayed the reality of caregiving in advanced disease by describing common problems that result from caring for the patient such as fatigue or physical strain exacerbated by providing care. Examples would be chronic problems in the family member such as hypertension or arthritis that become exacerbated by the intense physical demands of caregiving.

One of the issues symbolic of caring for the patient in the current health care system is the increased burden of care at home. This physical care encompasses administering medications, managing side effects of medications, providing help with or actually performing activities of daily living, wound care, managing ambulatory infusion pumps, providing symptom management, and meeting nutritional needs.[10–13] The literature over the past decade has uniformly captured the impact on family members as care has shifted from the inpatient setting to home care.

Family caregivers are routinely asked to assume complete care of severely ill patients that was previously provided in the hospital setting.

Interestingly, studies have also demonstrated that basic caregiving tasks also are very demanding and burdensome. In a recent study by Ferrell et al.,[7,14] family caregivers of advanced cancer patients recognized the stress of high-tech, complex care but these caregivers also voiced distress and feelings of inadequacy with providing basic intimate care such as bathing and toileting. Many caregivers felt as though they were violating a boundary of intimacy. Such private, personal care of a parent or spouse, was viewed as out of the realm of normal intimacy.

Another major issue commonly cited for family caregivers is management of the patient's pain, especially if not well controlled.[3,14–18] Several factors contribute to this issue. Family caregivers often hold incorrect knowledge and inappropriate beliefs about pain such as the fear of addiction and respiratory depression. They also withhold pain medications in order to save medications for later if anticipating that the pain will become worse.[14,17] Family caregivers frequently voice concerns of not wanting the patient to be "out of it" as they do not want the remaining time to be spent groggy from medication. The caregiver struggle between providing adequate pain management and their desire to have quality interaction during the time left, is profound during any life threatening illness but becomes intensified as the disease progresses and death becomes imminent.[16]

Family caregivers have been found to exhibit multiple symptoms themselves including fatigue, appetite disturbance, pain, and lack of sleep. Fatigue is cited in the literature as one of the predominant problems for the caregiver. Many family caregivers have reported that they did not realize the enormity of caring for their loved one at home.[3] Jensen and Given[19] found a direct correlation between the number of hours spent on caregiving, the impact on their daily schedule, and the amount of fatigue experienced. Physical symptoms such as fatigue are also exacerbated by psychological strain. Boland and Sims[4] evaluated 17 families to describe caregiver burden and related concepts. Caregivers described their care as a "duty without any break" and viewed themselves as a "24-hour-care person."

Family members entering the phase of advanced disease are often already exhausted by the preceding months or years of the patient's active treatment or chronic illness demands. Many studies have described the toll of chronic illness care.[3,4,13] In Ferrell et al.'s[16] study of 231 family caregivers of older cancer patients receiving home care, the greatest problems were sleep changes, followed by fatigue, appetite changes, overall physical condition, and pain. Many caregivers themselves face declining health[9,13] and many elderly spouses with health problems serve as the primary or sole caregiver of the patient. In addition, it is estimated that 10% of the elderly have a child aged 65 years and older,[20] thus there is a higher probability of caregivers having health problems themselves.

Psychological well-being

The literature reveals many psychological issues faced by family caregivers such as anxiety, depression, feelings of helplessness, and fear. Many caregivers feel overwhelmed and have difficulty coping with their loved one's illness because of all that is required of them. For some family caregivers, change may be the only consistent variable in their lives during advanced disease as they seek to maintain stability through coping with the many demands, mourning losses they have already incurred, and carrying on routine family functions.[6]

Family caregivers are usually novices in providing health care to someone with an advanced disease and not well prepared for the final course of the disease progression. Watching the patients suffering during the disease progression causes tremendous anxiety and family caregiver distress often exceeds that of the patient.[4,12,13] Prior coping methods and the caregiver's role in the family effect their ability to cope in the present situation.[9] In a study of 28 caregivers of cancer patients, Perry and Roades de Menses[21] found that 77% of subjects reported an inability to cope and 55% reported withdrawing emotionally. Ferrell et al.[16] reported difficulty coping, anxiety, depression, lack of happiness, and loss of control as the main psychological issues for 231 family caregivers of older cancer patients at home.

A review of the psychiatric literature and physical morbidity effects on caregivers by Schulz et al.[22] revealed higher levels of psychiatric symptomatology and illness when compared to the general population. A study of 21 family caregivers of dementia patients conducted by Szabo and Strang,[23] revealed that those who experienced a lack of control were unable to recognize their need to ask for help, identified negative internal resources such as doubts about their own ability to manage as a caregiver, and had not anticipated the future with regards to what would be required of them by the patient. Having a sense of control possibly lessens the emotional impact of not being able to slow down the disease's progress in a way that provides meaning.[3]

Social well-being

In the social context, the most common issues for family caregivers found in the literature are lack of family support, lack of professional support, changes and adjustments in role responsibilities, and financial concerns.[4,10,16,24,25] Real or perceived lack of support by family caregivers has been found to correlate with high levels of physical exhaustion.[3] However, they are so involved with the present situation that socialization is rare if nonexistent.[3] According to Hinds,[26] community resources are ignored because of fatigue and low morale.

Advanced disease impacts, to varying degrees, the roles each family member has performed. Now, role requirements are both unpredictable and ambiguous[27] and to some degree, continue changing until the death of their loved ones. As a result, feelings of inadequacy are common among family caregivers as well as feelings of failure in that asking for help somehow implies a lack of commitment to care for their loved ones.[13] In addition, family caregivers often perceive that they are an imposition on the health care professional, resulting in a belief that help is then prioritized according to health care entitlement rather than according to need.[28] The crisis of heightened demands for support accompanied by the perception of less access to such support contributes to feelings of inadequacy with performing an unfamiliar role. The foundation of the family structure may fragment or collapse in disharmony at a time when they need each other the most.[3]

Distress from assuming care in advanced disease was found by Ferrell et al.[16] to be the greatest disruption to their social well-being. Family caregivers of a patient with an advanced disease have been found to experience equal or greater distress than the patient.[29] The family caregiver's distress needs to be assessed in context of the family's life as a whole. Caregivers may be dealing with other pre-existing issues that have been exacerbated by the present illness[30] such as financial concerns that are multiplied by illness.

Spiritual well-being

Spirituality is the process by which one attempts to make meaning in a personal way that transcends self. A frequently cited issue for caregivers is questioning the meaning of the illness. Caregivers, like patients, are faced with their own vulnerability and mortality and struggle to find meaning in the midst of suffering. Questions asked by caregivers often represent deeper underlying questions concerning death.[6] Caregivers may or may not be struggling with the same spiritual issues as the patient, and they may place similar or divergent values on those issues. The fact that caregivers search for meaning is a positive step in coping and healing. Zika and Chamberlain[31] reported that "meaning in life is consistently related to positive mental health outcomes, while meaninglessness is associated with pathological outcomes."[31] This is especially true for those caring for a loved one with an advanced disease. Noonan and Tennstedt[32] found overall sense of meaning in caregiving to be positively related to the search for meaning, in that the more caregivers searched for meaning, higher levels of meaning were reported. In a study of seven family caregivers of patients who died from terminal diseases, Enyert and Burman,[33] found that experiencing meaning came from the belief that what they were doing, no matter how difficult it was, was important to their loved one.

A connection or closeness to God is also important to family caregivers. Pollner[34] found that a divine relationship or closeness to God had a significant effect on several areas of well-being. Feeling supported and comforted by one's faith was associated with positive emotional outcomes.[35] When caregivers perceive forgiveness from God and are able to reframe caregiving into a positive experience, spirituality becomes therapeutic in that it can affirm their senses of well-being.[36] Forbes,[37] studied 17 patients with chronic illnesses and their caregivers and found that religious commitment and a relationship with God, self, environment, as well as an ability to find meaning and purpose, were crucial to transcending the situation. Harrington et al.[38] evaluated the needs of both clinic and hospice caregivers of cancer patients. Caregivers of clinic patients identified "hope for the future" and "a strong faith in God," as important spiritual needs. "Prayers from others" and "a strong faith in God" were identified as priority spiritual needs among caregivers of hospice patients. The common theme being, "a strong faith in God."

Spiritual needs are universal because spiritual care is not bound to a specific religion or faith. Instead, spiritual care is connected to transcendent values of love, faithfulness, generosity, and selflessness.[39] Another issue faced by family caregivers is uncertainty about the future.[16] The uncertainty of what will happen to their loved one or what will happen to themselves after their loved one dies are difficult issues to confront. These thoughts and feelings may intensify as caregivers watch the disease progression. Uncertainty has been documented as a priority concern for all caregivers including parents of terminally ill children as well as caregivers of the elderly.[14]

The concept of hope, or lack of hope, is also important to family caregivers. Yates and Stetz[40] interviewed 20 family caregivers and identified two stages to hoping. Hope almost always started as a hope for cure, many times continuing until the very end. As the disease progressed, hope sometimes shifted from hope for cure to hope for relief from suffering. Hope also ties in closely with uncertainty in that hope dwells in the future. Caregivers facing a loss of the future in ways not intended or expected experience feelings of uncertainty and sometimes despair.[12,41] Dufault and Martocchio[42] reported that hope becomes an anesthetic or an insulation during difficult times. Given that hope is dependent on finding meaning and purpose in life, it becomes a life jacket of security in that no matter what happens, the caregiver can find meaning in the midst of all that is happening.[12]

In summary, advanced disease has been documented to greatly influence all dimensions of quality of life. Caregiving is physically strenuous, creates intense psychological distress, and impacts family structure and function. Caregiving challenges spiritual beliefs at a time when spiritual support is needed. Optimum care of the patient is enhanced by attention to caregivers.

Caregiver Perceptions of Cancer Care

In order to further illustrate the needs of caregivers in advanced disease, data will be presented from a recently completed study involving caregivers of cancer patients. Ferrell et al.[16] conducted a study "Pain Education for Elderly Cancer Patients at Home," funded by the National Cancer Institute. The overall purpose of the study was to test the impact of a structured pain education program on elderly cancer patients and their family caregivers. The study was guided by the conceptual model of quality of life (QOL)[43] applied to family caregivers. Of the 231 patient—caregiver dyads, 10 caregivers ($N = 10$) were invited to participate in an in-depth interview as a component of a masters thesis of Tami Borneman. The purpose of this companion study was to further understand the demands of family caregiving.

Data were collected by the research nurse with open-ended questions during a taped interview session. The interview followed the conclusion of the family caregivers participation in the larger study mentioned above. Interview questions included assessing the caregivers involvement in providing care (i.e., physical care and decision making), changes in the health care system affecting care at home, how their role differed from others in the family in providing care, what aspects of care they felt most and least confident in providing, the most difficult care given, satisfaction with care, and their own quality of life (i.e., physical, psychological, social, and spiritual well-being).

Data was analyzed using content analysis methods[44] to identify major themes of family caregiving based on the quality of life model. Findings revealed several major themes in each domain. Predominant themes in the Physical Well-Being domain included "Total Care," "Physical Demands," and "Distress from Providing Intimate, Personal Care." In the Psychological Well-Being domain, major themes included "Observing the Patient's Decline," "Losing Control," and "The Need to be Valued and Heard." Major themes in the Social Well-Being domain included "Caregiver Isolation" and "Reluctance in Asking for Help." The fourth domain, Spiritual Well-Being, was characterized by themes of "Trusting an Unjust God," "Spirituality as a Source of Support," and "Seeking a Purpose."

These themes demonstrate the importance of educating health care providers about the identified needs of family caregivers, how the shift in health care to the home adds further responsibility and burden on an already overwhelmed family caregiver, and the need for further research to identify effective ways to meet the needs of family caregivers. Examples of family caregiver comments illustrating these themes are included in Tables 5.1–5.4.

Clinical Implications

The issues addressed in this chapter demonstrate that family caregivers have multiple and sometimes complex needs requiring assistance from health care professionals. Family members must constantly adapt to the results of the disease progression and, the changing needs of their loved one. Health care professionals need to make a united effort to identify and implement more effective interventions for supporting family caregivers caring for those with an advanced disease. While the issues cannot be eradicated, interventions to support the family in coping with the situation are vital to improving health care practice. Table 5.5 summarizes potential interventions useful for supporting family caregivers.

Table 5.1. Physical well-being

Theme	Example caregiver comments
Total physical care	"Constant care. I mean I do everything. I bathe her . . . I prepare her meals. Real caretaker is a real good descriptive word . . . I help her down the stairs, I help her to the bathroom, I get her water, I go back down the stairs some days and feels like 50 times a day!"
Pain management	"Some nights we'd be at a motel room and he'd be so full of pain he could not stand it and it wasn't doing a lot of good. He'd be up in the middle of the night most of the nights. Just pain. And the pain, they're trying to control that. That's pretty good. If you don't move him"
Aspects of care felt most confident about	"Making sure that she feels that she is not creating a big burden—or is an imposition on me or things like that. If that's a part of caregiving, and I really believe it is,—then I think that's what I feel most confident about, the fact that there's nothing in my demeanor that conveys in any way—that I'm, that I feel handcuffed—or that I feel cheated or anything like that."
Aspects of care felt least confident about	"I don't like the bathing part. I don't know. I'm not sure. Maybe I feel that I'm not as good at it as, as maybe I could be or should be. But that gives me a little, that gives me a little, makes me a little uncomfortable. But I guess having to take her to the bathroom, and that's, it seems so unnatural to me I guess."
Fatigue	"I was beginning to get worn out. Really physically and mentally worn out. Uh, there was not enough help. I'm still tired. I guess I'll be tired . . . until I can stop worrying about her when I'm laying in bed and picking my head up every ten minutes, 'Did I hear a bell?'"
Appetite changes	"I've put on weight because I sit more with him and eat with him and eat the things he likes."
Own pain	"I have a lot of headaches all the time for the last two years. I had them before that too, but tension headaches, I can't get rid of them for several days."
Sleep changes	"I noticed that I shake a lot, and I don't know if that's from lack of sleep or lack of just everything, because I don't sleep that well. Um. Just probably the inner tension."
Own physical health	"I just have a problem right now. I'm going to have a biopsy on Monday. It's not a lump. It's something showed up in my mammogram."

While the needs of family caregivers have been studied over the years, most of the literature has focused on practical support with very little regard to addressing the issues of emotional support such as anticipatory grieving, dealing with feelings of guilt and inadequacy, and being left behind.[40,45] These caregiver issues are found not only within the walls of the hospital, but are also found across

Table 5.2. Psychological well-being

Theme	Example caregiver comments
Difficulty coping	"She's just a shell of what she used to be. Lot of weight, yeah, very feeble. Really difficult, difficult—And, you know, for me that is by far the toughest part of this whole thing, seeing the effects of the disease, how it ravages, you know,—ravages the body. I feel a great deal of sadness. Being unable to do anything to control what's happening, you know. Being unable to stop this—thing that's happening to her. It's not, it doesn't relate to being able to prevent her death. It relates to being able to prevent all the suffering—or to stop the suffering and the—just the agonizingly slow deterioration."
Happiness/satisfaction	"He's the best thing that happened in my whole life. And, my kids can tell you that too . . . Yes. It is a beautiful life. And just going everywhere with him. Whatever we did, we just sat together. It was fine."
Ability to Concentrate/remember	"Bad. I, I have forgotten so many things. Like, I'll start out to go somewhere to do something, in the middle of it, I forget, and then . . . What did we start out with, what was that question that you started asking?"
Professional insensitivity	"The Tuesday that we went in and told him about the shortness of breath in the wheelchair, he said at that time, well we could get on hospice and get O_2 at home and they could pay for it. Mark was very upset by that comment because he figured at that point that he said he felt like they'd, the doctor, had just thrown rocks in his coffin."
Decision making	"As far as her, um, personal aspect, personal things, I basically have made all the decisions on everything. I'm her executor, I have to keep everything, um, intact and running. Checking account, bills, that kind of stuff."
Methods of coping	"What I try to do is, is get to the gym—and just go over and do weights and stuff and, you know, I find that to be very, very therapeutic—because you don't have to think. It's just physical exertion and, you know, that just tends to, ah, I don't know,—wash away, yeah, just wash away the, the stressful feelings."
Sense of control	"Why would I be in control? God is in control. Or not God. His disease is in control. I don't know if that's what you mean by control. But, I remember that was on that questionnaire I filled out somewhere too. And I don't feel I'm in control. If I was in control, everything would be fine. He wouldn't have what he's got. But, I don't have any control over that. So, I'm not in control . . . Something else is controlling my life. Not me."
Overall quality of life	"It's the pits."

Table 5.3. Social well-being

Theme	Example caregiver comments
Feeling isolated	"I feel that like I could be doing so much more than I need to do for him if I could get out. But, I don't want to be out for long periods of time . . . one time I was trying to go find a pan for him 'cause they were coming but there was nobody here. So he couldn't go. Or, he ran out of bread. I gotta plan things so carefully because I don't have any time to go out and do these errands."
Patient/family caregiver relationship	"My dad dedicated his life to make it to where I could live mine. And, um, so basically I mean he and I were teammates and, ah, you know when one of your team members are going, it's, that's hard for the other one to go on. And I had to reassure him that I would be okay."
Communications with the patient	"I don't know what to say sometimes . . . Sometimes we don't know what to say. I'm so surprised when he has his eyes opened so long and he's looking, and I'm thinking, 'Oh my goodness, what are we going to talk about now?'"
Interference with employment/ activities at home	"If I'm at the computer, then I worry about him and I go check on him. Then I get distracted by doing something for him, and I don't get back to the computer. Or then somebody calls and asks how he is. Or, then the hospice comes in. Or, then it's time for a bowel movement. And, then it's time just to decide what he wants to eat."
Support from others	"There's nobody else to help. I'm the only one with her all day, and there just isn't anybody else. And, it wears me out. I'm 71 years old now. And, it, it sort of wears me out."
Support from home care	"The . . . people I've met. The doctors, the nurses, the therapists, the receptionist, they've all been great. They all still call. I guess that makes me happy. They were so helpful to my husband. They were so caring. They understood my pain. And they reached out and I remember them sharing. That's so important because you're not a statistic. You know, you're a person with feelings, and scared, and you're concerned about a loved one. And what's going to happen to him. And so when somebody is kind and concerned and helpful oh, it's the best therapy in the world. Kindness."
Unmet needs	"It's like, again, you're trying to maintain your normal life but there's always demands there. So, it's that struggle."
Advice to others	"Do your best. Don't feel guilty if your best is not as good as somebody else's, and don't be afraid to ask for help. That's about the only advice I can give."

Table 5.4. Spiritual well-being

Theme	Example caregiver comments
Meaning	"It doesn't mean religion. I'll tell you that. I don't think it does, and I guess it means having a connection with something other than just material things, um, knowing that we have a physical body but then there's that spark, whatever, whatever that thing is that makes us live."
Importance of spirituality	"Because to me that is what makes the person. You know, you're the kind of person who cares for other people who, who is sensitive to the needs of other people, who believes there is a right way and a wrong way, moral, immoral, ethical, unethical, all those sort of things. To me all those things relate to the spirit of the real person."
Spiritual needs	"I've had a lot of spiritual needs. And, I, ah, I have found that, ah, going to church has been a very emotional thing for me. I've needed a lot of spiritual help. And, sometimes the pastor's message . . . It's like it was just to me."
Spiritual activities	"I've been reading my Bible a lot more. And praying a lot."
Death awareness	"Sometimes I go back and forth. This is torture. This is torture for two years. But there's the good moments that you wouldn't have. You, you have a chance to say good-bye even if he doesn't understand it. You don't say good-bye, but you have a chance to be with him."
Anger at God	"I just don't care to pray to Him today. Because He hasn't helped me yet. Yes, He has in the past, I am sure. And, I know He's there. And I know He cares, and, I just am on a little break from God."
Hope	"I think it's crucial to have (faith) in other life because unless you believe that there are things that you can accomplish whatever they may be, which relates to hope, then you're just simply not going to have a good life . . . and without that there's, you're just nothing, and I think you can see the results of that when you drive down in skid row and other places where people have just given up. They've lost hope."

health care settings. Those caregivers in the home have the added burden and responsibility of the patient's physical care as well as other life demands.

Families caring for a loved one with an advanced disease are emotionally vulnerable. Issues surrounding the illness become the primary topic of thought and discussion for which they give health care professionals significant importance and authority.[6,46] The family observes the health care professionals for any sign of the patient's condition and also embraces the health care team's unspoken beliefs and rules.[6] With such informal power, health care professionals need to be sensitive to their influence given the vulnerable state of the caregivers. The goal is not to fix the problem because the root problem cannot be fixed. The patient's disease is not going away and the inevitable, death, will occur. What is important is the human support health care professionals can offer the family

Table 5.5. Summary of potential interventions for support of family caregivers

Domain	Intervention
Physical	1. Provide resources for help in physical care and respite 2. Offer home health aides to help with personal hygiene 3. Offer occupational therapists to teach work simplification and energy conversation skills 4. Monitor the caregiver's health status, and known acute or chronic health problems.
Psychological	1. Facilitate discussion of concerns regarding future care 2. Offer services of psychiatric personnel or licensed clinical social workers 3. Offer respite care 4. Assess for caregiver depression 5. Facilitate sharing of feelings
Social	1. Help minimize isolation and loneliness by facilitating the use of the family network 2. Provide a resource list of support groups 3. Offer volunteer services 4. Facilitate family discussion regarding concerns, and help them create realistic schedules for sharing caregiving duties 5. Validate caregivers feelings about what they are experiencing 6. Offer support of social service to evaluate financial needs
Spiritual	1. Use active listening and presence 2. Facilitate discussion about finding meaning in the experience 3. Assess past spiritual support, religious practices, and resources 4. Help to construct a sense of hope 5. Offer prayer and religious readings 6. Involve chaplaincy

caregiver both practically and emotionally. Presencing, being fully present to another, can diminish feelings of isolation, increase feelings of connectedness, increase the sense of being valued, and decrease feelings of vulnerability.[47] Professionals can be a catalyst for healing, and healing takes place in many forms. The professional's role is not just a matter of being there to provide answers, but rather being there to share the questions.

Conclusions

This chapter reviews issues faced by family caregivers caring for a loved one with an advanced disease. It truly is a difficult journey. While the goal of health care is often described as patient focused, it also must be family centered. For care in advanced disease, it is important to remember that the whole is greater than the sum of its parts. Consistent literature findings reinforce the need for improved interventions for family caregivers. As Lederberg[6] states, they are second-order patients requiring as much support if not more, than the patient.

Acknowledgments

This research was conducted as the masters thesis of Tami Borneman from Azusa Pacific University.

References

1. Mor V, Greer DS, Kaastenbaum R. *The Hospice Experience.* Baltimore: Johns Hopkins University Press, 1988.
2. Corr C. Death in modern society. In: Koyle D, Hanks G, and MacDonald N, eds. *Oxford Textbook of Palliative Medicine.* 2nd ed. Oxford: Oxford University Press; 1998:31–40.
3. Schachter S and Coyle N. Palliative home care—impact on families. In: Holland J, ed. *Psycho-oncology.* New York: Oxford University Press; 1998:1004–1015.
4. Boland D and Sims S. Family care giving at home as a solitary journey. *Image: J Nurs Scholarship* 1996; 28:55–58.
5. Nijboer C, Tempelaar R, Sanderman R, Triemstra M, Spruijt R, Van Den Bos G. Cancer and caregiving: the impact on the caregiver's health. *Psycho-oncology* 1998; 3–13.
6. Lederberg M. The family of the cancer patient. In: Holland J, ed. *Psycho-oncology.* New York: Oxford University Press; 1998:981–993.
7. Ferrell B. The family. In: Doyle D, Hanks G, MacDonald N, eds. *Oxford Textbook of Palliative Medicine.* 2nd ed. Oxford: Oxford University Press; 1998:909–917.
8. Kemp C. *Terminal Illness: A Guide to Nursing Care.* Philadelphia: J. B. Lippincott; 1995:29–42.
9. Vachon M, Kristjanson L, Higginson I. Psychosocial issues in palliative care: the patient, the family, and the process and outcome of care. *J Pain Symp Manage* 1995; 10:142–150.
10. Ferrell B, Grant M, Rhiner M, Padilla G. Home care: maintaining quality of life for patient and family. *Oncology* 1992; 6:136–140.
11. Silveira J, Winstead-Fry P. The needs of patients with cancer and their caregivers in rural areas. *Oncol Nurs Forum* 1997; 24:71–76.
12. Borneman T. Caring for cancer patients at home: the effect on family caregivers. *Home Health Care Management & Practice* 1998; 10:25–33.
13. Steele R, Fitch M. Needs of family caregivers of patients receiving home hospice care for cancer. *Oncol Nurs Forum* 1996; 23:823–828.
14. Ferrell B, Borneman T. Pain and suffering at the end of life (EOL) for older patients and their families. *Generations* 1999; 28:12–17.
15. Ferrell B, Juarez G, Borneman T, ter Veer A. Outcomes of pain education in community. *Home care. J Hospice Palliat Nursing* 1999; 1:141–150.
16. Ferrell B, Grant M, Borneman T, ter Veer A. Family caregiving in cancer pain management. *J Palliat Med* 1999; 2:185–195.

17. Gorman L. The psychosocial impact of cancer on the individual, family, and society. In: Carroll-Johnson R, Gorman L, Bush N, eds. *Psychosocial Nursing Care Along the Cancer Continuum.* Pittsburgh: Oncology Nursing Press; 1998:3–25.

18. Rhiner M, Coluzzi P. Family issues influencing management of cancer pain. In: McGuire D, Yarbro C, Ferrell B, eds. *Cancer Pain Management.* Boston: Jones and Bartlett Publishers; 1995:207–230.

19. Jensen S, Given B. Fatigue affecting family caregivers of cancer patients. *Cancer Nurs* 1991; 14:181–187.

20. Reich W. ed. *Encyclopedia of Bioethics.* New York: Simon & Schuster; 1995.

21. Perry G, Roades de Menses M. Cancer patients at home: needs and coping styles of primary caregivers. *Home Health Nurs* 1991; 7:27–30.

22. Schultz R, Vistainer P, Williamson G. Psychiatric and physical morbidity effects of caregiving. *J Gerontology: Psychol Sci* 1990; 45:181–191.

23. Szabo V, Strang V. Experiencing control in cargiving. *Image: J Nurs Scholarship* 1999; 31:71–75.

24. Northouse L, Peters-Golden H. Cancer and the family: strategies to assist spouses. *Semin Oncol Nurs* 1993; 9:74–82.

25. Ruppert R. Caring for the lay caregiver. *Am J Nurs* 1996; 96;40–46.

26. Hinds, C. The needs of families who care for patients with cancer at home. Are we meeting them? *J Adv Nurs* 1985; 10:575–581.

27. Schumacher K. Reconceptualizing family caregiver: family-based illness care during chemotherapy. *Res Nurs Health* 1996; 19:261–271.

28. Grande G, Todd C, Barclay S. Support needs in the last year of life: patient and carer dilemmas. *Palliat Med* 1997; 11:202–208.

29. Vachon M. Emotional problems in palliative medicine: patient, family and professional. In: Doyle D, Hands G, MacDonald N, eds. *Oxford Textbook of Palliative Medicine.* Oxford: Oxford University Press; 1993:577–605.

30. Ferszt G, Houck P. The family. In: Amenta, M, Bohnet N, eds. *Nursing Care of the Terminally Ill.* Boston: Little, Brown and Company; 1986:173–190.

31. Zika S, chanberlain K. On the relation between meaning in life and psychological well-being. *Br J Psychol* 1992; 83:135–145.

32. Noonan A, Tennstedt S. Meaning in caregiving and its contribution to caregiver well-being. *The Gerontologist* 1997; 37:785–794.

33. Enyert G, Burman M. A qualitative study of self-transcendence in caregivers of terminally ill patients. *Am J Hospice & Palliat Care* 1999; 16:455–462.

34. Pollner M. Divine relations, social relations, and well-being. *J Health Soc Behav* 1989; 30:92–104.

35. Rabins P, Fitting M, Eastham J, Fetting J. The emotional impact of caring for the chronically ill. *Psychosomatics* 1990; 31:331–336.

36. Kaye J, Robinson K. Spirituality among caregivers. *Image: J Nurs Scholarship* 1994; 26:218–221.

37. Forbes E. Spirituality, aging, and the community dwelling caregiver and care recipient. *Geriatric Nurs* 1994; 15:297–302.

38. Harrington V, Lackey N, Gates M. Needs of caregivers of clinic and hospice cancer patients. *Cancer Nurs* 1996; 19:118–125.

39. Carson V. Spiritual care: the needs of the caregiver. *Semin Oncol Nurs* 1997; 13:271–274.

40. Yates P, Stetz K. Families' awareness of and response to dying. *Oncol Nurs Forum* 1999; 26:113–120.
41. Amenta M. Spiritual concerns. In: Amenta M, Bohnet N, eds. *Nursing Care of the Terminally Ill.* Boston: Little, Brown and Company; 1986:115–161.
42. Dufault K, Martocchio B. Hope: its spheres and dimensions. *Nurs Clin North Am* 1985; 20:379–391.
43. Ferrell B, Grant M, Padilla G, Rhiner M. The experience of pain and perceptions of quality of life: validation of a conceptual model. *Hospice J* 1991; 7:9–24.
44. Krippendorff K. *Content Analysis: An Introduction to its Methodology.* Newbury Park: SAGE Publications; 1980.
45. Stewart A, Teno J, Patrick D, Lynn J. The concept of quality of life of dying persons in the context of health care. *J Pain Symp Manage* 1999; 17:93–108.
46. Cassileth B. *The Cancer Patient: Social and Medical Aspects of Care.* Philadelphia: Lea and Febiger; 1979.
47. Pettigrew J. Intensive nursing care: the ministry of presence. *Crit Care Nurs Clin North Am* 1990; 2:503–508.

III
COMMUNICATION ISSUES
IN PALLIATIVE CARE

6

Truth-Telling and Reciprocity in the Doctor–Patient Relationship: A North American Perspective

JOSEPH J. FINS

During a visit to a bioethics program in Europe, I recognized how far North American practice has strayed from global norms. In talking about truth-telling and the importance of providing patients with diagnostic information that would allow them to make important life decisions, I was asked how information about a grave diagnosis could possibly be helpful to a dying patient. After being accused of being a proponent of a cruel and brutal North American ethic, based more on patient autonomy than physician beneficence, I was proudly told of an act of deception to spare a dying patient the truth.

As it was shared with me, a senior physician at a leading hospital was dying of adenocarcinoma of the pancreas. The tumor, at the head of the pancreas, was causing biliary obstruction and marked jaundice. The patient, who was a gastroenterologist, suspected the worst and feared that he had either hepatocellular or pancreatic cancer. When he asked to see his computerized axial tomography (CAT) scan, his residents and fellows wanted to spare him any additional grief. They substituted the scan of another patient and told him that the cause of his jaundice was hepatitis. This blatant act of deception was told to me not with the regret of hindsight, but shared proudly. In their view, the professor's clinical heirs had done their chief a great service by protecting him from the harm that would follow from disclosing the unvarnished truth.

Although the actions of these European physicians seems deviant from the North American perspective, North Americans are actually the ones who have deviated from global norms in embracing an autonomy ethic far more expansive than our colleagues around the world.[1] In doing so, we have also departed from medical tradition. Throughout the history of medicine, palliation and truth-telling have been at odds. If palliation was seen as a way to preserve hope, then the truth was the enemy of hope and frequently hidden from the patient's view. Palliation was not about disclosure, as its seventeenth century usage suggests, but rather about cloaking or disguising the truth.[2] Traditionally, as Jay Katz has observed, the doctor–patient relationship was silent when it came to sharing the truth.[3] Patients were felt to be served by less, not more information—especially when the news was bad and there was little to offer.

Practice patterns in the United States might even be said to be counterintuitive. Our clinical intuitions tell us that sharing a grave diagnosis with a patient has to be antithetical to the promotion of palliation. If the goals of palliation are to relieve pain, minimize suffering, and protect vulnerable patients from unnecessary burdens, it would seem unlikely that the truth could be comforting.

And yet, physicians in the United States now overwhelmingly believe that patients have the right to know their diagnoses, even if they are grave and terminal.[4] Are we cruel and insensitive practitioners, as our international colleagues quietly allege? Or is it that we are products of a different culture? As a practitioner in North America, I cannot believe that we are either cruel or inhumane. I have seen acts of kindness and charity in the clinic that might even restore the faith of a cynic. I would prefer, instead, to believe that our actions reflect our nation's history and social transformation in this century. These forces have shaped medical practice. They have helped us appreciate palliation as something more than the mere protection of patients from pain or harm or the provision of symptom relief.

The most progressive of North American practitioners have taken a more expansive view of palliative care. They understand it as an opportunity for patients to reflect on life experiences and perhaps reach closure. The idea is to help the patient live as fully as possible even as they experience the dying process. But for a patient to live fully, they need to be fully informed of their situation. Self-reflection and authentic encounters with loved ones cannot be accomplished through a veil of deception. A dying patient cannot find meaning in the dying process if he does not know he is dying. Indeed if we value meaning, we must also value the truth. Understood this way, the truth is not the enemy of hope, it is a palliative.

The Evolution of Practice in the United States

It might be argued that our practice patterns began to break from tradition in 1914 when the great American jurist Benjamin Cardozo articulated the right of adult competent patients to consent to treatments. Writing as a judge on the New York State Court of Appeals in *Schloendorff vs. the Society of The New York Hospital*, Cardozo opined that ". . . Every human being of adult years in sound mind has a right to determine what shall be done with his own body; and a surgeon who performs an operation without the patient's consent commits an assault for which he is liable for damages. . . . This is true except in cases of emergency when the patient is unconscious and when it is necessary to operate before consent can be obtained."[5]

Although this historic decision prefigured the notion of informed consent, which would later guide medical practice in the United States, its significance was not immediately recognized. In fact, jurists honoring Cardozo's legacy a year after his death did not even mention informed consent in a commemorative law review volume jointly sponsored by the Harvard, Columbia, and Yale Law schools.[6] This 1939 collection does cite *Schloendorff* but only an aspect of the opinion, which has since been overruled.

Ten years later a text on legal medicine cites *Schloendorff*, but offers a traditional vision of medical decision-making. While giving lip-service to informed consent, the author suggests that patients will be best served by a paternalistic doctor–patient relationship. Commenting on patient consent for surgery, the author advises that patients place their faith in the physician, as a child might entrust a parent. He writes that, ". . . The relationship of physician and patient is one of trust and confidence. It is submitted that the best interest of the patient is served in trusting his welfare to the skill and integrity of the physician."[7]

Medical practice patterns changed little during the 1950s even though cancer patients were beginning to express a strong desire to know their diagnoses.[8] Despite these early rumblings, the prevailing medical ethic remained paternalistic. This is illustrated by Oken's study of physicians at Michael Reese Hospital, which was published in 1961.[9] Oken observed that 90% of physicians reported that they withheld the diagnosis when their patients had cancer. When information was shared, disclosure was limited or deliberately misleading in order to ". . . sustain and bolster the patient's hope." Although earlier patient surveys demonstrated that patients wanted to know their diagnosis, Oken observed that the physicians he studied disagreed. He wrote that, "The vast majority of these doctors feel that almost all patients really do not want to know, *regardless of what people say.* (italics added) They approach the issue with the view that disclosure should be avoided unless there are positive indications, rather than the reverse."

The status quo began to change dramatically in the years after Oken conducted his study.[10] By 1979, Novack et al. found that 97% of practitioners ". . . indicated a preference for telling a cancer patient his diagnosis." The authors characterized this change as a "complete reversal of attitude" since Oken made his observations.[11]

The Emergence of the Truth

Tracing the evolution of practice patterns is a far easier task than attempting to explain why these changes occurred. Some have maintained that disclosure of the truth has been made easier by improvements in treatment. When the truth was not directly equated with the erosion of all hope it became easier to be forth-coming.[12]

Although technological advances surely played a role in these changes, the emergence of truth-telling in medical practice was influenced more by factors outside of medicine. In many respects, the decline of physician paternalism was a broader reflection of the times and the social turbulence that convulsed the nation in the 1960s. These forces, external to medicine, reconfigured all aspects of American life and influenced how physicians and patients communicated with each other. The emergence of assorted rights movements, which asserted the rights of minorities, women, and consumers, inevitably led to a broader articulation of patient rights. If citizens enjoyed new rights in civil life, and consumers had increased protections in the marketplace, then patients were also logically entitled to know about their medical condition if they became ill.

America's preoccupation with rights in the 1960s also led to the birth of modern medical ethics. Like other rights movements of that era, medical ethics sought to minimize hierarchies and promote the individual's self-determination. But in illustrating the possibilities of patient self-determination, medical ethics more importantly demonstrated the limitations of physician paternalism. Medical ethics suggested that some clinical decisions were more than technical determinations: they were value choices that drew upon a patient's beliefs and mores. Because these values were highly personal—and at times idiosyncratic—the patient was best positioned to make these decisions. However well-intentioned a physician might be, he could not decide what was in the patient's best interest or what counted as a "good."[13] These decisions were outside the purview of the physician's expertise and thus the inappropriate object of paternalism. Patients had to make these judgements for themselves and be given the necessary information they would need to make these decisions. Simply put, patients would need to know the truth. For, as Pellegrino has noted, the ". . . human capability for autonomous choices cannot function if truth is withheld, falsified, or otherwise manipulated."[14]

Structural changes in the delivery of care during this period also fostered an autonomy ethic. During the 1960s medical care became more impersonal and anonymous. The rise of medical technology, coupled with the restructuring of health care financing, moved care from the home to the hospital. Care became increasingly institutionalized. The local physician who made house calls and took care of the entire family's medical needs was replaced by a team of doctors working in offices and clinics outside the neighborhood. Gone were the days of the general practitioner who delivered your parents and took care of your ear infections when you were in grade school. He was replaced by specialists of all stripes. Overall patient care became more fragmented.

Although I am generationally removed from the era of the general practitioner, I had the good fortune to observe one at close range during the mid-1970s, when he worked as an emergency room physician in my community.[15] Ten years after closing his practice, his patients continued to come to the ER for his care and counsel. He gave advice in that setting just as he did 30 years earlier in the office in the back of his home: generously and knowingly. It was obvious he knew these people and their personal histories. Although today we might critique his style as paternalistic, it wasn't authoritarian. It was informed by years of altruistic hard work caring for patients who trusted him. He did give direction and advice, but it had a certain kind of moral authority that came from knowing patients and nurturing *entire* families back to health.

As the general practitioner was replaced by a new generation of doctors, his style of doctor–patient communication also went out of fashion. The guidance that seemed appropriate and sensitive from a trusted neighborhood physician seemed increasingly directive when it came from a virtual stranger who did not know you, much less your parents or grandparents. Advice that was once appreciated from one source seemed to be an intrusion when it came from another. Such counsel was soon labeled pejoratively as paternalistic, and it probably was.

These physicians did not know their patients as their predecessors in general practice did. When this younger generation of physicians tried to use their own values as a proxy for their patients, it became increasingly clear that doctor and patient now inhabited different worlds. With the fragmentation of care, the broader institutionalization of medical practice, and the rapid escalation of physician incomes beginning in the 1960s, physician and patient were less likely to hail from the same cultural background, pray in the same congregation, or share the same socioeconomic class. This social dislocation made old-style paternalism increasingly untenable, if not impossible.

In this emerging environment, the patient's voice had to be heard. Physicians who did not know their patients could not speak for them. Empirical studies demonstrate that the more modern doctor–patient relationship did not provide physicians with the information they would need to make the care decisions that their patients would make for themselves.[16] If the physician could no longer speak for their patients, patients had to speak for themselves.

But patient self-determination became more than a vehicle for self-expression. It soon became a protection against vestigial paternalism and a defense against the beliefs, values, or prejudices of the practitioner. This became especially important when people of different cultural and faith traditions began to come together to provide and receive health care. Today, it is not unusual to observe a Muslim physician caring for a Jewish patient in a hospital sponsored by the Catholic church. Mayor Rudolph W. Giuliani of New York captured this diversity in a speech celebrating the 50th anniversary of the United Nations. Giuliani observed that ". . . whatever part of the world you're from, you can find people in New York City who speak your language, share your cultural traditions, practice your religion, and enjoy your cuisine."[17]

Although this diversity enriches America's cultural life, this same diversity can create challenges when moral dilemmas arise in the practice of medicine. Unlike other nations with a dominant religion, we do not have a single religious tradition to turn to for guidance. Instead, we have a plurality of traditions capable of responding to ethical dilemmas in patient care. A secular ethic, with its emphasis on patient autonomy was especially well-suited to this situation. Stressing patient self-determination as its overriding principle, secular bioethics laid the ground rules for adjudicating moral dilemmas in patient care when cultural mores clash. Tolerance would prevail and the patient's values would have primacy. Although the stakeholders did not have to agree with the patient's beliefs, all would come to the table accepting the importance of pluralism and accommodation. In a complicated world, secular bioethics allowed a diversity of peoples to pursue their beliefs and be different without being deviant.[18]

The Law and the Rise of Patient Self-Determination

A consideration of the forces that advanced truth-telling in North American medicine would be incomplete without acknowledging the important role played by the law over the past 35 years. Broader social changes, like the emerging rights movements of the 1960s, were able to infiltrate the sequestered world of medical practice through the growing influence of the courts. Judicial activism of this period dramatically altered the clinical landscape with decisions advancing the centrality of informed consent and patient autonomy. Indeed, it would not be an exaggeration to suggest that the legal system became the vector by which the old paternalism was breached and replaced by a new strain of patient self-determination.

Patient self-determination was promoted through a new genus of informed consent cases, which considered both the patient's right to medical information and his/her place in medical decision-making. Early cases from this period hinged upon questions of disclosure.[19,20] These cases first articulated the physician's affirmative obligation to share important information with the patient.[21] Subsequent cases specified what constituted *reasonable* disclosure about a patient's illness and treatment options.[22–24] More stringent requirements for disclosure naturally led to greater patient involvement in medical decision-making. As patients became more knowledgeable about their circumstances, they came to expect a greater role in medical decision-making.

Over the past 15 years, patient self-determination flourished. During this period, disclosure and truth-telling was promoted by the courts, and patients have achieved a wealth of new rights, most notably in end-of-life decision-making. Since 1980, patients have gained an ability to forego life-sustaining therapy and the right to consent to do-not-resuscitate-orders.[25–27]

Patient autonomy became so ingrained in our nation's consciousness that a federal law was passed in 1990 mandating that health care institutions provide patients with the means to articulate end-of-life preferences in an advance directive.[28] Appropriate to an era marked by the rise of patient autonomy, this law was entitled the Patient Self-Determination Act. Its passage codified autonomy's displacement of physician beneficence that had been slowly evolving since *Schloendorff.*

Backlash

If the Patient Self-Determination Act represented the legal codification of patient autonomy, it also heralded a new era when some would ask whether there were limits to patient self-determination. Since its passage, the broad societal consensus that had advanced patient self-determination began to splinter. Prominent commentators, many of whom were instrumental to the growth of the bioethics movement, began to question whether our national embrace of self-determination had gone too far.

Old fault lines that had been obscured by the rights movements of the 1960s began to resurface as autonomy arguments were pushed to their limits, most notably in the physician-assisted suicide debate.[29] This stress proved to be too much and the bioethics movement split on this contentious issue.[30] Arguments advancing physician-assisted suicide as the logical extension of a patient's autonomy[31,32] were opposed by equally articulate observers. They asserted that in extending the patient's right to be left alone to an affirmative obligation to assist in dying "patient self-determination had run amok."[33] In a matter of a few short years, many who had agreed on the reasonableness of the Patient Self-Determination Act,[34] found themselves on opposite sides of the physician-assisted suicide question.[35]

The emerging critique of our autonomy ethic, however, has not been limited to the divisive assisted suicide debate. There is a new genre in bioethics noting the costs associated with the prizing of autonomy over other social goods.[36] Viewing autonomy as an end to be achieved—and not as a means to other important goods—has led to distortions in health care policy that are unique to our country. Our preoccupation with the rights of individuals has distracted us from efforts to foster broader societal solidarity and the just distribution of health care resources. Indeed, it is plausible to assert that our nation's singular failure to universalize access to health care is a consequence of our focus on the individual and not the broader community of which he or she is a part. This systemic inattention to the common good was especially apparent in recent federal circuit court decisions that asserted an individual's constitutionally protected right to physician assisted suicide even though collectively Americans do not yet have a right to health care.[37,38]

At the bedside, even the seemingly settled question of truth-telling has been reopened for debate. In what could be described only as a clinical backlash against an ethic dominated by self-determination, some have begun to wonder whether patients are always served by absolute and total disclosure. These commentators appeal for compassion and clinical common sense over a theoretical or legal obligation to respect a patient's autonomy. Their views echo the criticisms heard from abroad that cast the North American penchant for truth-telling as cruel and even inhumane.

The journalist Martha Weinman Lear captured this sentiment in her essay, "Should doctors tell the truth? The case against terminal candor." Published in *The New York Times Magazine*, her piece depicts how the aggressive promotion of truth-telling can often disable the patient under a mound of information.[39] Noting the psychoanalyst Willard Gaylin's description of excessively robust disclosure as truth-dumping, Weinman Lear offers a trenchant critique of a mechanical notion of informed consent and patient autonomy. She suggests that there is something terribly wrong—even iatrogenic—when the doctor–patient relationship is a conduit for information but not a vehicle for healing. When this occurs, physicians become functionaries who neither comfort, nor instruct. Simply put, they impose the truth.

Acknowledging the Doctor–Patient Relationship

Although Weinmann Lear's criticism could be understood as an appeal for a return to an era of physician beneficence, it illustrates that in responding to one extreme in practice we have created another. It is hard to disagree with her criticism of physicians who are insensitive with the truth, but it is equally difficult to endorse practitioners who withhold the truth from patients who might be served by it. Neither deception nor insensitive disclosure seems worthy of patients or the physicians entrusted to serve them.

Although full disclosure has been advanced as a way to remedy the deception that had traditionally marked the doctor–patient relationship, each practice falls short because it isolates the physician and the patient from each other. The judgement necessary to titrate the proper amount of disclosure to a particular clinical situation does not reside solely in the physician. It emerges from the relationship between the physician and the patient.

The irony of our embrace of disclosure as a response to the moral excesses of deception is that both actions fail to acknowledge the doctor–patient encounter as a relationship. Just as the paternalist views the relationship as amenable to his unilateral decision making, the autonomist views medical decision-making as the domain of the patient. Both views are misconstruals. The doctor–patient relationship is a dialectic. Each partner influences the other. Neither operates alone or in isolation. Instead, the relationship is a dyad, that imposes limits on both the autonomy of the patient and the clinical discretion of the physician. The failure to acknowledge the interdependency of the patient and physician on each other fosters the excesses of patient self-determination on the one hand and paternalism on the other.

It is impossible to escape the interdependency that marks the doctor–patient relationship, even though we speak of clinical autonomy or patient self-determination. Because the encounter between the doctor and patient involves the other, neither can be completely self-determining. Complete self-determination in any sort of relationship is a fictional construct. This is especially true of patients when they enter into a doctor–patient relationship. Patients are neither alone, nor fully self-determining but subjected to an element of dependency, which cannot be ignored. Their choices and options are framed by how the physician presents information. Although they may make choices based on what they have been told, they do not have control over the information that they are given.

Consider the physician who describes an intensive care unit to a critically ill patient who must decide whether to pursue aggressive treatment. A physician who wanted to steer his patient away from intensive care might describe the intensive care unit (ICU) as follows:

> If we take you down to the ICU we will put you on a ventilator. Some patients find the tube that we will put down your throat uncomfortable, but it is necessary for the breathing machine. We will also put a large intravenous line into your neck. This will limit your ability to turn your head and neck. Visiting hours are limited in the ICU, so your family can only see you for 10 minutes twice a day.

Contrast this description with that of a physician hoping to persuade a patient to accept a recommendation for an ICU transfer:

> We will take you down to the ICU and put you on a breathing machine. Although you'll have a tube in your throat, you should be less short of breath. If you are uncomfortable we can give you pain medicine. We will also put an intravenous line in your neck, which will limit your ability to turn your neck—but we'll bandage it securely. We'll use that special intravenous to give you medicines that will make your heart pump better. Although visiting hours are just 10 minutes twice a day, there is one nurse for every two patients in the unit and part of her job is to keep your family apprised of your progress.

While the law mandates that patients be told what a reasonable person would need to know to make an informed decision,[40] these descriptions of the ICU illustrate the difficulty of translating theoretical guidelines into clinical practice. Both of these descriptions are accurate portrayals of the technologies used in an ICU. Yet, neither one is entirely truthful or forthcoming.

Each discussion betrays the bias of the physician's treatment recommendations. The first narrative describes side effects of technologies employed in the ICU without explaining the rationale for these interventions or how their associated morbidities might be softened. The second description provides this additional information but may be misleading about the discomfort the patient may experience.

A close reading of these narratives illustrates that the line is pretty thin between disclosure and distortion. Each bit of information that is shared reflects a decision to disclose one part of the story, perhaps at the expense of another. Such editorial decisions can influence the choices made by patients illustrating that even when a physician discloses information, he has the ability to be authoritarian.

Even this fairly routine example illustrates that doctor and patient are in a relationship and that the structure of the power dynamics within that encounter are asymmetrical.[41] The physician controls the information that might be disclosed and crafts the way the information is shared.

It is important to recognize the power that the physician can wield if we hope to avoid the excesses of paternalism or truth-dumping. Curiously, both are abuses of the physician's power. Paternalism, with its unilateral decision-making is an error of commission in which power is authoritarian and solely within the hands of the physician. Truth-dumping is a more subtle abuse. It is an error of omission and represents the physician's failure to use his therapeutic power to help the patient make sense of the medical facts. It is nothing less than an abdication and the abandonment of the patient.

Reciprocity and Truth-Telling

Both paternalism and truth-dumping are threats to the doctor–patient relationship. Each mistakenly consolidates decision-making power in an individual at the expense of the relationship between doctor and patient. This undermines the potential for collaboration and obscures the fact that neither member of the doctor–patient partnership alone possesses the judgement to properly titrate the truth. There is no escaping the reciprocity of physician and patient when considering how the truth is shared and employed.

It is, in fact, the acknowledgement of this reciprocity that prevents abuses. The physician is less likely to abdicate his authority or act in an authoritarian manner when he appreciates that the patient depends upon him for medical information and that he must, in turn, look to the patient for guidance. When this is acknowledged, advice and information can be given in a way that is tempered. The physician can provide guidance without being so determinative that the patient is forced to agree with the physician's recommendation. Information can be shared in a manner that is attentive to the patient's ability to apprehend and comprehend.

Such reciprocity can be fostered when the physician emulates what Brody has termed transparency.[42] Brody suggests that when a physician is transparent and thinking out loud, he shares both his thoughts and power with the patient. This exercise in explication allows the physician to use his therapeutic power without becoming authoritarian. In this dynamic, physician and patient empower each other. The patient enfranchises the physician to provide guidance and comfort. The physician, in turn, empowers the patient with information that only he can provide.

It is a *reciprocal* relationship that is unequal but still collaborative. Physician and patient make different, yet mutually enhancing, contributions to make the relationship successful. The physician's greater technical knowledge is balanced by the fact that the patient has a greater stake in the decisions that are made. The patient values this technical information but needs to interpret it in light of life experiences and personal values.

Reciprocity and the Therapeutic Exception

Viewing the doctor–patient relationship as a reciprocal relationship is most helpful in deciding whether or not it is appropriate to withhold the truth and invoke the therapeutic exception. Although patients should be engaged in as much of their care decisions as possible, patients' levels of involvement must be weighed against their abilities to actively interact in their relationships with their physicians. Generally, a physician invokes the therapeutic exception when disclosure would be disproportionately burdensome or dangerous. The therapeutic exception, as its name would imply, is a departure from the general norm to disclose the truth. Exceptional circumstances are needed for a physician to invoke his therapeutic privilege and withhold the truth.

Patients who cannot collaborate with a physician because of cognitive limitations or psychological distress should be the object of a therapeutic exception because they cannot engage in reciprocal decision making with their physicians. They should neither have the truth imposed upon them nor be asked to participate in relationships when they are unable to do so. Instead, decisions should be made for them by the appropriate surrogate decision makers. In these cases, disclosure will neither empower the patient nor foster self-determination.

Viewing truth-telling through the prism of reciprocity suggests that the truth itself is not an absolute good. Instead, it is an instrumental good that is valued because it generally leads to greater goods. Truth-telling is a good that needs to be contextualized within the broader provision of patient care. When disclosure leads to reciprocity in the doctor–patient relationship, it is a good to be sanctioned and promoted. But when truth-telling does not lead to an enhanced ability for patients to make important life choices it can be abridged.

Palliation, Reciprocity, and the Truth

If we return to the case of the European physician dying of pancreatic cancer, we will recall that his colleagues, intending to protect him from harm, invoked the therapeutic exception and withheld the truth about his diagnosis. Were his colleagues protecting him from a harm he could not bear or depriving him of an opportunity to share in a reciprocal relationship with them?

From what I heard of the story, there was every indication to suggest that the physician–patient was in a position to participate in a reciprocal doctor–patient relationship. He was, after all, a gastroentereologist who had cared for patients with the very disease that was taking his own life. He had been witness to their deaths and might have been able to use this experience to make sense of his own situation had he known his diagnosis. Beyond that, it appeared that he wanted to know about his medical condition. His request to see his computerized axial tomography (CAT) scan suggests that he wanted to know his diagnosis and indicates that he suspected that the truth was being hidden. He was, after all, still the teacher of his students and he knew how they had been trained when it came to sharing bad news.

It would be ironic, and tragic, if this physician lay dying wondering about his diagnosis and the likelihood of whether his well-intentioned colleagues were deceiving him. We can only imagine the loneliness and private concerns as he sought to engage his colleagues, his family, and the truth. Although we can only speculate from this distance, it is quite possible that the desire to protect this physician–patient from harm had only fostered his suspicion and amplified his isolation.

It appears that the truth, as tragic as it was, might have been comforting to this patient who was asking for it. His colleagues failed him because they failed to appreciate that their teacher could have been engaged in a reciprocal relationship with them. Although we might remain sympathetic to their well-intentioned beneficence, their failure to recognize the potential for reciprocity led to a paternalistic abuse of the therapeutic privilege depriving the patient empowerment by information that should have been shared with him.

In this case the truth should have been shared. Even though his doctors knew the patient's diagnosis and prognosis, they could not know what would invest the dying process with meaning. Only the patient was positioned to understand the significance of his illness in light of prior life experiences as physician, teacher, husband, and father. It was presumptuous of his colleagues to believe that they could interpret these facts for the patient.

The search for meaning begins with the medical facts of the case. It does not end there. If a patient does not know he is dying, he will not be able to find meaning in the dying process. Patients who are deprived of the truth about their illness are also deprived of a genuine opportunity to participate in life's culminating experience.

Deception robs the patient of the opportunity to stay engaged in life's drama. The dying patient who remains unaware of a truth known by everyone else is isolated in his ignorance. Those who make visits intended to comfort must be careful in choosing their words. The patient, in turn, who suspects the worst is similarly constrained and may not impose his burden on those who do not yet know that he is dying. Mutual deception, at the expense of more productive reciprocity, only serves to further sequester the dying from the living. In short, it isolates the dying patient and makes a palliative embrace impossible.

Acknowledgments

Dr. Fins is a Soros Faculty Scholar of the Project on Death in America of the Open Society Institute. The author acknowledges Sara Gill for research assistance on the Schloendorff case.

References

1. Surbone A. Truth telling to the patient. *JAMA* 1992; 268:1661–1662.
2. Fins JJ. Palliation in the age of chronic disease. *Hastings Cent Rep* 1992; 22(1):41–42. Reprinted in *Cases in Bioethics: Selections from the Hastings Center Report*. 2nd Edition. New York: St. Martin's Press, 1993.
3. Katz J. *The Silent World of Doctor and Patient.* New York: The Free Press, 1984.
4. Novack DH, Plummer R, Smith RL, et al. Changes in physicians' attitudes toward telling the cancer patient. *JAMA* 1979; 241:897–900.
5. Schloendorff v Society of New York Hosp., 211 N.Y. 125 (1914).
6. Essays dedicated to Mr. Justice Cardozo. *Columbia Law Review* vol. XXXIX, no. 1; *Harvard Law Review* LII, no. 3; *Yale Law Journal* XLVIII, no. 3. January 1939.
7. Regan LJ. *Doctor and Patient and the Law.* 2nd Edition. St. Louis: The C.V. Mosby Company, 1949.
8. Kelly WD, Friesen SR. Do cancer patients want to be told? *Surgery* 1950; 27:822–826.
9. Oken D. What to tell cancer patients. *JAMA* 1961; 175:1120–1128.
10. Klenow DJ, Youngs GA. Changes in doctor/patient communication of a terminal prognosis: A selective review and critique. *Death Studies* 1987; 11:263–277. Hemisphere Press.
11. Novack DH, Plummer R, Smith RL, et al. Changes in physicians' attitudes toward telling the cancer patient. *JAMA* 1979; 241:897–900.
12. Pentz R. Hope. Presented at the Eight Annual Bioethics Summer Retreat. Copper Mountain Resort, Colorado. June 21, 1996.
13. Veatch RM. Why physicians cannot determine if care is futile. *J Am Geriatr Soc* 1994; 42:871–874.
14. Pellegrino ED. Is truth-telling to the patient a cultural artifact? *JAMA* 1992; 268:1734–1735.
15. John L. Battenfeld, M.D. 1911–1987.
16. Pearlman RA, Uhlmann RF. Quality of life in chronic disease: Perceptions of elderly patients. *J Gerontol* 1988; 43:1125–1130.
17. Giuliani RW. Speech commemorating the 50th Anniversary of the United Nations. June–1995. Personal Communication, Colleen Roach, Press Secretary to the Mayor.
18. Fins JJ. Encountering diversity: medical ethics and pluralism. *J Religion Health* 1994; 33(1):23–27.
19. Montange CH. Informed consent and the dying patient. *The Yale Law Journal* 1974; 83(8):1632–1664.
20. Zaubler TS, Viederman M, Fins JJ. Ethical, legal, and psychiatric issues in capacity, competence, and informed consent: An annotated bibliography. *Gen Hosp Psychiatry* 1996; 18:155–172.

21. Salgo v. Leland Stanford Jr. Univ. Bd. of Trustees, 317 P.2d 170 (Cal. Ct. App. 1957).
22. Natanson v Kline, 350 P 2d 1093, 1960.
23. Canterbury v Spence, 464 F 2d 772, 1972.
24. Annas G. Informed consent, cancer, and truth in prognosis. *N Engl J Med* 1994; 330:223–225.
25. President's Commission for the Study of Ethical Problems in Medicine and Biomedical and Behavioral Research. *Deciding to Forego Life-Sustaining Treatment.* Washington, D.C. US Government Printing Office, 1983.
26. The Hastings Center. *Guidelines on the Termination of Life Sustaining Treatment and the Care of the Dying.* Bloomington. Indiana University Press. 1987.
27. Cruzan v Director, Missouri Department of Health, 110 S. Ct. 2841 (1990).
28. The Patient Self-Determination Act (OBRA 1990). Public Law 101-508, Sect 4206, 4751, (OBRA), 42 USC 1395 cc(a) et seq. (1990).
29. Fins JJ. Physician-assisted suicide and the right to care. *Cancer Control* 1996; 3(3):272–278.
30. Fins JJ, Bacchetta MD. Framing the physician-assisted suicide and voluntary active euthanasia debate: The role of deontology, consequentialism, and clinical pragmatism. *J Am Geriatr Soc* 1995; 43.563–568.
31. Brock DW. Voluntary active euthanasia. *Hastings Cent Rep* 1992; 22:10–22.
32. Compassion in Dying v. Washington, 850 F. Supp. 1455 (W.D. Wash. 1994).
33. Callahan D. When self-determination runs amok. *Hastings Cent Rep* 1992; 22:52–55.
34. Wolf SM. Mercy, murder, & morality: perspectives on euthanasia. Holding the line on euthanasia. *Hastings Cent Rep* 1989; 19(1):suppl 13–15.
35. Fins JJ, Bacchetta MD. Physician-assisted suicide and euthanasia debate: an annotated bibliography of representative articles. *J Clin Ethics* 1994; 5(4):329–340.
36. Gaylin W, Jennings B. *The Perversion of Autonomy.* New York, The Free Press, 1996.
37. Compassion in Dying v Washington. 79 F.3d 790 (9th Cir. 1996) (en banc).
38. Quill v Vacco. 80 F.3d 716 (2d Cir. 1996).
39. Lear MW. Should doctors tell the truth? The case against terminal candor. *The New York Times Magazine.* January 24, 1993, page 17.
40. Salgo v Leland Stanford Jr. Univ. Bd. of Trustees, 317 P.2d 170 (Cal. Ct. App. 1957).
41. Brody H. *The Healer's Power.* New Haven: Yale University Press, 1992.
42. Brody H. Transparency: Informed consent in primary care. *Hastings Cent Rep* 1989; 19(5):5–9.

7

Truth-Telling in Cancer Care: The Japanese Perspective

YOSUKE UCHITOMI

During the 1990s, the Japanese people talked more openly about cancer and death. Some high profile public figures disclosed their own battle with cancer, and bereaved family members and journalists wrote about dying cancer patients.

In 1989, a Japanese Ministry of Health and Welfare (JMHW) task force recommended the practice of telling the truth to terminally ill patients,[1] and in 1995, JMHW promoted the practice of obtaining the patients' informed consent before every medical practice.[2] Since April 1996, it has been permitted for the physician to charge a fee for giving the patient information about their cancer treatment plan. However, a survey of bereaved family members, conducted in 1994, showed that only 20.2% of the cancer patients had been told the true diagnosis.[3] Hence, the move toward full disclosure is advancing slowly. The Japanese population may prefer slow advances in truth-telling practice in cancer care.

The ethical aspects of truth-telling in Japan can be discussed on the basis of a systematic review of the literature and the other material. Surveys of the general population, cancer patients and their families, and physicians and other medical professionals provide important information related to ethics, and to the medical and psychosocial aspects of the issue.

Cancer Epidemiology in Japan

Before 1953, the leading causes of death in Japan were infectious diseases, such as tuberculosis. The advent of antibiotics and improvements in the public health system have reduced the death rates from such diseases.[4] The lifestyle and diet of the Japanese people became Westernized after World War II and so-called lifestyle illnesses, such as cerebrovascular and heart diseases and cancer, have become the leading causes of death. In 1981, the cancer rate overtook the rate of cerebrovascular disease. The number of cancer-related deaths in Japan in 1996 was 271,094 (217.4 per 100,000 population), which accounted for 30.2% of the total number of deaths. The death rates of some cancers, such as lung, colorectal, and breast cancer, have been increasing whereas those of other cancers, such as stomach and uterine cancer, have clearly decreased. These trends in the cancer-related death rates are similar to those observed in Western countries.

Telling the Truth in Cancer Care in Japan

General population survey

Reports of 1981–1990 surveys conducted by newspapers of randomly selected sample populations in Japan show that 53%–56% of the respondents would want to be informed truthfully if they were diagnosed as having cancer[5] (Table 7.1). Recent reports have shown a rapid increase in the percentage of the general population who would wish to know the true diagnosis, to 86%, although only 69% wished to be told if they had incurable cancer.[6]

The data from a survey on Health and Daily Life, which was conducted in 1995,[7] show that 86.2% of the respondents wished to be informed of the diagnosis if they had early stage cancer and 66.7% wished to be informed if they had terminal cancer. Logistic regression analysis showed that the wish not to be informed of the cancer diagnosis significantly correlated with older age and female gender, probably reflecting the groups of people who have been accustomed to paternalistic physicians.

Despite these trends toward the disclosure of a diagnosis of cancer, there are still some people who do not wish to be informed of their condition. Furthermore, some people indicated that they would wish to know the diagnosis, but would want the decisions about treatments to be made by their families and physicians rather than by themselves. This trend has also been observed in other non-Western societies, which are more likely to have a family-centered model of medical decision-making than the patient-autonomy model favored by most Western countries.[8]

Patient survey

Surveys of Japanese patients with cancer, noncancerous disease, or suspected cancer were conducted in 1989–1995; 55.9% to 83% of the respondents wished to be informed of a diagnosis of cancer[9–11] (Table 7.1). However, as in the general population survey,[5–7] a small number of patients did not wish to be informed of a diagnosis of cancer.[11] This group included some who were being treated in a cancer center hospital.[11]

Table 7.1. Wishes and policies toward cancer disclosure in Japan

Study	Year of survey	Respondents	Findings
General Population Surveys			
Mainichi Shinbun[5]	1981–1990	Approximately 2900 randomly sampled people aged over 20 years in Japan. Survey repeated 7 times during the period.	53%–56% wished to be informed of the cancer diagnosis; 17%–23% not; 24%–26% wished case by case. If a family member had cancer, 10%–13% would disclose the truth.
Matsumura et al.[7]	1995	3395 randomly sampled people aged over 16 years in Japan.	86.2% wished to be informed of the diagnosis and 81.7% of prognosis if they had early-stage cancer. 66.7% wished to know the diagnosis and 62.9% the prognosis if they had terminal cancer.
Mainichi Shinbun[6]	1997	2913 randomly sampled people aged over 20 years in Japan.	86% wished to be informed of the diagnosis if they had curable cancer. 69% wished to be informed of the diagnosis if having incurable cancer
Patient Surveys			
Mizushima et al.[9]	1989	789 outpatients from one rural university hospital.	55.9% wished to be informed of cancer diagnosis. If a family member had a cancer, 31.2% would disclose this.
Tanida[10]	1991	221 first-visit outpatients and 210 clients before stomach endoscopy from one urban college hospital.	72% and 83% wished to be informed of cancer diagnosis. If a family member had cancer, 27% and 21% would disclose this.
Hamajima et al.[11]	1995	293 first-visit outpatients, revisit outpatients and inpatients in good condition at discharge from 1 urban Cancer Center hospital.	74% wished to be informed of the cancer diagnosis irrespective of circumstances.
Sasaki[29]	1997	1215 stomach, colon, or lung cancer inpatients from 24 Cancer Center hospitals after obtaining informed consent of cancer therapy.	75.1% of cancer patients were informed.

(Continued)

Table 7.1. Wishes and policies toward cancer disclosure in Japan (*continued*)

Study	Year of survey	Respondents	Findings
Bereaved Family Caregiver Surveys			
Ministry of Health and Welfare[15]	1992	1918 bereaved family caregivers who had cared for the patients aged between 40 and 64 in Japan.	18.2% reported that the patients were informed of the cancer diagnosis. 42.5% were not informed, but might have suspected that they had cancer.
Ministry of Health and Welfare[3]	1994	1590 bereaved family caregivers who had cared for patients aged over 40 in Japan.	20.2% reported that the patients were informed of the cancer diagnosis. 43.8% were not informed, but might have suspected that they had cancer. 28.6% reported that patients aged between 40 and 64 were informed.
Physician Surveys			
Mizushima et al.[9]	1989	116 physicians and 206 paramedical professionals from 1 rural university hospital.	62.9% of physicians and 53.9% of other medical professionals wished to be informed of cancer diagnoses. If a family member had cancer, 32.8% and 22.8% would disclose this.
Suzuki et al.[12]	1990	278 primary physicians from urban clinics.	16% of physicians preferred the usual truth-telling policy for patients with incurable advanced cancer; 67% preferred to inform patients with early curable cancer. 77% of physicians wished to be informed if they had incurable advanced cancer; 87% wished to be informed if they had curable early cancer.
Uchitomi et al.[20]	1989	329 physicians from 21 cancer center hospitals and 10 teaching hospitals in Japan.	14% of physicians told the truth to half or more of their terminally ill cancer patients.
Tanida[10]	1991	179 physicians from one urban College hospital.	13% of physicians preferred the usual truth-telling policy for cancer patients.
Elwyn et al.[21]	1995	77 physicians from one university hospital and one affiliated hospital in a rural area.	40% of physicians preferred the usual truth-telling policy for cancer patients. If the patients wished to know, but the family was against disclosure, 35% of physicians preferred truth-telling and 35% did not.

Physician and other medical professionals survey

Would the physicians wish to be told if they had cancer? Of the physicians surveyed at a rural university hospital in 1989, only 62.9% said they would want to be informed, 25.3% said their preference would depend on the specific circumstances and 7.8% would not want to be told.[9] Furthermore, 53.9% of other medical professionals wished to be told, which is similar to proportion of the patients who gave the same response (55.9%). In a survey conducted in 1990,[12] 77% of 278 primary physicians from private clinics and hospitals said they would wish to be told if they had incurable advanced cancer and the number rose to 87% for early-stage cancer. Surprisingly, some of the physicians said they would not wish to be told.

One reason for wanting not to be told is the strong belief in Japanese culture that the knowledge of the cancer diagnosis would make the patient feel helpless and without hope.[13] Furthermore, some Japanese people feel that being a terminally ill cancer patient will cause them to be isolated and treated as outsiders,[14] which may be why some people said that they would not wish to be informed of their true diagnoses if they had terminal cancer.

Family wishes

If a member of your family had cancer, would you want the diagnosis to be disclosed to the patient? Ten to thirteen percent of the general population,[5] 27% of the patients, 32.8% of the physicians and 22.8% of other medical professionals[9] said that they would want the truth to be told to their family members (Table 7.1). Therefore, many Japanese would not want a family member to be given a truthful diagnosis, even though they would want to be told the truth if they themselves were diagnosed with cancer. Thus, even some medical professionals seem to believe that the disclosure of the diagnosis will bring only a loss of hope and a fear of death, and that withholding the truth may protect the patient from emotional distress. It is believed that disclosure of the true diagnosis may result in only a loss of hope for terminally ill cancer patients.

Decision Making in Truth-Telling Practice

Family involvement in the decision to disclose or withhold the truth

In surveys of bereaved families conducted by JMHW in 1992,[15] only 18.2% of family members who had cared for a terminally ill cancer patient (28.6% of the age-adjusted sample in 1994[3]) reported that the cancer patient was given the true diagnosis (Table 7.1). Although a clear trend toward disclosure has been observed between the two surveys, 42.5% (43.8% in 1994) of caregivers reported that the patient might have suspected cancer, 25.1% (28.8% in 1994) reported that the patient was not aware of the diagnosis, and 12.6% (3.2% in 1994) had no idea whether the patient was aware of the diagnosis. The 1992 survey did show a significantly higher rate of disclosure for younger patients than for older patients, and for patients living in urban areas compared to those living in rural districts. Details of the treatment plan were known by 98.1% (93.8% in 1994) of the families, although only 22.5% (43.7% in 1994) of the patients were informed, respectively.

In Japan, the principle family members (e.g., spouse and children) are usually informed by the physician of the cancer patient's diagnosis, prognosis, and the treatment plan before the cancer patient is told the truth.[16] Then, the family member(s) decide whether the patient should be told, usually after discussions with other family members (e.g., the patient's siblings, uncles, and aunts).

The family's decision is usually accepted by the physician. At the time of the diagnosis, rapid treatment will probably be needed to improve the patient's chance of survival. Thus, most cancer patients who are not informed of the diagnosis probably suspect that they have cancer.[13] Usually, the patient never says the word cancer to their family or physician.[13,14] Therefore, Japanese people seem to fear that disclosure of the truth would cause tension and distress among the family members, including the patient, and between the family and the physician, and that the patient may not accept the family's and physician's decision to withhold the cancer diagnosis.

This practice of family decision making is common in Japan and can be traced to the aspects of Japanese culture that guide interpersonal relations, which probably originated in the traditional agricultural society of Japan.[17] Group decision-making is more common than the individual making his/her own decisions because the sense of belonging to the family is strong. Cancer patients who are not informed of the diagnosis but who nevertheless suspect that they have cancer may accept the family's decision because they think that their family hopes to protect them from disappointment. Hosaka[18] reported that, in Japan, the rate of psychiatric morbidity (e.g., adjustment disorder with depressed mood) in cancer patients who knew the true diagnosis was higher than for those who did not know the truth. A similar observation has been made in Indian society.[19]

Thus, Japanese cancer patients may accept their families' decisions to withhold the diagnoses in order to avoid distress and tension within the family. They may want to be informed about their diseases step by step, rather than all at once. The family may buffer the psychological impact of the cancer on the patient. Further research regarding the relationship between the patient's wish and the family's decision is required.

The physician's policy toward truth disclosure

Japanese physicians are taught to interpret the Hippocratic oath as requiring them to do that which is expected to have the best consequences for the patient; they usually consider themselves the final authority regarding the medical treatment of their cancer patients. However, the decision of whether to disclose a cancer diagnosis is left to the family members, who usually did not tell the truth prior to the 1980s.

During 1989–1991, three surveys of Japanese physicians reported that only 13%–16% had a standard policy of disclosing the truth to their cancer patients.[10,12,20] However, a 1995 survey showed the rapid adoption of a more open attitude; 40% of the physicians had a standard policy of telling the truth.[21] Surprisingly, the 1995 survey also showed that physicians are now more likely to make exceptions when deciding whether to tell the patient the truth. The Japanese physicians reported considering more factors when making their decisions than physicians in the United States. Seventy percent or more of Japanese physicians consider the patient's intelligence and age, the patient's wish, the relative's wishes, the patient's desire to have hope, the available family support, the type and stage of cancer, the length of expected survival, and anticipated suicide.

The 1995 survey also revealed the physician's attitude toward conflict between the wish of the patient and that of his or her family about disclosure; 35% reported that they tell the patient the truth and 35% do not. Therefore, Japanese physicians do not always adopt the family's decision,[21] which suggests that they are moving from a policy of nondisclosure to a case-by-case assessment of the drawbacks and benefits of disclosure. Kai et al.[22] studied patient–physician communication about terminal care in Japan and reported that the concordance between the patient's preference and the physician's estimation was close to the figure expected by chance alone. Whether decision making on a case-by-case basis really helps the patients and their families should be examined further.

Court rulings

On April 25, 1995, the Japanese Supreme Court issued its decision regarding whether patients should be told the true diagnosis.[23] The case involved K. Makino, a 50-year-old nurse. She was examined at a hospital in January 1983 and died of gall bladder cancer in December 1983 after having been told by her physician in March that she had a gallstone. Her physician suspected cancer and recommended hospitalization for surgery. She promised to return to the hospital after a trip planned for the end of March, but she did not return to the hospital immediately and by June the cancer had spread to her liver.

The Supreme Court ruled that the doctor's practice was acceptable. The doctor had undertaken a detailed examination of the patient and not told her of his suspicion of cancer at her first attendance for two reasons: the doctor did not know the patient well at the time of the first visit and concealment of the truth was the usual practice in 1983 in Japan.[23]

Earlier, the Supreme Court upheld the decision of a lower Court in the same case. The District Court in 1989 ruled that, although it is a doctor's duty to explain to the patient his or her illness accurately and concretely, it is up to the doctor to decide to whom, and when, what, and how much to explain because the disclosure can affect the patient's recovery.[24,25] In 1990, the High Court stated that the patient's decision may be respected in certain circumstances but that the doctor's decision overrides the patient's decision.[16] Ms. Makino was solely responsible for the outcome because she had not followed her doctor's instructions.[26]

This Supreme Court ruling has met with heavy criticism from Western countries, which adopt universal cancer diagnosis disclosure. Although in 1983 the vast majority of patients in Japan were not told of their cancer diagnosis, this case had a great impact on the attitudes of Japanese physicians as well as those of Japanese people.

Promotion of Truth-Telling by the Japanese Ministry of Health and Welfare Task Force

In 1989, a JMHW task force on care for terminally ill patients advocated informing patients of their limited life expectancy, as well as of the cancer diagnosis.[1] The task force recommended that telling the truth to such patients should be considered a necessity. Guidelines for informing terminally ill patients of their limited life expectancy have been published. The physician is advised to inform the patient of the true diagnosis if the following criteria are met: (1) the physician expects that the patient will maintain a stable psychological state after the disclosure of the truth, for example, the patient has a desire to know the diagnosis, the patient will be able to deal with family affairs and to continue working, the patient will be able to avoid a quarrel over inheritance, the patient will be able to cope with and adapt to the emotional distress, and the patient will comply with treatment; (2) the physician expects that the patient will be able to make decisions related to their own care; (3) the physician is aware of the prior existence of a good relationship between the health care providers, the patient and the patient's family; and (4) a good support system is available to help the patient manage the physical and psychological aspects of the illness.

In 1995, a JMHW task force on informed consent promoted the practice of obtaining the patients' informed consent before beginning every medical practice.[2] However, these reports did not recommend that obtaining the patients' informed consent, or telling the truth to cancer patients, should be made a legal requirement, because a balance has not yet been established in Japan between the patients' desire for detailed information of their illnesses and the physicians' belief that providing the patient with that information is not beneficial. The task force stressed the beneficial aspects of informed consent and suggested that the Japanese general public, as well as the cancer patients and medical professionals, would use the information to achieve a better quality of life.

The levying of a fee by the physician for providing information about the patient's treatment plan to the patient was endorsed by JMHW in 1996. It was an epoch-making event for the practice of telling the truth because a consultation with a physician in Japan used to be free or extremely inexpensive compared to Western countries.[27]

Conclusion

During a 1995 clinical trial at National Cancer Center Hospital in Tokyo, one of the leading cancer center hospitals, cancer patients were always told the true diagnosis and patients were only enrolled in the trial after their written consent had been obtained.[28] In 1997, 75% of 1215 stomach, colon, or lung cancer in-patients treated at 24 of the 26 cancer center hospitals in Japan reported (anonymously by mail) that they had been diagnosed with cancer and had given their informed consent for cancer therapy.[29] The truth-telling practice has been introduced only in the cancer center hospitals in recent years.

Education about communication between medical professionals and cancer patients and their families is required, especially in medical schools (although an oncology department has not yet been established), and should be run in cooperation with the Cancer Center hospitals.[30] It would also be beneficial to establish a mental health service run by psycho-oncology professionals to support the communication between physicians and their cancer patients.[31,32]

A survey of bereaved family members that was conducted in 1994 showed a slow but steady move toward disclosure.[2] The predominant ethical principles in Japan are thought to be based not only on respecting the patient's right to know but also on protecting the patient from the emotional distress of tense family relationships. We conclude that Japanese people may prefer small changes to the truth-telling practice in cancer care to avoid the psychological impact of the cancer on the patient and to respect the family's and physician's decisions as well as the patient's wishes, without legalizing the requirement for truth-telling in cancer care.

Acknowledgments

This work was supported in part by a Grant-in-Aid for Cancer Research (9–31) and by the Second Term Comprehensive 10-Year Strategy for Cancer Control from the Ministry of Health and Welfare of Japan.

References

1. Japanese Ministry of Health and Welfare and the Japan Medical Association. *The Report for Terminal Care*. Tokyo: Chuo Hoki Shuppan, 1989 (in Japanese).
2. Japanese Ministry of Health and Welfare, Yanagida K. *The Report for Informed Consent*. Tokyo: Chuo Hoki Shuppan, 1996 (in Japanese).

3. Japanese Ministry of Health and Welfare. *FY 1994 Report on the Socioeconomic Survey of Vital Statistics; Medical Treatment For Terminally Ill Patients*. Tokyo: Statistics and Information Department, Minister's Secretariat, Japanese Ministry of Health and Welfare, 1995 (in Japanese).

4. Japanese Ministry of Health and Welfare. *FY 1996 Report on Cancer Statistics*. Tokyo: Statistics and Information Department, Minister's Secretariat, Japanese Ministry of Health and Welfare, 1997 (in Japanese).

5. Mainichi Shinbun-sha. *The Report on Public Opinion Survey on "Cancer."* Tokyo: Public Opinion Center, Mainichi Shinbun-sha, 1990 (in Japanese).

6. Mainichi Shinbun-sha. *The Report on Public Opinion Survey on "Aged Society."* Tokyo: Public Opinion Center, Mainichi Shinbun-sha, 1998 (in Japanese).

7. Matsumura S, Fukuhara S, Bito S, Ohki M, Kurokawa K. Analysis of Japanese people's wish to be informed of cancer and correlated factors. *Nihon Iji Shinpo* 1997; 3830:37–42 (in Japanese).

8. Blackhall LJ, Murphy ST, Frank G, Michel V, Azen S. Ethnicity and attitudes toward patient autonomy. *JAMA* 1995; 13:820–825.

9. Mizushima Y, Kashii T, Hoshino K, et al. A survey regarding the disclosure of the diagnosis of cancer in Toyama prefecture, Japan. *Jpn J Med* 1990; 29:146–155.

10. Tanida N. Japanese attitudes towards truth disclosure in cancer. *Scand J Soc Med* 1994; 22:50–57.

11. Hamajima N, Tajima K, Morishita M, et al. Patients' expectations of information provided at cancer hospitals in Japan. *Jpn J Clin Oncol* 1996; 26:362–367.

12. Suzuki K, Kurosaka H, Kaneko S, et al. Telling the cancer. *Nihon Iji Shinpo* 1992; 3543:43–47 (in Japanese).

13. Long SO, Long BD. Curable cancers and fatal ulcers: attitudes toward cancer in Japan. *Soc Sci Med* 1982; 16:2101–2108.

14. Tsuji S. Psychological aspects of dying patients. In: Japan Soc Death Dying, eds. *Shi no Rinsho*. Tokyo: Ningen to Rekishi Sha, 1990:114–127 (in Japanese).

15. Japanese Ministry of Health and Welfare. *FY 1992 Report on the Socioeconomic Survey of Vital Statistics: Malignant Neoplasms*. Tokyo: Statistics and Information Department, Minister's Secretariat, Japanese Ministry of Health and Welfare, 1993 (in Japanese).

16. Hattori H, Salzberg SM, Kiang WP, Fujimiya T, Tejima Y, Furuno J. The patient's right to information in Japan: legal rules and doctors' opinions. *Soc Sci Med* 1991; 32:1007–1016.

17. Namihira E. *Brain Death, Organ Transplantation, and Telling the Truth to Cancer Patients: Anthropological Studies on Death and Medical Care*. Tokyo: Fukutake Shoten, 1988.

18. Hosaka T, Aoki T, Ichikawa Y. Emotional states of patients with hematological malignancies: preliminary study. *Jpn J Clin Oncol* 1994; 24:186–190.

19. Alexander PJ, Dinesh N, Vidyasagar MS. Psychiatric morbidity among cancer patients and its relationship with awareness of illness and expectations about treatment outcome. *Acta Oncol* 1993; 32:623–626.

20. Uchitomi Y, Okamura H, Minagawa H, et al. A survey of Japanese physicians' attitudes and practice in caring for terminally ill cancer patients. *Psychiatr Clin Neurosci* 1994; 49:53–57.

21. Elwyn TS, Fetters MD, Gorenflo W, Tsuda T. Cancer disclosure in Japan: historical comparisons, current practices. *Soc Sci Med* 1998; 46:1151–1163.

22. Kai I, Ohi G, Yano E, et al. Communication between patients and physicians about terminal care: a survey in Japan. *Soc Sci Med* 1993; 36:1151–1159.
23. Tanida N. Supreme Court's decision on patients' rights in Japan. *Lancet* 1995; 345:1176.
24. Brahams D. Right to know in Japan. *Lancet* 1989; 2:173.
25. Swinbanks D. Japanese doctors keep quiet. *Nature* 1989; 339:409.
26. Tanida N. Patients' rights in Japan. *Lancet* 1991; 337:242–243.
27. Mitsuya H. Truth-telling practice in cancer care in Japan. *Ann NY Acad Sci* 1997; 809:279–289.
28. Asahi Shinbun-sha. Clinical trials shall be explained through a written document. *Asahi shinbun* 1995; April 6.
29. Sasaki J. Survey on informed consent and truth-telling. In: Sasaki J, ed. *Annual Report of the Cancer Research (8–12) of the Japanese Ministry of Health and Welfare FY 1997*. Tokyo: Japanese Ministry of Health and Welfare, 1998 (in Japanese).
30. Okamura H, Uchitomi Y, Sasako M, Eguchi K, Kakizoe T. Guidelines for telling the truth to cancer patients. *Jpn J Clin Oncol* 1998; 28:1–4.
31. Uchitomi Y, Sugihara J, Fukue M, et al. Psychiatric liaison issues in cancer care in Japan. *J Pain Symp Manage* 1994; 9:319–324.
32. Uchitomi Y, Yamawaki S. Truth-telling practice in cancer care in Japan. *Ann NY Acad Sci* 1997; 809:290–299.

8

Advance Directives in Different Cultures

AKIRA AKABAYASHI AND RAYMOND VOLTZ

How can health care professionals communicate with patients effectively in the palliative care setting? How can we make better clinical decisions when a terminally ill patient can no longer give consent due to conditions like coma, anxiety, or incompetence?

One method used to resolve such dilemmas is the provision of an advance directive (AD), particularly in the United States. Such directives are made while the patient is still competent, and specify the forms of medical treatment to be provided by caregivers and/or designate someone to act as a proxy should the subject in question lose his or her capacity to make decisions.

The moral arguments supporting ADs in the United States are based primarily on the concept of autonomy or the patient's right to self-determination. Advance directives and the use of a health care proxy have been recommended as a means to improve communication about the patient's preferences in making health care decisions. Several articles indicate ADs should contain disease-specific information rather than general statements that do not offer much assistance in clinical situations, and should be seen as part of a more general plan for end-of-life decisions in which improved communication would be more important than a more formal preservation of rights, achieved by simply completing a document.[1-3] However, whether the disease-specific ADs really improve patient–physician relationship has not been confirmed yet.[4]

An important question remains. Are ADs accepted and desired by patients and health care professionals outside the United States, or even within a heterogeneous American culture? It is accepted to some degree, within all cultures that individuals should not be treated against their wills, and some form of the concept of informed consent is usually in evidence. Nevertheless, there is enough variation concerning perceptions of autonomy and informed consent to make cross cultural studies of ADs important.

The idea of institutions specializing in the care of the dying such as hospices or palliative care units, has spread to nearly all industrialized countries since their inception in 1967 in Great Britain. These institutions do not fight death but rather make dying as comfortable as possible. Once again, there is a question whether or not basic hospice tenants cross cultural boundaries. More specifically, how do ADs for palliative care work in institutions with diverse cultural backgrounds?

In order to explore this issue, international cross-cultural collaborative studies were conducted between 1994 to 1996 in the United States, Germany, and Japan (Note 1). This chapter reviews these studies and discusses their implications for the future development of ADs in palliative care.

A Multicultural Perspective on Advance Directives

The multicultural research under discussion took place in two phases. The first phase was a book project where contributors from legal, medical, and philosophical disciplines described each country's situation.[5] The second phase moved beyond the national perspective. People with disease-specific conditions (for example, cancer, end-stage renal disease, HIV, dementia, amyotrophic lateral sclerosis) as well as healthy people were examined by each multinational research team.

In the preface of the book, the accomplishment of the first phase was summarized by the editors, who stated:

> In modern societies, rich with diverse values and wishes manifest in individual expressions and convictions, there is no longer a uniform, general answer to the question of when life-supporting medical interventions should cease. The answer the physician might give if only his or her convictions mattered is not necessarily the answer for the patient, who most likely will have other religious beliefs, visions, personal expectations, hopes and fears. What is true for postmodern multicultural societies is even more true for the diversity of attitudes among different traditions, cultures, religions, and attitudes in the global village
>
> Sass et al.[5]

In the context of this diversity of values, the acceptability of ADs was assumed to be quite different in each culture or society. For example,

> In cultures where self-determination and individual autonomy and choices play a primary role in day-to-day life, competent and risk-aware adults will favor the execution of medical care directives in advance just as they write wills and employ other strategies, legal and nonlegal, to reduce future risk that their wishes will not be carried out.
>
> Sass et al.[5]

However, in some contexts there was less of a need for ADs:

> . . . there is a more traditional understanding of the individual person as a part of the family and community, and therefore self-determination must be defined within

the constraints and borders of family and community. In such a system, there is less motivation to make advance oral or written statements, as the family or community or the trusted medical professional is customarily trusted to "do the right thing."

Sass et al.[5]

It is worthwhile examining the Japanese situation. The numbers in the Japan Society for Death with Dignity who have signed living wills are steadily increasing, although they still represent less than 0.1% of the population. A survey conducted in 1996 of healthy subjects illustrates the Japanese situation more clearly.[6] In this study, 210 healthy men who visited two urban general hospitals for their physical check-ups were asked to fill out a self-administered questionnaire asking about their knowledge, experiences, and attitudes related to ADs. More than 80% of the respondents knew the term living will and wanted to express their preferences concerning future medical care. However, more than 80% answered that they would give a lot of authority to surrogates to represent their preferences, and did not feel the necessity for detailed, concrete directives such as an expressed preference for cardio-pulmonary resuscitation and the use of respirators. More than 60% answered that oral statements were enough, whereas about 30% recognized the necessity for written documents. Eighty percent stated that they would designate family or relatives, in most cases, a spouse as their surrogate decision maker. However, those who do not want to express their preferences in advance (18%) gave the following reasons: psychological resistance to talking about death and dying; difficulty in imagining such a future situation—a point that represents a serious theoretical limitation of ADs—and trust in their families (omakase, Note 2), etc.

In Japan, people know about ADs, but do not tend to make them. Tomoaki Tsuchida explains the reasons for this as follows:

> This limited utilization of advance directives is not just a result of slowness or "underdevelopment" in terms of human rights among Japanese. Certainly, however, the Japanese in general have yet to catch up with American and European counterparts in terms of being aware of and respecting individual human rights. In addition to the issue of rights, there are some basic differences in the Japanese concept of human life and death and in their view of "nature," and so on, which contribute to somewhat different attitudes among the Japanese toward advance directives.

Tsuchida[7]

Tsuchida further analyses the role of the family in Japan.

> . . . in the traditional context this attitude of entrusting vital decisions to others (family and/or physician) is interwoven with the Japanese view of the nature of human being . . . the Japanese concept of human being is embodied in the German word Mitsein, for example, that humans are human insofar as they live together with fellow humans and that one's life and death as a human renders one part of the whole community of humans. Life and death are not wholly private acts but rather concern the entire community of which one is a member. . . . It is the family

to whom people turn for crucial decisions, especially those concerning life and death.

Tsuchida[7]

There has been much written about the family in Japan. However, Tsuchida suggests that traditional views are now largely fragmented, and some have been consigned to oblivion (Note 3).

Throughout the book under discussion, Japan is considered to have a traditional culture still oriented to patterns of familial loyalty with social relationships based upon status. The United States is seen to be the opposite. Germany is located between these two extremes. The work also notes that different cultural and legal traditions are not the only factors that underlie advance health care planning. There is also a tension between different professional cultures (such as medicine and law) as well as between professional and individual lay cultures. Finally, five AD models (The Living Will Model, The Proxy Model, The Value History Model, The Medical Instruction Model, and the combination Model) were suggested. However, it is concluded that there is not and will not be one single best moral, legal, or medical model that ensures that patients are not treated against their interests, values, or plans for the future.

The work described above was a theoretical study, based upon literature that emphasized cultural differences. In the second phase of the project we tried to conduct an empirical study, based upon surveys that included hospice patients.

Advance Directives in the Palliative Care Setting: A Cross-Cultural Perspective Based Upon Questionnaires and Interviews of Patients and Health Care Professionals in the United States, Germany, and Japan

How relevant are ADs in the palliative care setting compared to other clinical situations? The Canadian bioethicist Peter A. Singer[8] attempts to answer this question as follows:

> ADs are at once more and less relevant in the palliative care setting than in health care generally. They are more relevant to palliative care because of the high likelihood of deterioration and death among palliative patients. At the same time, they are less relevant because palliative patients have already accepted a philosophy of care that probably predetermines many of the treatment choices that are usually made in the ADs. For this reason the AD concept should not be imported wholesale into the context of palliative care.

Singer[8]

To further explore this question, we will summarize briefly three papers resulting from the studies conducted during the second phase of the project under discussion.[9–11] These were exploratory studies, using convenience sampling, at several selected locations in the three countries in question. Although these samples are small, we believe the results have significant implications when we consider the use of ADs in palliative care. The topics investigated were (1) organization of palliative care in three countries; (2) the views and perceptions of patients in palliative care institutions concerning their end-of-life decisions, and attitudes towards ADs; (3) the attitudes of experienced health care professionals toward ADs in palliative care; and (4) the development of a method to help in the planning of end-of-life decisions.

Methods

Patient interviews in palliative care institutions
A total of 159 patients were recruited between 1994 and 1996 from convenience samples of specialized palliative care institutions in the United States (One institution, $N = 90$, mean age 68.0 years, 64% female, 51% diagnosed with cancer), Germany (five institutions, $N = 34$, mean age 62.6 years, 65% female, 97% cancer) and Japan (five institutions, $N = 34$, mean age 58.6 years, 65% female, 79% cancer). All of the patients suffered from a terminal illness. Patients were considered eligible if they could communicate and participate without distress and give informed consent. Structured interviews were performed and the answers given were coded by the interviewer into the preformulated categories.

Self-administered questionnaire to health care professionals
A total of 93 health care professionals (convenience sampling, physicians: the United States $N = 8$, Germany $N = 14$, Japan $N = 14$; nurses the United States $N = 18$, Germany $N = 15$, Japan $N = 24$) with at least part-time experience with palliative care patients were given or mailed a self-administered questionnaire. The questionnaire asked subjects their perceptions of the usefulness of ADs in palliative care settings. In order to investigate attitudes toward end-of-life clinical decisions related to ADs, a case vignette was used where six important decisions about care had to be made. (Appendix 1). At each critical point, the questionnaire asked "Was there adherence to the patient's wishes? Why or why not?" and "Was the decision which was taken correct? Why or why not?" In addition, at the end, the questionnaire asked "Did the patient accomplish what she wanted in her AD? Why or why not?"

Results

Patients' perception of palliative care
In all of the countries surveyed, two-thirds of the patients investigated were female. In the United States 34 patients (43%) had a non-cancer diagnosis, in contrast to only 1 patient in Germany (3%) and 1 patient in Japan (4%). More patients were cared for at home in the United States (69%) than in Germany (32%) or Japan (6%). In all participating centers, only palliative therapies were offered. These therapies included radiation, minor surgery, or chemotherapy if

these were indicated for the control of symptoms. No resuscitation measures were taken in the event of life-threatening complications.

In the participating centers in the United States, all patients or families were asked to sign a written informed consent sheet. This included statements like "hospice care is not designed to cure disease."[9] and that it "precludes the use of aggressive, curative, life-extending treatments." One paragraph read: "We understand that we have the right under federal/state Patient Self Determination laws to make health care decisions, accept and refuse treatments, and make advance directives. We understand that a completed Advance Directive is not a requirement for admission to Family Hospice."[9]

In Germany, no written informed consent forms were used. However, the palliative goals were stressed before admission and oral consent was obtained from patients in most cases. Similarly, in Japan, there was no procedure for written consent. A certain proportion of the patients did not know the way in which the disease they had would progress, or even their present medical condition at the time of admission. Members of the patients' families concerned, however, were usually well informed. Obtaining oral consent for end of life decisions from either the patients or their families is a common practice in Japan.

The vast majority of patients had been familiar with the concept of hospice care for quite some time. When asked who recommended the hospice, patients responded that the role of physicians in recommending palliative care was most important in Germany (56%) and least important in Japan (12%). Family members were most involved in Japan (35%). About 75% of patients in all three countries felt that the decision to go into hospice care had been very easy or easy. The vast majority of patients in all three countries felt that their expectations were fulfilled. The reasons for a positive attitude toward hospice care did not vary from country to country. The following comments were most frequent; "the help was needed" ($N = 49$); "services were well explained by the staff" ($N = 13$); "this was a relief of my symptoms" ($N = 10$); "I am not alone," "they have time for me" ($N = 8$).[9]

End-of-life decisions and advance directives in palliative care:
the patients' view

In order to assess patients' views about their end-of-life decisions, they were asked open-ended questions. Namely, what was the most important decision they had to make in the last days or weeks, and what important decision they expected to have to make in the near future. The answers were categorized in the following ways: location of care decisions, medical treatment decisions (continuation or discontinuation of therapy, etc.), coping with the dying process, (that is, to accept death, live life to the fullest), making an AD (signing an AD or appointing a proxy), and other personal organizational decisions. The response "I entrust the decisions to my family (omakase)" was given only by Japanese patients.

Past and future decisions about the location of care and medical therapy ranged between 3% and 45% without clear differences between the countries surveyed. In Japan, fewer patients (16%) than in the United States (49%) or Germany (52%) indicated a concern about coping with future decisions. About 10% of the past decisions in the United States and Germany concerned formalizing the patients' wishes through the use of an AD. However, no Japanese patients answered so.

When asked how they felt when they faced future decisions, patients discussed a wide range of emotions. In the United States and Germany, more than 80% of the patients mentioned negative feelings. In Japan, 17% of patients said they felt no emotions when facing their future decisions. Only 45% of Japanese patients talked about experiencing negative emotions, this percentage being lower than in the United States or Germany.

Turning specifically to the role of ADs in palliative care, patients were asked whether they had signed an AD, and whether they had appointed a proxy. In the United States many more patients had written an AD ($N = 69$, 79%). Some patients in Germany and Japan had given an oral AD. In all three countries, about 25% of those not having an AD wanted more information. When asked what the signed ADs said, patients only mentioned general statements. None of the ADs were disease- or patient-specific.

More American patients had appointed a proxy (had given durable power of attorney according to the U.S. law) than in Germany (Betreuungsverfugung). This possibility does not exist according to Japanese law. However, an informal entrusting of everything to the family (omakase) was prevalent in Japan.

Advance directives in palliative care: the health care professionals' view
There was a 100% agreement in the United States and Germany that ADs were useful in palliative care. In Japan, fewer agreed with this view ($N = 27$, 71%). In Germany and Japan, health care professionals felt less comfortable in helping patients with their ADs than in the United States. In Germany, although 100% ($N = 29$) had agreed that ADs were useful, only 62% ($N = 18$) of the professionals questioned felt comfortable helping patients in setting up an AD.

When asked about their views on appointing a proxy in palliative care, fewer professionals agreed that appointing a proxy was useful when compared to the writing of an AD (the United States $N = 20$, 78%, Germany $N = 17$, 41%, Japan $N = 17$, 55%). The proportion of health care professionals who felt comfortable in helping patients was similar to those who answered that appointing a proxy was useful. The health care professionals responded by saying "the proxy becomes the patient's advocate" ($N = 23$), "it is a duty for health care professionals to help with naming a proxy" ($N = 10$), "a proxy cannot know patients' real wishes" ($N = 9$).[10]

Attitudes toward clinical decision: a case vignette study
In general, this study (see Appendix 1) revealed only small differences between the countries surveyed. At decision point A, a patient Ms. O., who is not actually suffering, deliberately does not want to drink fluid although her general

practitioner (GP) has asked her to do so. In the United States and Germany, 90%–92% of professionals felt this was in accordance with Ms. O.'s wishes, slightly less (83%–85%) thought this was a correct decision. In Japan, only 66% of the health care professionals agreed with this decision. Many professionals suggested that communication between the members of the health care team should be improved. At decision point B, Ms. O. develops symptoms due to suspected nerve root involvement, but no further diagnostic tests were performed. Fewer Japanese (42%) than American (85%) or German (76%) health care professionals felt that this decision was in accordance with Ms. O.'s wishes.

At decision point C, Ms. O. is helped by the hospice nurse to set up an AD, which is Ms. O.'s wish and brings her much relief. There was 100% agreement from the health care professionals surveyed from all three countries that this was in accordance with her wishes. At decision point D, while in the hospital for palliative laser therapy, the resident follows Ms. O.'s wish not to perform any further investigations or administer iv fluids. The majority of health care professionals from all three countries agreed that this was in accordance with her wishes and the correct decision. Some remarked that both admission to the hospital and laser therapy should have been included in a specific AD for Ms. O.

At decision point E, Ms. O.'s GP admits her to the hospital because of confusion due to suspected pneumonia. The majority of American and German and half the Japanese health care professionals thought that the hospital admission was against her wishes. Similarly, only about 10% of those questioned from each country thought that this decision was correct. Most would have preferred treatment of the suspected pneumonia with oral administration of antibiotics at home. At decision point F, no further diagnostic tests were performed, and no iv fluid was given. The vast majority of those questioned thought that this was in adherence with Ms. O.'s wishes; slightly fewer agreed that this was the correct decision (79%–89%).

When asked whether Ms. O. had accomplished overall what she wanted in her AD, the majority of professionals from all countries said yes: (the United States $N = 14$ [54%], Germany $N = 17$ [59%], Japan $N = 30$ [79%]). Fewer professionals disagreed, although the health care professionals from (the United States contested the statement in greater numbers the United States $N = 12$ [46%], Germany $N = 11$ [38%], Japan $N = 7$ [18%]). It was felt that Ms. O. had indeed reached her aims as expressed in her AD, because she died peacefully, without receiving further diagnostic tests or life-prolonging therapy. Some others felt that she did not achieve her aim, however, because she died in the hospital, and she had expressed a wish to die at home. In addition they felt that her wishes were not fully understood by the family physician. Again, it was remarked upon that her AD had not been specific enough.

Planning for end-of-life decisions: a checklist

The most important findings of this study are that palliative care patients face their decisions with mostly negative feelings and rely heavily on advice from their health care professionals. The health care professionals' survey revealed that they think ADs are useful in palliative care settings, and that the ADs used by patients were not as specific as they would like them to be. We feel that these findings indicate that ADs could be instrumental in aiding health care professionals, especially those who do not specialize in palliative care, in planning for end-of-life decisions. Therefore, we have compiled a checklist from the answers obtained in this study (see Appendix 2). Since writing an AD and naming a proxy were considered important by patients and health care professionals, these categories are included in Part A. The procedure for writing an AD in the palliative care setting was then extrapolated for the comments made by the health care professionals that we interviewed, and these are included in Part B.

Comments

Patients' views
In this cross-cultural comparison, we found no differences in basic hospice tenets, these being better care for dying patients, a focus on palliative care, and no resuscitation. Small differences between the countries surveyed were seen in the patients' diagnoses and the location of patients. The types of end-of-life decisions were also similar in all three countries. The number of coping decisions were relatively lower in Japan, probably because more than 50% of the respondents had already made all relevant decisions or entrusted them to their families.

Clear differences were seen when we examined how hospices gain consent. In the United States, an explicitly written consent form is signed by the patients before admission. In Germany, an explicit oral consent from the patient is obtained in most instances, whereas in Japan, explicit oral consent is mostly obtained from the families. Signing of an AD form and appointing a proxy (durable power of attorney according to the U.S. law) is highly prevalent in the palliative care setting in the United States.

Views of health care professionals
There was a unequivocal agreement among the health care professionals in the United States and Germany that ADs were useful in palliative care. In contrast to current practice, however, the professionals wanted ADs to be specific. In Germany and Japan, there was an obvious discrepancy between the low prevalence of ADs and the relative readiness of health care professionals to use them.

The study based upon the vignette also illustrated similarities rather than differences. At all the points where decisions had to be made, there was a clear majority opinion with a 10%–20% minority opinion. The majority of those interviewed thought it was wrong to admit Ms. O. to the hospital because she was suffering from confusion due to suspected pneumonia. It was felt that this decision was clearly against Ms. O.'s wishes, although she did not specify hospital admissions in her AD. The greatest agreement in all decisions taken in this case report was that it was important to help Ms. O. to set up an AD.

It has been shown in many studies that one's cultural background affects one's values. In this study, however, we did not observe any major cultural differences in attitude. Why then did we not find differences in attitudes that we might have expected? Although there is the widely held and commonsensical theory that one's culture affects one's values, there are some scholars who hold a different position on this issue. For example, Tom Beauchamp insists that there is a universal code of morality, that goes beyond culture, which he describes "morality in a narrow sense,"[13] while Edmund Pellegrino supports valuing "something close to autonomy"[14,15] as universal (Notes 4, 5).

In sum, patients in all three countries perceive that these diverse palliative care programs satisfy fundamental medical and social needs. There are some differences between the countries under discussion based upon this investigation. These may be organizational or related to cultural factors, such as the strong role of the family and commumication style in Japan.[15,16] This combination of addressing fundamental needs and flexibility in practical terms may explain the success of the hospice idea in many countries. Moreover, our study supports the concept of a universal "palliative care culture," which emphasizes a universally accepted good, the core concepts of which are shared by ordinary people in many cultures. The unity of opinion between health care professionals and patients that we found in our study upon issues like not using fluid substitution, restricting diagnostic procedures to a minimum, and emphasizing home care, are, we believe, all part of a palliative care culture that is seen as a universally accepted good. This somewhat counter-intuitive lack of cultural difference may be a sign that certain attitudes toward death and dying transcend cultural boundaries.

Checklist

The results discussed above imply that ADs have a use in many societies, when they are modified to fit the cultural context. The checklist provided in Appendix 2 can be used as a guide for discussion on how to establish a procedure if a written AD or a formal appointment of a proxy is desired by the patient. If, however, it is felt that a written formal AD is not necessary, ADs can be made orally. Then, however, the health care professionals involved with the case should record the patient's wishes in the treatment notes. An implicit, culturally based appointment of a proxy should also be recognized and noted in the records. Each advance care plan has to take into account the specific situation of each patient, according to the patient's medical condition and cultural background.

If a written AD appears useful in a given situation, the checklist may be used to set up an individually tailored specific AD. We suggest that this checklist may also be used in the future to develop and validate an easy-to-use instrument for physicians, especially non-palliative care specialists. This instrument might prove useful to enhance communication between patients and health care professionals.

Advanced Directives and Palliative Care: A Global Perspective

Our discussion is based on our study conducted in three industrialized countries, the United States, Germany, and Japan. We have tentatively concluded that ADs are useful to some extent when they are modified to fit the cultural setting, although only randomized intervention studies will prove their usefulness in these industrialized countries.[4] However, we realize these findings may not apply to the important area of care in developing countries. Jan Stjernsward and Sandro Pampallona movingly describe the problems of suffering in the developing world.[12] In countries where basic access to health care is not guaranteed, the modern Western hospice philosophy is rendered somewhat useless. Crucially, there is an obvious injustice concerning the means of palliation, chief among these being the availability of morphine. Morphine consumption seems to have a positive correlation with the gross domestic product (GDP) of each nation. Palliative care for children is becoming a topic of concern in industrialized countries. However, infants are dying without adequate comfort in regions where the infant mortality rate is particularly high. Palliative care for HIV/AIDS patients is also an important issue, although major pandemics are occurring in the world's poorest countries.

Our assertion that basic hospice tenets cross cultural boundaries may seem somewhat naive if we consider these urgent medical problems that face many developing countries. As Tsuchida states:

> [t]he onslaught of modern Western values, embedded in technoscientific culture and society, ranged from the maternal view of the human body to a belief in the autonomy of individuals. . . . Today, advanced medical technoscience has forced us to face the need to determine, in the name of individual rights and autonomy, the kind of medicine we desire or can afford. This advanced technological force, backed by the capitalist principles of free enterprise and cost-benefit analysis and counterbalanced by socialized medicine in differing degrees from one developed country to another, of course promises us much in the way of lessening or obscure our pain and suffering. . . . Advance directives are necessary part of this type of medicine and the society that enables it to flourish.
>
> Tsuchida[7]

This is one perspective on ADs. Nevertheless, ADs in palliative care can be a useful tool in many different cultures, particularly in those cultures that have adopted Western medical practices. However, it is hard to imagine ADs in a palliative care setting in places that do not even have the capacity to provide basic health care. If the day arrives when all people are able to access modern medicine, and especially palliative care, then ADs may well have a universal role to play.

Acknowledgments

The authors thank Drs. Deborah Zion, Monash University, and Todd S. Elwyn, University of Hawaii, for their insightful comments on the manuscript.

Notes

Note 1. This study was funded in part by an international grant from the Volkswagen Foundation to the Kennedy Institute of Ethics, Georgetown University, Washington DC and the Institute of Philosophy, Ruhr University, Bochum, Germany. It was also supported by a grant-in-aid for scientific research nos. 0867259 and 09672297 by the Ministry of Education, Science, Sports and Culture, Japan. The results of this study is published in a book,[5] Jahrbuch fur Recht und Ethik (Annual Review of Law and Ethics, Berlin: Duncker and Humblot) vol. 4, 1996, and in other peer reviewed journals.

Note 2. Omakase: an attitude of dependency frequently observed among the Japanese. This attitude entails entrusting one's care to one's family and physician, assuming that they will give the patient the most beneficial or appropriate care. The patient would, thus, defer to his or her family and the physician in charge for decisions about continuing or foregoing treatment, a matter that is very likely to affect his or her life and death.[7] It should be noted that omakase patients defer decision making authority when they are still competent.

Note 3. Tsuchida also notes that ". . . [w]hat has been said above may not be peculiar to the Japanese but may be rather common among non-Western peoples. There are important factors other than mere economics that must be considered if people living in the North are willing to reflect on the significance of advance directives in a global health care context."[7]

Note 4. Beauchamp states as follows. "Many today believe that secular pluralism has created a so-called postmodern world in which we should give up our robust past beliefs in the universality of moral precepts. I will maintain, however, that a body of general ethical precepts constitutes morality wherever it is found. I will call this shared, universal system of beliefs 'morality in the narrow sense.'"[13] These beliefs included: obtain consent before invading another person's body, do not kill, do not cause pain, do not cause offense, remove conditions that will cause harm to others, and help persons with disabilities. Many of these beliefs are applicable to the hospice care setting, and more generally, to the modern practice of medicine across the world.

Note 5. Pellegrino argues that autonomy is a universal principle and is not just a cultural artifact.[14] He maintains that the democratic ideals that lie behind the contemporary North American concept of autonomy will spread and that something close to it will be the choice of many individuals in other countries as well. He suggests that a nation can enjoy the benefits of medical progress only by dealing constructively with the conflict between traditional values and modern medical progress. However, it is clear that Pellegrino is not simply arguing for the American version of autonomy.[15]

References

1. Miles SH, Koepp R, Weber EP. Advance end-of-life treatment planning. A research review. *Arch Intern Med* 1996; 156:1062–1068.
2. Emanuel L. Advance directives: What have we learned so far? *J Clin Ethics* 1993; 4:8–16.
3. Teno JM, Nelson HL, Lynn J. Advance care planning. Priorities for ethical and empirical research. *Hastings Center Report* 1994; S32–S36.

4. Teno JM. Lessons learned and not learned from the SUPPORT project. *Palliat Med* 1999; 13:91–93.

5. Sass HM, Veatch RM, Kimura R, eds. *Advance Directives and Surrogate Decision Making in Health Care: United States, Germany, and Japan*. Baltimore: Johns Hopkins University Press, 1998.

6. Akabayashi A, Kai I, Itoh K, Tsukui K. The acceptability of advance directives in Japanese society: A questionnaire study for healthy people in the physical check-up settings. *J Japan Association for Bioethics* 1997; 7(1):31–40. (in Japanese)

7. Tsuchida T. A differing perspectives on advance directives. In: Sass HM, Veatch RM, Kimura R, eds. *Advance Directives and Surrogate Decision Making in Health Care: United States, Germany, and Japan*. Baltimore: Johns Hopkins University Press, 1998:209–221.

8. Singer PA. Advance directives in palliative care. *J Palliat Care* 1994; 10:111–116.

9. Voltz R, Akabayashi A, Reese C, et al. Organization and patients' perception of palliative care: a cross-cultural comparison. *Palliat Med* 1997; 11:351–357.

10. Voltz R, Akabayashi A, Reese C, et al. End-of-life decisions and advance directives in palliative care: A cross-cultural survey of patients and health-care professionals. *J Pain Symp Manage* 1997; 16(3):153–162.

11. Voltz R, Akabayashi A, Reese C, et al. Attitudes of health-care professionals towards clinical decisions in palliative care: a cross-cultural comparison. *J Clin Ethics* 1999; 10:309–315.

12. Stjernsward J, Pampallona S. Palliative medicine—a global perspective. In: Doyle D, Hanks GWC, MacDonald N, eds. *Oxford Textbook of Palliative Medicine, 2nd ed.*, Oxford: Oxford Medical Publications, 1998:1227–1245.

13. Beauchamp TL. Comparative studies: Japan and America, In: Hoshino K, ed. *Japanese and Western Bioethics—Studies in Moral Diversity. Philosophy and Medicine, Volume 54*. Dordrecht: Kluwer Academic Publishers, 1994:25–47.

14. Pellegrino ED. Is truth telling to the patient a cultural artifact? *JAMA* 1992; 268:1734–1735.

15. Akabayashi A, Fetters MD, Elwyn TS. Family consent, communication, and advance directives for cancer disclosure: A Japanese case and discussion. *J Med Ethics*, 1999; 25:296–301.

16. Akabayashi A, Kai I, Takemura H, Okazaki H. Truth telling in the case of a pessimistic diagnosis in Japan. *Lancet* 1999; 354:1263.

Appendix 1. Case Vignette[11]

Ms. O. is 84 years old and has been diagnosed with advanced-stage rectal carcinoma. She receives regular palliative laser therapy for which she has to be admitted to the hospital for several days. The last time she suffered a bowel perforation, and has now been in the hospital for several weeks. She desperately wants to go home. Her daughter contacts a hospice home care service (offering nurses and volunteers, but no full-time medical doctors), which she has heard of through friends. Ms. O. is constantly getting weaker, refuses to drink, and becomes confused, which resolves with intravenous (iv) fluid replacement. Help is organized, and Ms. O. is discharged home with medical advice to drink as much as possible and take her medications (digitalis and diuretics for heart failure). Ms. O. is feeling well back home, and her general practitioner (GP), who knows Ms. O. for years, is now in charge.

After 1 week at home Ms. O. refuses to drink or take her medication. Thereafter her nights are calmer than before and even without medication she has no pain or other discomfort. Her GP urges her to drink more and take her medication. Despite her not drinking, no action is taken (Decision point A). A few days later Ms. O. feels that both her legs do not belong to her, and she has pins and needles in them. Her GP suspects tumor infiltration of the nerves. Because of Ms. O.'s declining state, no further investigation is pursued (Decision point B). Two days later, the GP calls in again: Ms. O.'s legs are feeling better. The GP is angry with Ms. O., as she has not followed the instructions to drink or take her medication. Ms. O. says repeatedly: I do not want to drink so much, this is awful for me. Confronted with the possibility of kidney damage, Ms. O. says: I want it to be finished as soon as possible. According to her wish and with the help of the hospice nurse, an advance directive (AD) is set up, which includes her statements against fluid intake and the wish not to have life-prolonging therapy or any other investigations. Having such an AD eases Ms. O. very much (Decision point C).

A week later, Ms. O. is admitted to the hospital for another laser therapy. She has no further studies and is not given iv fluids (Decision point D). Four days later, Ms. O. is discharged home. On the last visit by the hospice nurse, Ms. O. sits in front of her TV watching a soccer game, drinking Rebenbrau beer. On the next day, Ms. O.'s condition suddenly deteriorates. She is confused. Her GP admits Ms. O. to the hospital because of a suspected pneumonia (Decision point E). The resident respects Ms. O.'s AD, no further investigations are done and no iv fluids given (Decision point F). She improves slightly. Ms. O. dies peacefully the day before her planned discharge.

Appendix 2. Checklist for Planning of End-of-life Decisions in Patients with a Terminal Disease[10]

A. *What should be discussed?*

1. Medical therapy decisions, such as

- disease modifying treatments—cardio-pulmonary resuscitation
- use of respirator—parenteral artificial nutrition
- enteral nutrition and hydration (for example, through percutaneous entero Gastrostomy)—anticoagulation
- antibiotics—specific emergency treatments (e.g., for pain, dyspnea, bleeding, epileptic seizure, restlessness, delirium)

2. What is the preferred locus of care?

- stay at home?
- admission to hospital?—which hospital?—hospice care?

3. Who is the patient's source of support?
for example, family, friends, emergency phone numbers, physicians, nurses, social worker, other professionals, technical help, hospice group, proxy

4. How is the patient coping?

- Is professional help in communication with relatives wanted?
- Is spiritual help wanted?

5. Are there personal organizational decisions where the patient may need help?

- for example, financial?—writing a will?—funeral details?

6. Does the patient want to give an advance directive (AD)?

- Does the patient express preferences for future decisions on any decisions mentioned above?
- Does the patient want information on how to set up a written AD?

7. Does the patient want to appoint a proxy?

- Is there an informal or culturally implicit appointment?
- Does the patient want information on a formal appointment?

B. How to proceed, if the patient wishes to express preferences in advance?

Any expression of preferences should be the result of an intensive and long-standing communication between patients, health care professionals, and relatives.

1. Advance directives

- note orally expressed ADs in the medical record
- help in writing an AD:
    should know patient well
    patient must be fully informed about diagnosis, prognosis, options
    patient must be mentally clear (statement of treating physician included)
    should be as specific and individualized as possible
    regular (for example, monthly) revision
    avoid influencing the wording, but give all necessary information

- patient must know that AD may be changed any time
- witness should be present when signing

2. *Appointing a proxy*

- Has the patient informally or (culturally) implicitly named a proxy already?
- help in formally appointing a proxy according to national laws
   proxy must be trustworthy, fully informed, and available
   try to avoid obvious conflicts of interests
   regular revision and discussions
- witness present when signing

9

Assessment of Symptoms in the Cognitively Impaired

WENDY M. STEIN

This chapter focuses on symptom assessment in the cognitively impaired, one of the more challenging assessment problems faced by clinicians in the practice of palliative medicine. Pain is the symptom best researched to date in cognitively impaired patients, and the majority of the data presented pertains to this symptom. The challenge in assessment predominantly affects the elderly; this chapter emphasizes research in this rapidly growing segment of the population. Clinical suggestions for cogent treatment strategies will be offered on the basis of the data presented and recent clinical trials.

Folstein and Folstein defined cognitive impairment or altered mental state as "a change in the patient's usual premorbid state of mind".[1] This can include delirium and dementia, as well as altered emotions and behaviors. Acute and subacute changes in mental status have been documented in as many as 20%–30% of medical inpatients and 50%–90% of nursing home residents.[1] These changes impact significantly upon an individual's ability to participate actively in both initial symptom assessment and evaluation of treatment efficacy. The first step in assessment is to establish the patient's premorbid mental status, and the nature and association of any clinical changes that may have occurred. The presence of vision or hearing impairments must be determined because either may further complicate both the assessment and treatment of pain and nonpain symptoms in the cognitively impaired.

The Graying of America

By the year 2020, the population over the age of 60 years is expected to increase by 69%; those older than 85 years represent the most rapidly growing subsegment of this population.[2] Many scientific and technological breakthroughs have contributed to the growth of an older, chronically ill elderly population. Prevalence rates of many of the dementias, and specifically Alzheimer's disease, rise exponentially after age 65 years.[3] Rates of Alzheimer's disease have ranged as high as 50% in those over the age of 90.[2] Rates of delirium are also higher in those affected by dementia.[4] As a result of these trends, there is a very large and growing population of elderly individuals suffering from delirium and dementing illnesses.

Pain Prevalence in the Elderly

Population-based studies of community dwelling elderly have noted a two-fold increase in important pain problems among those over age 60.[5] Important pain problems were defined as those significant enough to prompt patients to take a pain medication daily or impair functional status. Among nursing home residents, studies have estimated a pain prevalence of 45%–80%. It is common for these individuals to suffer from more than one kind of pain, with musculoskeletal sources of pain being the most common.[6] Elderly individuals, when compared with their younger counterparts, are also disproportionately affected by painful syndromes such as peripheral vascular disease, temporal arteritis and polymyalgia rheumatica, peripheral neuropathy, herpes zoster (and the postherpetic neuralgia that follows), and many types of cancer. These demographics suggest that individuals suffering from dementia and delirium are likely to be disproportionately affected by these painful syndromes. There are a large number of cognitively impaired elderly in need of aggressive and appropriate pain assessment and treatment.

Dementia

Folstein and Folstein define dementia as "a syndrome characterized by a decline in multiple cognitive functions occurring in clear consciousness".[7] An estimated 10%–15% of elderly surgical patients, one-third of elderly medical inpatients, and more than 50% of nursing home residents develop dementia.[7] There are over 50 causes of dementia. Primary dementia has no other associated disease; secondary dementia is related to an underlying neurologic condition such neoplasm, movement disorders, motor neuron disease, multiple sclerosis, vascular disease, chronic infection, brain trauma, toxic exposures, endocrine disorders, and vitamin deficiencies. Psychiatric disorders such as chronic schizophrenia or pseudodementia, can mimic dementia. Conditions largely affecting adolescents or young adults such as Wilson's disease, progressive myoclonic epilepsy, tuberous sclerosis, and the metabolic storage diseases can cause dementia as well.

The first etiologies to be excluded in the course of a comprehensive dementia evaluation are depression, which can mimic dementia, and the potentially reversible dementias. The effort to reverse brain pathology might involve changing or eliminating drugs; treating infection; anemia, or metabolic impairments such as hypothyroidism and B$_{12}$ deficiency; and managing structural disorders such as normal pressure hydrocephalus, tumors, and subdural hematomas.[8] The primary concern in identifying these phenomena is to limit further deleterious consequences, not to reverse the degree of cognitive impairment that has already occurred, as this is generally permanent in nature.

Dementia has been separated on clinical grounds into subcortical and cortical categories. Subcortical dementias include Huntington's disease, Parkinson's disease, and hydrocephalus. These characteristically exhibit amnesia, slowness of thought, apathy and lack of initiative in all aspects of cognitive function, and early disorders of movement.[7] Cortical dementias such as Alzheimer's disease, Jacob-Creutzfeldt disease, Pick's disease and multi-infarct dementia feature aphasia, apraxia, agnosia, prominent amnesia, and in Alzheimer's disease specifically, preservation of fine motor movement until late in the illness.[7]

Delirium

Lipowski defined delirium as "an organic mental syndrome featuring global cognitive impairment, disturbances of attention, reduced level of consciousness, increased or reduced psycho-motor activity, and disorganized sleep-wake cycle."[4] Symptoms can include difficulty in thinking coherently, anxiety, restlessness, insomnia, disturbing dreams as well as fleeting hallucinations. Psychological stress, sleep loss, and sensory deprivation or sensory overload can all facilitate and maintain delirium. Factors such as age greater than 65, brain damage, and chronic cerebral disease are the primary predisposing characteristics.[4]

Delirium has been well described in the cancer literature,[9,10] but is actually common in all elderly populations, especially those with underlying dementia. Rates of delirium have ranged as high as 50% in hospitalized patients with previously diagnosed dementia;[8] in reality, figures may be even higher as a large number of community dwelling individuals often go undiagnosed for long periods of time as their loved ones naturally begin to compensate for the mental deficits. Obviously, accurate diagnosis is extremely challenging.[4]

Ouslander et al. suggest the word DELIRIUMS as a way to recall its etiologies.[8] D represents drugs, especially those with anticholinergic properties, as well as drug overdose or withdrawal. E suggests emotional causes such as mania or agitated depression. L stands for low oxygenatic includes hypoxia as occurs in cardiac ischemia, congestive heart failure, chronic pulmonary disease, or pulmonary embolism. I represents infection of any sort, and in hospitalized elderly most often is urosepsis or pneumonia. "I" includes ictal states. R refers to retention of either urine or feces. U represents undernutrition and dehydration that occur commonly in community-dwelling as well as instituionalized elderly. *M* includes metabolic causes such as hypo- or hyperthyroidism, or organ failure. And finally, S suggest possible stroke or subdural hematoma. Each of these possible etiologies need to be carefully contemplated when investigating a diagnosis of delirium.

Differentiating Delirium From Dementia

It is vital to differentiate between delirium and dementia. This can be challenging, particularly when they occur simultaneously. Rates of delirium run as high as 50% among hospitalized patients with previously diagnosed dementia.[8]

Dementias, excluding vascular dementia, which follows a stepwise progression, usually evolve insidiously over time. Patients exhibit a normal sleep-wake cycle and level of consciousness with stable and persistent symptoms. In early dementia, the ability to attend to task is not yet affected. Orientation is most often impaired, and aphasia and apathy are quite common. Autonomic or other physical changes are unusual and EEG is normal, or at worst may exhibit mild slowing.

Delirium presents acutely over days to weeks, fluctuating over time with waxing and waning levels of consciousness. Sleep-wake cycle may be disturbed. Ability to attend to task is impaired as well as orientation. Autonomic changes are common and EEGs show diffuse slow waves. Language may be incoherent and the patient may be fearful and agitated.

The Additional Burden of Sensory Impairment

Auditory and visual impairments occur commonly with aging and often complicate both symptom assessment and management. Additionally, when uncompensated, sensory impairment can negatively affect mood, function, sociability, and gait and balance.

Hearing loss is the third most commonly reported chronic problem in individuals over age 65.[11] Prevalence statistics for hearing loss in nursing home patients range between 50% and 100%, with prevalence figures rising with advancing age.[12] Hearing impairment is composed of sensorineural disease (cranial nerve VIII damage from noise, cochlear damage, ototoxic drugs such as gentamycin, presbycusis, trauma, infarction, and acoustic neuroma), conductive disorders (cerumen impaction, middle ear disease, and otosclerosis), and mixed and central hearing loss. Mixed hearing loss itself affects 50% of those ages 51–91.[12] Data from the Framingham Heart Study show that although 41% of those over age 65 had some level of hearing impairment, only 10% of these individuals had ever tried hearing aids.[12] This is a significant problem among the elderly, which can seriously impede the clinicians ability to conduct meaningful symptom assessment.

Presbyopia, senile miosis, and age-related changes in color vision can occur with normal aging. The four most common causes of blindness in older persons are cataracts, glaucoma, age-related macular degeneration, and diabetic retinopathy. These disorders affect 9% of adults 65–74 years old, and the prevalence in those over 75 years old rises to greater than 50%.[13] These impediments, then, pose significant challenges to be overcome if the clinician is to conduct valid and meaningful symptom assessments.

Studies of Pain in the Cognitively Impaired

Of the more than 50 documented symptoms occurring commonly at the end of life, pain is the single symptom which has been best described in the cognitively impaired. Sengstaken and King[14] studied physicians' abilities to detect pain among geriatric nursing home residents and found that 66% of those able to communicate were identified as having pain by both chart review and patient interview. Only 34% of these patients, however, had pain identified by their treating physicians. When the noncommunicative residents were compared to those able to communicate, the physicians were found to have identified pain less frequently in those who were noncommunicative. The groups were matched with regards to demographics and medical diagnoses other than dementia, and although they would be equally likely to suffer pain, treating physicians identified chronic pain more than twice as frequently in those who were able to communicate.[14]

Parmalee et al.[15,16] studied self-reported pain in 758 nursing home and residential housing residents with mild to moderate levels of cognitive impairment, as documented by the Blessed Memory Information Concentration Test. This study showed that, in general, pain complaints decreased with increasing levels of cognitive impairment. Severely impaired subjects reported both less intense pain and a smaller number of pain complaints than those who had either intact cognition or mild impairment. However, when cognitively impaired individuals reported pain, their pain complaints were no less valid.

Ferrell et al.[17] examined the utility of currently existing pain scales for cognitively impaired nursing home residents, drawing study patients drawn from 10 different Los Angeles nursing homes. The study population consisted of patients with moderate to severe degrees of cognitive impairment (mean 12.1 +/- 7.9 on the Folstein Mini Mental Status Examination).[18] The five scales included the McGill Present Pain Intensity Subscale (0 to 5 with word anchors), the 10 cm. Visual Analog Scale, the Rand Coop Chart (cartoon figures with word anchors), the Memorial Pain Assessment Card Subscale, and a verbal 0 to 10 scale. All scales were presented in enlarged format and with adequate amounts of light and hearing augmentation if required. Of the five scales presented, the Present

Pain Intensity Subscale had the highest rate of completion (65%). Although only 32% of patients could complete all five scales presented, 83% of these individuals with significant degrees of cognitive impairment could complete at least one of the existing scales presented. These findings validate the utility of attempting to utilize established pain assessment tools in communicative, cognitively impaired elderly. The study participants were also able to communicate qualitatively their present pain intensity, but were unable to convey a sense of their pain intensity in the past.

Porter et al.[19] studied of 51 cognitively intact and 44 cognitively impaired patients, and found that dementia significantly impacted upon the subjects' ability to respond to questions about pain. Likewise, in a study of anti-inflammatory use in patients with Alzheimer's Disease, Scherder and Bouma[20] found a lower percentage of patients with Alzheimer's Disease using analgesics than in controls despite similar percentages with a painful condition (69.7% and 78.6% respectively). The inability to communicate is likely the major explanation for this discrepancy.[14] Additionally, it remains unknown as to whether the experience of the dementing illness itself might further exacerbate a patient's perceived suffering,[21] making the above disparity all the more tragic.

Pain in Noncommunicative Cognitively Impaired Patients

Many of the studies of pain assessment in the noncommunicative cognitively impaired focused on the use of pediatric instruments, and specifically those developed for neonates.[22] There are some fundamental issues to address when contemplating the use of pediatric assessment tools in elderly patients. First, pediatric tools were developed to measure acute, and often externally induced, procedure-related pain; in the cognitively impaired elderly, clinicians are most often evaluating chronic pain, or acute on chronic pain, which might be expected to present differently. In acute pain, the clinician might anticipate changes in facial expression, vocalization, increased muscle tension, and autonomic discharge resulting in elevations of heart rate, blood pressure, and respiratory rate. Although in chronic somatic pain states such as arthritis, which is highly prevalent in both community-dwelling and institutionalized elderly, clinicians may witness vocalizations and increased muscle tension, chronic pain may just as likely present as depression, or more likely as a change from the individual's baseline mental status. Second, infants have no wealth of pain memory to influence their pain interpretation, and therefore cannot attach any meaning to induced pain. It is currently unknown whether cognitively impaired elderly retain this ability. Yet, nonverbal behavior, vocalizations, changes in function, and caregiver reports are often used as indicators of pain in the noncommunicative cognitively impaired elderly.[23]

Marzinski[24] studied 60 patients living in a dementia unit. Forty-three percent had potentially painful conditions based on chart review. Only 3 of these patients received routinely scheduled analgesics. The most clinically interesting finding of this study was that the nursing staff could identify what amounted to normative behavior for individual patients. Once deviations were identified, they were noted and acted upon.

Empiric Treatment Studies in the Cognitively Impaired

Several studies have sought to initiate pain interventions empirically in non-communicative cognitively impaired demented elders. Of this group of studies, the most detailed to date, in terms of extensive physical assessments and chart reviews before medications are initiated, is that of Kovach et al.[25] In a pilot study that was part of a larger program to improve pain management practices in 57 Wisconsin facilities, researchers studied 104 noncommunicative residents with dementia who resided at 32 participating long-term care facilities and had signs or symptoms of pain or discomfort. The residents had a mean age of 85 years and a variety of dementing illnesses. The nursing staffs were instructed to initiate a newly developed protocol entitled The Assessment of Discomfort in Dementia (ADD) Protocol if a patient displayed signs or symptoms of possible physical or affective discomfort. The first step was excluding common physical causes for discomfort, such as occult infection or impaction, by thorough physical assessment and review of history, including consultations with family and/or physicians. If the assessment was negative, nonpharmacologic comfort interventions were undertaken. If non-drug interventions were unsuccessful in ameliorating the symptom in question, the nurses were educated to administer an non-opioid analgesic as needed. The nurses had asked the physicians for an analgesic of their choice; in the event that none were available, the nurse requested an order for a scheduled analgesic, such as 500 mg of acetaminophen routinely administered three times per day. If there was no response to the last step, the nurse could consult with the study personnel and request an order for a stronger analgesic agent, according to the World Health Organization three-step ladder approach to the treatment of pain. The sample population went from an average of 32.85 behavioral symptoms associated with discomfort in the 7 days prior to initiating the ADD Protocol, to 23.47 symptoms on protocol, which was a statistically significant clinical change. Of particular interest was the fact that 88% of the nurses involved felt that the protocol was somewhat to very helpful.

Non-Pain Symptoms in the Cognitively Impaired

Despite the reasonably high prevalence of non-pain symptoms such as dyspnea and cough in both cognitively intact and cognitively impaired elderly, there is little or no information in the scientific literature.[26,27] Most of the information available is usually in the form of case studies or case series.[27]

Table 9.1. Recommendations for symptom assessment

1. Give adequate time for the cognitively impaired patient to think about and respond to questions.
2. Provide large print visual cues, adequate ambient light, hearing aids or pocket amplification devices and refractive lenses as needed.
3. Spread some portions of the assessment over time in the case of patients with limited attention spans.
4. When using standardized assessment tools, establish the best single tool for use with that patient and document this information in the chart.
5. Ensure each team member utilizes the same assessment tool.
6. Conduct more frequent symptom assessment in the cognitively impaired patient; he or she can tell you the degree of symptom severity at the moment but not in the past.
7. Enlist the support of the family member(s)/caregiver(s) to journal pain assessments.

Some symptoms are relatively easily assessed because objective findings can suggest symptom distress. These include constipation, diarrhea, nausea and vomiting, decubiti, dry mouth, edema, insomnia, itching, seizures, urinary retention, and anorexia and weight loss.

The prime considerations in the management of non-pain symptoms are to start only one drug at a time to judge both efficacy and possible side-effects, to prevent their occurrence whenever possible (such as rectifying constipation before initiating opioids), and to avoid pharmacological agents with the potential to cause delirium, especially those with strong anticholinergic properties. Repeated assessment is key to safe and effective therapy.

Guidelines for Symptom Assessment and Management

The clinician must create an optimal physical situation in order to adequately assess pain and non-pain symptoms in the cognitively impaired who are able to communicate (Table 9.1). Extra time should be provided for the patient to assimilate questions. Large print visual cues, adequate ambient light, and the use hearing aids or pocket amplification devices and refractive lenses are vital. Limited attention span may necessitate performing symptom assessments in portions over time. Subjective responses must carry equal weight with fixed answers to standardized tools. In the case of pain, multiple tools should be presented upon initial assessment if standardized instruments are being utilized. Whichever standardized pain tool is most clinically useful with a particular patient should be carefully recorded in the chart and this information communicated to other members of the interdisciplinary team. A large print version of the particular tool can be physically placed in the clinical chart or over the patient's bed. This procedure will ensure that each subsequent assessment is performed exactly the same way regardless of the team member asking the questions. As the cognitively impaired elderly are often able to report on pain at the time of, but not

Table 9.2. Recommendations for symptom management

1. Any deviation from the patient's usual behavior should trigger a thorough chart review for recently added medications, physical examination for evidence of occult infection, impaction, ischemia, or hypoxia, and tests appropriate to the patient's/proxy's goals of care.
2. If the above does not yield results, contemplate a trial of short-acting Step 1 non-opioid analgesics administered on a routine basis and for an adequate trial period.
3. If the patient appears to respond to an empiric analgesic trial, discuss this response with family members and caregivers, and document the discussion carefully in the medical record.
4. Reassess intervention efficacy in terms of effects on function, mood, and sleep and document in the medical record consistently and continuously.
5. Ensure that any potential analgesic side-effects are part of the ongoing monitoring process for that patient.

previous to, the pain assessment, pain assessment should be conducted more frequently than would be necessary with a cognitively intact patient.

When caring for the non-communicative cognitively impaired, the single most important sign is deviation from what is considered baseline or normal behavior for that particular individual (Table 9.2). If this should occur, a complete and thorough bedside examination should be conducted, with laboratory and imaging studies consistent with the patient and family's wishes. Physical examination should focus specifically on occult sources or atypical presentations of infection in the elderly, such as pneumonia or urinary tract infections. The input of nursing and other staff should be sought to exclude alterations in sleeping, eating, or elimination as the source of change in behavior. Chart review should exclude changes in medications, doses, or dose intervals as a possible etiology. After all of the above have been completed and reviewed carefully with family members and staff, and informed consent obtained from involved family members, there may be a role for a well-defined empiric trial of short acting pain medication with consistent and continual reassessment.[28]

References

1. Folstein MF, Folstein SE. Neuropsychiatric assessment of syndromes of altered mental state. In: Hazzard WB, Bierman EL, Blass JP, Ettinger Jr. WH, Halter JB, eds. *Principles of Geriatric Medicine and Gerontology*. New York: McGraw-Hill, Inc., 1994:221–228.
2. Mittlemark MB. The epidemiology of aging. In: Hazzard WB, Bierman EL, Blass JP, Ettinger Jr. WH, Halter JB, eds. *Principles of Geriatric Medicine and Gerontology*. New York: McGraw-Hill, Inc., 1994:135–151.
3. Albert MS. Cognition and aging. In: Hazzard WB, Bierman EL, Blass JP, Ettinger Jr. WH, Halter JB, eds. *Principles of Geriatric Medicine and Gerontology*. New York: McGraw-Hill, Inc., 1994:1013–1019.

4. Lipowski ZJ. Delirium (acute confusional states). In: Hazzard WB, Bierman EL, Blass JP, Ettinger Jr. WH, Halter JB, eds. *Principles of Geriatric Medicine and Gerontology*. New York: McGraw-Hill, Inc., 1994:1021–1026.

5. Crook J, Rideout E, Browne G. The prevalence of pain complaints among a general population. *Pain* 1984; 18:299–314.

6. Ferrell BA. Pain in elderly people. *J Am Geriatr Soc* 1991; 39:64–73.

7. Folstein MF, Folstein SE. Syndromes of altered mental state. In: Hazzard WB, Bierman EL, Blass JP, Ettinger Jr. WH, Halter JB, eds. *Principles of Geriatric Medicine and Gerontology*. New York: McGraw-Hill, Inc., 1994:1197–1204.

8. Ouslander JG, Osterweil D, Morley J. Delirium and dementia. *Medical Care in the Nursing Home*. New York: McGraw-Hill, Inc., 1997:147–162.

9. Derogatis LR, Morrow GR, Fetting J, Penman D, Piasetsky S, Schmale AM, et al. The prevalence of psychiatric disorders among cancer patients. *JAMA* 1983; 249:751–757.

10. Stiefel F, Fainsinger R, Bruera E. *J Pain Symptom Manage* 1992; 7:94–98.

11. Rees TS, Duckert LG, Milczuk HA. Auditory and vestibular dysfunction. In: Hazzard WB, Bierman EL, Blass JP, Ettinger Jr. WH, Halter JB, eds. *Principles of Geriatric Medicine and Gerontology*. New York: McGraw-Hill, Inc., 1994:457–472.

12. Mangione CM. Vision and hearing: screening and treatment efficacy. lecture. *Proceedings of the Intensive Course in Geriatric Medicine*. UCLA Multicampus Program in Geriatrics and Gerontology, 1997:267–276.

13. Michaels DD. The eye. In: Hazzard WB, Bierman EL, Blass JP, Ettinger Jr. WH, Halter JB, eds. *Principles of Geriatric Medicine and Gerontology*. New York: McGraw-Hill, Inc., 1994:441–456.

14. Sengstaken EA, King SA. The problems of pain and its detection among geriatric nursing home residents. *J Am Geriatr Soc* 1993; 41:541–544.

15. Parmalee PA. Pain in cognitively impaired older persons. In: Ferrell B, ed. *Clinics in Geriatric Medicine*. Philadelphia: WB Saunders Company, 1996:473–485.

16. Parmalee PA, Smith B, Katz IR. Pain complaints and cognitive status among elderly institution residents. *J Am Geriatr Soc* 1993; 41:517–522.

17. Ferrell BA, Ferrell BR, Rivera L. Pain in cognitively impaired nursing home patients. *J Pain Symptom Manage* 1995; 10:591–598.

18. Folstein MF, Folstein SE, McHugh PR. Mini-Mental State. *J Psychiatr Res* 1975; 12:189–198.

19. Porter FL, Malhotra KM, Wolf CM, Morris JC, Miller JP, Smith MC. Dementia and response to pain in the elderly. *Pain* 1996; 68:413–421.

20. Scherder EJ, Bouma A. Is decreased use of analgesics in Alzheimer Disease due to a change in the affective component of pain? *Alzheimer Dis Related Disord* 1997; 11:171–174.

21. Farrell MJ, Katz B, Helme RD. The impact of dementia on the pain experience. *Pain* 1996; 67:7–15.

22. Craig KD, Prkachin KM, Grunau RVE. The facial expressions of pain. In: Turk DC, Melzack R, eds. *Handbook of Pain Assessment*. New York: The Guilford Press, 1992:257–276.

23. American Geriatric Society Panel on Chronic Pain in Older Persons. The management of chronic pain in older persons. *J Am Geriatr Soc* 1998; 46:635–651.

24. Marzinski LR. The tragedy of dementia: clinically assessing pain in the confused, nonverbal elderly. *J Gerontol Nurs* 1991; 17:25–28.

25. Kovach CR, Weissman DE, Griffie J, Matson S, Muchka S. Assessment and treatment of discomfort for people with late-stage dementia. *J Pain Symptom Manage* 1999; 18:412–419.

26. Stein WM. Cancer pain in the elderly. In: Ferrell BR, Ferrell BA, eds. *Pain in the Elderly*. Seattle: IASP Press, 1996:69–80.

27. Stein WM, Min YK. Nebulized morphine for paroxysmal cough and dyspnea in a nursing home resident with metastatic cancer. *Am J Hospice Palliat Care* 1997; 3/4:52–56.

28. Stein WM. Palliative care in the cognitively impaired. In: Doyle D, Hanks GWC, MacDonald N, eds. *Oxford Textbook of Palliative Medicine*. 3rd ed. Oxford: Oxford University Press, in press.

Other Related Readings

Gagliese L, Melzack R. Chronic pain in elderly people. *Pain* 1997; 70:3–14.

Ingham J, Portenoy RK. The measurement of pain and other symptoms. In: Doyle D, Hanks GWC, MacDonald N, eds. *Oxford Textbook of Palliative Medicine*. 2nd ed. Oxford: Oxford University Press, 1998:211–215.

IV

RESEARCH OUTCOMES IN PALLIATIVE CARE

10

Defining and Measuring Quality of Life in Palliative Care

S. ROBIN COHEN

Palliative care is "the active total care of patients whose disease is not responsive to curative treatment. Control of pain, of other symptoms, and of psychological, social, and spiritual problems, is paramount. The goal of palliative care is achievement of the best quality of life (QOL) for patients and their families."[1] Therefore, if palliative care providers wish to evaluate the full impact of their care, they must measure changes in QOL as well as improvements in areas specifically targeted by particular interventions (e.g., pain; depression). Since palliative care considers the family as the unit of care,[1] patient QOL, family member QOL, and the QOL of the family unit are all primary outcomes of palliative care. Although problems in specific areas are important to address with specific interventions and specific measures, the best indicator of the quality of whole person care is the QOL of the care recipients.

The importance of measuring QOL has been widely recognized in the health care literature in the last 2 decades. Unfortunately, this has led to a great pressure to measure QOL at all phases of cancer and HIV disease, even though the measures are not adequately developed to be primary outcomes. We can do harm if we base treatment and funding decisions on data obtained from instruments that are not valid, reliable, and responsive to change. We would not consider making important decisions based on a blood test that had not been shown to have these properties, and we should not do so in the case of QOL. However, just as in the case of blood tests that are accurate, accurate QOL measures can help us to provide the most appropriate care or to detect problems sooner, when they may be treated more easily. Therefore, we will also do harm if we do not work to develop these measures that can be of great benefit in ensuring patient- and family-centered care and can help us to reach our goal to achieve the best QOL possible for them.

Conceptualizing Quality of Life

In their 1989 review of the QOL literature, Donovan and colleagues[2] state that an accepted general definition of QOL is "a person's subjective sense of well-being derived from current experience of life as a whole." Based on some large studies of the QOL of Americans[3,4] and more recent qualitative work asking people with cancer or HIV disease to describe what health or QOL means to them,[5-8] I believe that their definition of QOL is an excellent one, but unfortunately I cannot agree that this definition is generally accepted, especially in the health care literature.

Depending on how people use the terms, QOL is very much like or identical to the concepts of life satisfaction and happiness, although all three terms require clarification.[3,9,10] In 1965, Cantril[3] wrote that our satisfaction with our lives is determined by the discrepancy between the lives we perceive ourselves to have and the lives to which we aspire. Others have since produced evidence supporting this hypothesis.[4,11] More recently this hypothesis was used to define QOL in the health care setting by Calman,[12] and it is sometimes referred to as "Calman's gap."

When measuring QOL, both positive and negative contributors must be considered. Bradburn's large study on psychological well-being showed, to his surprise, that positive and negative affect are not two ends of a continuum.[13] The amount of negative affect people feel is not related to the amount of positive affect they feel, and these two constructs must be measured separately. Similarly, a high QOL will not necessarily result from the absence of problems, and instruments that attempt to measure QOL only through determination of the degree to which certain problems are present ignore the reality that QOL is the balance between positive and negative contributors.[2,12,14]

There has been a movement in the health care setting to ignore the broader implications of QOL and focus instead on that part of QOL that the investigators believe is directly related to health care by studying "health-related QOL". "Health-related QOL refers to the extent to which one's usual or expected physical, emotional, and social well-being are affected by a medical condition or its treatment."[15] The term "health-related QOL" was created because constructs such as life satisfaction and happiness are said to be "so distal to the goals and objectives of health care that it would seem inappropriate to apply them as criteria against which to judge the efficacy of medical intervention."[16] The term QOL has been labeled a "misnomer" and "imprecise" because "it conjures up images of religiosity, life satisfaction, and ambition, and makes pretense of representing deeper philosophical notions underlying living."[17]

Investigators choosing to measure "health-related QOL" seem to want to measure the impact of health care on QOL as though there is a direct relationship between them. A QOL measure is not an outcome measure that reflects the quality of the health care service alone, or the effect of an intervention alone. Instead, QOL is a measure of the outcome of the *interaction* between the health care service or intervention and the person or family whose QOL is being measured. We cannot separate out a health-related component of QOL from QOL as QOL is determined by who we are as well as the objective situation we are in.[18–20] It is evident that adding the word "health" before QOL does not allow us to disregard some aspects of the person such as spiritual well-being if we consider that people with cancer and HIV disease define *health* as a sense of personal integrity[6] consisting of physical, psychological, and spiritual domains.[5] Changes within the person, family and their life outside of the health care system are not a bothersome problem in QOL measurement[21] but rather an integral part of the equation that results in QOL. That is why QOL is truly a respondent-centered outcome measure and will help us to provide patient- and family-centered care. Many investigators make the mistake of thinking that contributors to QOL represent QOL. Surely severe physical symptoms contribute to QOL, but the extent of that contribution will depend on many factors. Therefore if QOL rather than the symptoms is of interest, it is important to determine how much of an impact the symptom has on the respondent, rather than its intensity. If the symptoms themselves are of interest, then a symptom assessment tool rather than a QOL instrument should be used.

If we are measuring QOL rather than symptoms we should expect that shifts in expectations will affect the score. For example, even if a person's functional capabilities decline, if that person also has lowered expectations, QOL may remain the same or even improve since the difference between the lived experience and the situation aspired to (the 'gap') may be the same or reduced. Social comparison theory predicts this kind of shift in expectations as we seek to compare our abilities with those perceived to have abilities similar to ours and tend not to compare ourselves to those whose abilities we perceive to be very different from our own.[22] Therefore, we would expect that when considering their QOL, patients will begin to compare themselves to other patients rather than those without a similar diagnosis, and family members who are exposed to other families going through a similar experience may compare their situation to that of those other families rather than their previous life situation.

Calman[12] hypothesized that those who are seriously physically ill focus on areas other than the physical when they are evaluating their QOL. Kreitler and colleagues[23] built on these ideas. They demonstrated that head and neck cancer patients had a similar degree of life satisfaction to orthopedic patients and physically healthy people. However, the cancer patients derived their life satisfaction from many more domains than the other subjects (10 versus 3 domains). Furthermore, the domains related to health had a decreased contribution to the life satisfaction of the cancer patients compared to the other subjects, while the domains not related to health made a relatively increased contribution.

Before we go any further with QOL studies, we need to reach a consensus as to what QOL is and what we need to consider when measuring QOL.[14,19–20] The confusion over the definition of QOL has resulted in investigations to assess the effect of specific interventions where overall QOL is measured but differences are expected only for a few physical symptoms or in the psycholog-ical domain. Unless there is a huge effect (for example, someone with very severe pain reduced to mild pain) it is unlikely that a difference in overall QOL will be detected. Failure to choose an instrument appropriate to measure the expected effect of the intervention has led and will continue to lead, I believe, to many studies that give us very little useful information. Ultimately this will lead some to the erroneous conclusion that QOL measures are of little value. I am con-cerned that this misuse will lead to a backlash where people refuse to use QOL measures, a situation that will be detrimental to care of the whole person or family. To determine what we should be including in measures of QOL for pal-liative care patients, family members, and families, we need to ask them what is important to their QOL. If we choose or create our measures based on what the respondents say is important to their QOL then the instruments are likely to have content validity.

Studies Defining Patient Quality of Life

We are partway to our goal of defining what is important to the QOL of pallia-tive care patients. There are now several studies wherein people who were ter-minally ill or had advanced cancer were asked to explain what is most important to their QOL. The earliest relevant study of which I am aware is that of Padilla and colleagues[24] carried out in the United States although the study population is not necessarily a palliative care one. Thirty-eight of their 41 subjects had advanced cancer. In order to learn what is important to the QOL of people with cancer pain, the investigators asked them to describe what QOL meant to them, what contributes to a good QOL and what contributes to a bad QOL, and how pain influenced their QOL. However, many were still receiving chemotherapy or radiation therapy, and it is not indicated whether the subjects believed that the goal of these treatments was to extend life or palliation. This situation and the fact that they all had chronic pain means that these subjects may differ somewhat from the typical palliative care patient. Content analysis of the responses revealed the three broad domains of physical, psychological, and inter-personal well-being. The physical well-being domain was broken into the sub-categories of general functioning and disease/treatment specific attributes. The psychological well-being domain included the subcategories affective-cognitive; coping ability; meaning of pain and cancer; and accomplishments. The inter-personal well-being domain included the subcategories social support and social/role functioning. Negative and positive attributes were described in each subcategory.

Chaturvedi[25] developed a list of 10 themes identified as important to QOL based on a few interviews with patients with metastatic cancer and health care professionals, as well as from two instruments: the Functional Living Index Cancer[26] and the European Organization for Research and Treatment in Cancer (EORTC) instrument available at the time.[27] The themes were: peace of mind;

spiritual tasks and satisfaction with them; satisfaction with religious tasks; happiness with family/relatives; fulfillment of basic needs; self esteem, self respect; satisfaction with functioning; physical health; psychological health; and level of individual functioning. He presented this list to 18 Indians with metastatic cancer, 20 relatives of people with metastatic cancer, and 3 doctors, 5 nurses, and 4 psychologists and asked them to rate the importance to QOL of each of the items/issues on the list. The themes rated as most important were: peace of mind; spiritual tasks and satisfaction with them; satisfaction with religious acts; happiness with family/relatives; and fulfillment of basic needs. He also developed a list of four domains, each with the aspects of functioning and satisfaction (marital functioning; marital satisfaction; occupational functioning; occupational satisfaction; social functioning; social satisfaction; self care functioning; and satisfaction with self) and had the same subjects judge their importance. Satisfaction in each of the domains was considered important, while functioning in each of these domains was deemed not important by at least 75% of the subjects. He concluded that "subjects in our study quite clearly have shifted the emphasis from physical functioning to spiritual ones. The existing scales on QOL in fact measure quality of functioning . . . QOL measurements were first made for patients undergoing active chemotherapy . . . and may not meet the needs of patients with a terminal illness adequately" (p. 93).

More recently the developers of two widely used QOL instruments, the Functional Assessment of Cancer Therapy (FACT)[28] and the EORTC QOL Questionnaire (EORTC-QLQ)[29] have recognized that their core QOL questionnaires are missing some contributors to QOL that are important for those with a terminal illness. Both questionnaires consist of a core questionnaire and modules that are disease specific that can be added to the core questionnaire. Greisinger and colleagues have been developing a palliative care module for the FACT.[30,31] They asked 74 cancer patients in the United States who were deemed to have less than 6 months to live and 39 of their family caregivers to identify the major concerns and needs of the people with advanced cancer, and to talk about all areas of their lives that had been changed by cancer. In addition, subjects were specifically asked to discuss physical well-being, emotional well-being, family issues, sexuality/intimacy, social relations, work status, and spirituality if they had not mentioned these spontaneously. A list of 104 concerns was generated, and a new group of 120 patients was asked to rate the importance of each concern on the list. The most important concerns were in the existential, spiritual, family, physical symptoms, and emotional domains. Interestingly, the items listed as most important in the physical symptoms domain concerned information: knowing what symptoms I might experience; knowing my prognosis; talking to my doctor truthfully about my prognosis. This study is enlightening, but it does not comprehensively address QOL. The focus of the questions used to elicit the themes was not on QOL as a whole, but rather on "health-related QOL", that is on negative contributors to QOL (concerns) and on changes in QOL since diagnosis, which excludes aspects of life that continue to affect QOL but were important before diagnosis.[31]

The EORTC-QLQ palliative care module is being developed based on interviews with 29 patients in Europe. Domains that emerged as needing to be added to the core questionnaire were: symptom control; information; communication; decision-making; social support; spirituality (religious and existential aspects).[32] Using the Schedule for Evaluation of Individual Quality of Life (SEIQoL), Waldron and colleagues[33,34] interviewed 80 patients receiving palliative care. The 10 areas most commonly listed as important to their QOL were: family; health; social life/activities; spiritual life/religion; friendship/relationships; contentment/happiness; work; finances; marriage; mobility; being pain free.

Together with Dr. Balfour Mount, I developed the McGill Quality of Life Questionnaire (MQOL) for people with a life-threatening illness, based on a literature review, clinical experience, and informal conversations with palliative care patients regarding QOL.[35-38] MQOL includes the physical, psychological, existential/spiritual, and support domains. Based on my sense that MQOL is missing some relevant domains, my colleagues and I, of the Sociobehavioral Cancer Research Network (SCRN) of the National Cancer Institute of Canada, interviewed (in English and in French) 60 palliative care patients with cancer in three Canadian cities to determine what is important to their QOL so that MQOL could be revised if required. We used questions similar to those of Padilla and colleagues[24] and asked them to tell us what was important to their QOL, what made for a good day, and what made for a bad day. To ensure that the content of the revised instrument would be valid both at home and in the hospital, half of the subjects were living at home and half were on a palliative care unit. Content analysis of verbatim transcripts of the interviews showed the following broad domains to be important: own state; quality of palliative care; relationships; outlook; environment. Domains and subcategories are shown in Table 10.1[7,39]

There is a lot of consensus among the results of these studies asking people with advanced disease to define what is important to their QOL. The domains concerning the spiritual/existential; social/family relationships; psychological; and physical symptoms/functioning were listed in all six studies. Information/communication was listed as important to QOL in two-thirds of the studies. Both Padilla and colleagues[24] and Cohen and colleagues[7] found control, coping, enjoyment of life, and cognitive function to be important to QOL. Cohen and colleagues[7] also include the concept of uncertainty and the domain of environment, while Kaasa and Ahlner-Elmquist[32] mentioned decision-making. The results of these studies show the domains important to the QOL of palliative care patients to be quite similar to those found to be important to the general population in a large international study by the World Health Organization Quality of Life Working Group (physical; psychological; level of independence; social relationships; environmental health; spirituality, religion, and personal beliefs).[40] This list of domains is more comprehensive than that included in most instruments designed to measure the "health-related QOL" of people with cancer or AIDS.[26,28,29,41-43]

Table 10.1. Domains and subcategories relevant to the quality of life of palliative care patients

Own state

Physical condition
Physical functioning
Cognitive functioning
Psychological

Quality of palliative care

Feeling secure/vulnerable
Feeling cared for/being treated with respect
Spiritual care
Continuity of care/staff
Availability/acceptance of limitations of health care staff

Environment

Right place to be: home/hospital
Indoors (does/does not meet psychosocial needs; does/does not meet physical/functional needs)
Outdoors (access to nature; weather)

Relationships

Support
Communication
Change in roles
Being a burden
Grow closer/more distant through crisis

Outlook

Coping/enjoying
Control/uncertainty
Existential/spiritual/facing death

Sources: Cohen et al., 1997[7]; Leis and Cohen, 1999[39].

Review of Palliative Care Patient Quality of Life Instruments

Without content validity, it is of no use to consider other psychometric properties. If an instrument does not have content validity but its reliability and responsiveness are high, then it is measuring something well, but that something is not QOL as the patients define it. The content validity is obvious for instruments that require the respondent to list the areas of his or her life that are most important to his or her QOL, and then to rate his or her current functioning or satisfaction in those areas. This approach is used in the SEIQoL[33,34,44,45] and the Patient Evaluated Problem Score.[45] Although the latter is described as a QOL measure, the respondents are only asked to list their major problems, and therefore it does not really focus on overall QOL, although it is likely to provide other useful information to clinicians. The SEIQoL asks respondents to nominate the five life areas most important to their QOL. Following this, they rate their current functioning in each area. They are then asked to assign weights to each area, based on the relative importance of that area to their QOL. The SEIQoL was originally developed using judgement analysis to assign weights.[44] An alternate form of SEIQoL was recently developed, replacing the fairly complicated judgement analysis with the more simple direct weighting (DW) procedure (SEIQoL-DW), making it more useful for clinical care.[33,34,45,47] This measure may be very useful for clinical services trying to ensure that their patients receive individualized care that addresses those areas that are most important to their QOL. It has been used to measure the QOL of palliative care inpatients[34] and outpatients who were HIV positive.[45]

Standardized instruments, which measure QOL with the same set of questions for every respondent, will not address the specific concerns of each respondent, but can, if they have content validity, inform us about the QOL of the group as a whole. Unfortunately, no published QOL instruments include all the domains that are important for palliative care patient QOL as determined in the six studies described in the previous section. Therefore, I will only consider briefly the psychometric properties of those instruments that have the most content validity (they contain items that represent the physical symptoms/ functioning, psychological, social/family relationships and spiritual/existential domains) and are in a format acceptable to palliative care patients (not too long, able to be administered by being read aloud). Several published self-report QOL instruments include items from at least these four domains but have not been developed beyond the initial stage[48,49] or the psychometric properties have not been established in the palliative care setting.[50–54]

The MQOL's 16 items form 5 submeasures established through factor analysis in three studies: a single item measuring physical well-being and subscales for physical symptoms, psychological well-being; existential well-being, and support.[36–38] The MQOL submeasures showed convergent and divergent validity with the Spitzer Quality of Life Index,[55] although not completely as expected. The total score for MQOL predicted the score on a single-item scale measuring overall QOL better than did the total score of the Self-Administered Spitzer Quality of Life Index. The MQOL Total score and each submeasure have acceptable test-retest reliability over a period of 2 days. All MQOL scores (total and submeasures) change significantly when the patients say that their QOL has changed, with the exception of the Support subscale, where mean scores indicate a high degree of support at all times.[56,57] Recently the MQOL Total, Physical Symptoms, Physical Well-being, Psychological Well-being, and Existential Well-being scores were shown to improve significantly during the first week following admission to five Canadian palliative care units.[8] This demonstrates that the effect of palliative care can be measured if appropriate QOL instruments are used.

The McMaster Quality of Life Scale contains 32 items referring to the physical, psychological, cognitive, social, and spiritual/existential domains, but data suggest that the questions can reliably be divided into two subscales: physical and nonphysical QOL.[58] The total score showed the expected correlation with the Spitzer Quality of Life Index. Test-retest reliability was good at an interval of 3 hours but decreased with an interval of 1 week between tests. Responsiveness was appropriately tested against the patient's judgement that QOL (rather than disease status) had changed. The authors hypothesize and report some evidence that nonphysical QOL declines as death approaches, in contrast to an earlier report that many factors contributing to QOL remain stable or improve as death approaches.[59]

The Hospice Quality of Life Index contains 25 items concerning the physical, functional, psychological, social, spiritual, and financial domains as well as an item concerning environment.[60,61] The attempt to weight patient ratings of satisfaction by patient ratings of item importance is laudable, but the method of calculation described would have the counterintuitive result of a higher (better) score for items indicated to be important but about which the patient is dissatisfied than for unimportant items on which satisfaction is rated as low. Factor analysis of data from the Hospice Quality of Life Index showed that not all items load on the factors in a way that allows a clear conceptual distinction between subscales.[60] The overall QOL score and the subscale scores were not significantly different at admission to hospice and 3 weeks later.[61]

The revised MQOL being developed by the SCRN (renamed Quality of Life in Life-Threatening Illness—Patient Version or QOLLTI-P) and the palliative care modules in development for the EORTC-QLQ and the FACT may give these instruments complete content validity. However, given that the core EORTC-QLQ has 30–33 items (depending on the version used) and the FACT-General Questionnaire has 29 items, adding items to them to achieve content validity may render them too long to complete for many palliative care patients, if they are not already too long. The QOLLTI-P will be as brief as possible, with a maximum of 20 items. The psychometric properties of these new versions are presently being tested.

Studies Defining Family Member Quality of Life

There are two projects presently underway to develop QOL measures for the family caregivers of cancer patients that are based on the reports of family caregivers themselves as to what is important to them. Both groups are studying the QOL of the primary family caregiver only rather than the QOL of all family members. Weitzner and colleagues developed their Caregiver Quality of Life Index-Cancer (CQOLC) Questionnaire with family caregivers of patients in the anticancer treatment phase, and have recently tested it in a United States hospice setting.[62–64]

The content in CQOLC is based on interviews with 22 patient-caregiver dyads wherein they were asked to explain how the patient's illness had impacted on the family caregiver's physical, emotional, family, social, and other functioning.[62] One limitation of this approach is that the emphasis is not on overall QOL, but rather on changes affecting functioning since the patient was ill. Another limitation is that only family caregiver interviews where the patient also participated were used. Therefore none of the family caregivers in the study were caring for patients who were unable to participate due to their poor physical or mental condition, which represents a large part of the palliative care population. In addition, the family caregiver was excluded "if substances known to affect the central nervous system (i.e., narcotic analgesics, antiemetics, or steroids) were administered to the caregiver or patient 1 week or less before entry into the study." This exclusion criterion is likely to result in few family caregivers of advanced cancer patients being included. The 35-item CQOLC was tested for validity and test-retest reliability in the anticancer treatment setting, where its psychometric properties appear to be good.[62] Factor analysis has revealed five factors representing mental/emotional burden, lifestyle disruption, hopefulness, social support, and financial concerns.[63]

My SCRN colleagues and I are developing a measure of the QOL of family caregivers of palliative care patients, the Quality of Life in Life-Threatening Illness–Family Caregiver Version questionnaire (QOLLTI–F) to complement our QOLLTI-P. Fifty-nine family caregivers of palliative care patients from three Canadian cities were interviewed in either English or French. They were asked to describe what was important to their QOL at this time, what made a day good, and what made a day bad. In half the cases the patient was at home, in the other half the patient was admitted to a palliative care unit. Content analysis revealed many themes that we grouped into the seven domains and subcategories listed in Table 10.2: state of caregiver; patient well-being; quality of palliative care; outlook; environment; financial; relationships.[39,65] The domains of state of the caregiver, patient well-being, quality of palliative care, relationships, and sense of purpose in life (which falls under the outlook domain) have previously been shown to be important to family caregivers of advanced cancer and/or palliative care patients in other studies not focussed specifically on QOL.[66–74]

Review of Family Caregiver Quality of Life Measures

A recent review of the literature concerning families with a palliative care patient indicated a need to develop appropriate and psychometrically sound outcome measures concerning the family.[72] In view of the trend to have more health care take place in the home and the desire of most people to die at home,[75] these measures are urgently needed.

Most of the literature concerning family members of palliative care patients, or even of patients at earlier phases of the disease trajectory or with Alzheimer's disease, has focussed on the burden and stress of caregiving,[70,76–78] caregiver needs,[79–82] family satisfaction with care,[66,81,83,84] family member health,[66] and family insight and anxiety as assessed by staff.[85]

Table 10.2. Domains and subcategories relevant to the quality of life of family caregivers of palliative care patients

---

State of caregiver

   Interference with/maintaining normal life
   Caregiver condition

Patient well-being

   State of the patient
   Meet patient needs/goals/wishes

Quality of palliative care

   Comfort with decision-making process
   Quality of care

Environment

Finances

Relationships

   Support
   Communication
   Family
   Impact on relationships

Outlook

   Coping
   Control/helplessness/uncertainty
   Existential/spiritual
   Feeling about being a caregiver
   Preparing for the future
   Hope

Sources: Leis and Cohen, 1999[39], Cohen and Leis, 1999[66].

Few studies have examined family member QOL. Our SCRN study is the only one that directly asked family caregivers of palliative care patients what is important to their QOL. While this study identifies the domains that need to be included in a measure of family caregiver QOL, evidence from other studies is required to confirm these findings. Some investigators have used modifications of instruments designed for the patients.[61,69,86,87] Mohide[88] developed a QOL measure specific to family caregivers that used the time trade-off technique, but this was tested with family caregivers of disabled relatives with chronic degenerative disorders and measured only physical, psychological, and social functioning.

McMillan and Mahon[89,90] developed the four-item Caregiver Quality of Life Index for caregivers of palliative care patients, covering emotional, social, financial, and physical domains, each measured by a single item. Content was based on a literature review and verified by five people who had been the family caregivers of patients who had died 2 years previously. They rated all the items as highly important. Some important domains are missing, including all that are concerned with patient well-being and care. Furthermore, it remains to be determined whether the single item measuring each domain has sufficient test-retest reliability. The CQOLC of Weitzner does not address caregiver physical condition, and patient well-being and quality of care are not directly addressed. The appropriateness of the environment and control/helplessness are also not included in the CQOLC. Since QOLLTI-F is based on our own qualitative study, we have, of course, included all of the relevant domains, but as mentioned above, confirmatory evidence of its validity is required.

Studies of Family Quality of Life

The quality of family life is not directly addressed by studies focussing on the QOL of its individual members. Studies such as those described in previous sections have focused on the patient, the primary caregiver, or both. There are very few studies of whole families in the palliative care setting. I am not aware of any studies that have focussed specifically on family QOL. Davies and colleagues[91,92] have made an excellent start to understanding how the family manages with the illness and their perceptions of care received, but this was a small study (8 families) and the focus was not on overall QOL but rather on the impact of the illness and care. Kristjanson and colleagues[66,93] studied family functioning from the perspective of a single family member (the primary family caregiver). They found that the discrepancy between the family caregivers' expectations and perceptions of palliative care while the patient was alive significantly predicted family functioning during the bereavement phase. Family caregivers who were older or caring for a female patient assessed family functioning as better than did family caregivers who were younger or caring for a male patient. However, neither study sampled more than one family member's viewpoint, and there is evidence that individual members of the same family may have important differences in their assessment of family functioning.[94]

Measures of Family Quality of Life

Since we do not know the basics of what is important to the QOL of families where one member is dying, we cannot judge whether instruments developed to measure the state of the family in the general population are valid in the palliative care setting. To my knowledge, the only instruments that have been used as measures relevant to the family in the palliative care setting are the Self-Report Family Inventory[66,95] and the General Functioning subscale of the McMaster Family Assessment Device.[93,96] These studies provided some interesting information regarding family functioning and its relationship to family caregiver variables in the palliative care setting.

Individualized Versus Standardized Measures

The specific contributors to QOL vary tremendously from individual to individual or family to family. In consideration of these individual differences, the argument has been made that it is not useful to measure QOL with standardized instruments, and that QOL measures must be individualized, as in SEIQoL, to include the specific contributors that are important to the individual whose QOL is being measured. A similar case has been made that QOL measures must allow the individual to assign weights to each domain indicating its importance to him or her.[12,18,44,45,47] This may be the case if one is attempting to measure the QOL of an individual for clinical purposes (although I am not convinced that a questionnaire can ever replace an excellent clinical interview). It should be noted that if an instrument is to be used to inform us about the QOL of individuals, the measure must have a higher degree of stability (test-retest reliability) than that required to measure the QOL of groups, where somewhat more measurement error is tolerable because both positive and negative measurement errors will occur and tend to average toward zero. For purposes other than clinical care for an individual, such as determining the strengths and weaknesses of a palliative care service, assessing the overall impact of a particular intervention, comparing the effectiveness of palliative care services, and determining what QOL is related to in order to provide better care in the future, it is appropriate to measure the QOL of groups of people. For these purposes, if the questionnaire items have been selected to reflect the areas that palliative care recipients have said are important and are worded in general rather than specific terms, so that they are applicable to everyone, then it may not be necessary to have items specific for each person or have individual weighting of the domains.[20,38,97,98] For example, it may be sufficient to know the degree to which the group is physically comfortable rather than to know that one person has uncontrolled pain, another has a problem with fatigue, another has no physical problems, etc. Similarly, we need to know the degree to which the group feels a sense of meaning in their lives, rather than that one person obtains their sense of meaning from their faith in God and another obtains it from feeling a part of a family. If the data are to be grouped, the specifics will be lost in any case, and we can measure QOL in more general terms with standardized instruments so that we are comparing groups on the same domains. To date weighted data have not been used in published studies or have correlated so closely with unweighted data that they did not supply any additional or different information.[61,99] This is the result that would be expected if equal numbers of people weight each of the different domains highly, so that the group average weight of each domain is similar. In addition, while some items are inherently important (for example, depression), circumstances that may be important for some people but not others (such as feeling in control) can be phrased to implicitly include a rating of importance by asking "How much of a problem was X for you?" rather than "How much of X is present?" The importance of weighting needs to be tested directly in studies comparing weighted and unweighted scores.

I am doubtful about the utility of individualized measures when comparison of groups is required. With individualized measures, each respondent is evaluating his or her status in areas nominated by him or herself, so that different groups of respondents are not rating their status in the same areas. Therefore, these instruments provide an overall QOL score but do not have subscales. For most purposes, I believe that how the group is faring in different domains is important, and subscales are required. Valid and reliable subscales are particularly important for measuring QOL in the palliative care setting, where QOL related to physical functioning and physical symptoms such as fatigue will inevitably decline, but QOL in other domains may improve. Data from studies using MQOL show that the more advanced the disease, the greater the discrepancy between scores in different domains for both people with cancer and HIV disease.[36–38] The importance of measuring each domain with a separate subscale is therefore greater when the disease is more advanced.

We can and should test directly whether the total score obtained from individualized QOL measures is more valid than that obtained from standardized measures by comparing them to QOL scores obtained from a valid and reliable questionnaire that directly assesses overall QOL (that is, contains items such as "How has your QOL been?").

Who Should Rate Quality of Life? Limitations in the Palliative Care Setting

If we accept that QOL is subjective well-being, then it is best measured by the person(s) whose QOL is of interest. If you are trying to determine the impact of a particular intervention that is geared toward at least some palliative care patients who are able to complete a QOL questionnaire, then it is best to make sure to have those patients rate their own QOL. However, in the palliative care setting the physical or mental condition of many patients is so poor that they cannot complete even a brief QOL questionnaire. If your goal is to evaluate or compare palliative care services, then you must collect information concerning all the patients treated by those services, not only those who can complete a QOL questionnaire. Different methods must be found for evaluating the care of those who cannot speak for themselves. Interested readers are referred to published work by Dr. Irene Higginson on audit in palliative care.

Conclusion

Since the goal of palliative care is to achieve the best QOL possible for patients and their families, measures of patient, family member, and family QOL are critically important as outcome measures in this field. The availability of valid, acceptable, reliable, and responsive QOL measures will enable studies to ensure that the palliative care delivered is perceived by the recipients as whole-person care. Considerable thought, time, and energy has been expended and will continue to be needed to define what is important to the QOL of palliative care patients, their family members, and their families in order to create measures that have content validity. These studies are also helping us to define whole-person care, a term widely used but not always understood, particularly by those outside the field or who are new to it. We are well on the way to having the patient QOL measures we need. The process has begun for the QOL of family members. We are still waiting for someone to take up the formidable challenge of understanding and measuring family QOL.

References

1. World Health Organization Expert Committee. *Cancer Pain Relief and Palliative Care*. WHO Technical Report Series 804. Geneva: World Health Organization, 1990.
2. Donovan K, Sanson-Fisher RW, Redman S. Measuring quality of life in cancer patients. *J Clin Oncol* 1989; 7:959–968.
3. Cantril H. *The Pattern of Human Concerns*. New Jersey: Rutgers University Press, 1965.
4. Campbell A, Converse PE, Rodgers WL. *The Quality of American Life*. New York: Russell Sage Foundation, 1976.
5. Fryback PB. Health for people with a terminal diagnosis. *Nurs Sci Quarterly* 1993; 6:147–159.
6. Kagawa-Singer M. Redefining health: living with cancer. *Social Science and Medicine* 1993; 37:295–304.
7. Cohen SR, Bunston T, Leis A, et al. Domains relevant to the quality of life of palliative care patients with cancer. Presentation at the 7th Canadian National Palliative Care Conference, Saskatoon, Saskatchewan, Sept. 28–Oct. 1, 1997.
8. Cohen SR, Boston P, Farley J, et al. Changes in quality of life following admission to palliative care units. *J Palliat Care* 1998; 14:104.
9. Campbell A. Subjective measures of well-being. *American Psychology* 1976; 31:117–124.
10. Kingwell M. Better living. *Pursuit of Happiness from Plato to Prozac*. Middlesex, U.K., Penguin Books Canada Ltd., 1998.
11. Najman JM, Levine S. Evaluating the impact of medical care and technologies on the quality of life: a review and critique. *Soc Sci Med* 1981; 15:107–115.
12. Calman KC. Quality of life in cancer patients: An hypothesis. *J Med Ethics* 1994; 10:124–127.
13. Bradburn NM. *The Structure of Psychological Well-Being*. Chicago: Aldine Publishing Company, 1969.
14. Cohen SR, Mount BM. Quality of life assessment in terminal illness: defining and measuring subjective well-being in the dying. *J Palliat Care* 1992; 8:40–45.
15. Cella DF. Measuring quality of life in palliative care. *Sem Oncol* 1995; 22:73–81.

16. Aaronson NK. Quality of life research in cancer clinical trials: a need for common rules and languages. *Oncology* 1990; 4:59–66.

17. Schipper H. Guidelines and caveats for quality of life measurement in clinical practice and research. *Oncology* 1990; 4:51–57.

18. Gill TM, Feinstein AR. A critical appraisal of the quality of quality-of-life measurements. *JAMA* 1994; 172:619–631.

19. Hunt SM. The problem of quality of life. *Qual Life Res* 1997; 6:205–212.

20. Mount BM, Cohen SR. Quality of life in patients with life-threatening illness. In: Stark S, ed. *Death and the Quest for Meaning*. New Jersey: Jason Aronson Inc., 1997:137–152.

21. Sprangers MAG. Response-shift bias: a challenge to the assessment of patients' quality of life in cancer clinical trials. *Cancer Treat Rev* 1996; 22(Suppl A):55–62.

22. Festinger L. A theory of social comparison processes. *Hum Relations* 1954; 7:117–140.

23. Kreitler S, Chaitchick S, Rapoport Y, et al. Life satisfaction and health in cancer patients, orthopedic patients and healthy individuals. *Soc Sci Med* 1993; 36:547–556.

24. Padilla GV, Ferrell B, Grant MM, Rhiner M. Defining the content domain of quality of life for cancer patients with pain. *Cancer Nurs* 1990; 13:108–115.

25. Chaturvedi SK. (1991). What's important for quality of life to Indians—in relation to cancer. *Soc Sci Med* 1991; 33:91–94.

26. Schipper H, Clinch J, McMurray A, Levitt M. Measuring the quality of life of cancer patients: the Functional Living Index—Cancer: development and validation. *J Clin Oncol* 1984; 2:472–483.

27. Aaronson NK, Bakker W, Stewart AL, et al. A multi-dimensional approach to the measurement of quality of life in lung cancer clinical trials. In: Aaronson NK, Beckman J, eds. *Quality of Life in Cancer Patients, EORTC Monograph Series*. New York: Raven Press, 1987.

28. Cella DF, Tulsky DS, Gray G, et al. The Functional Assessment of Cancer Therapy Scale: development and validation of a general measure. *J Clin Oncol* 1993; 11:570–579.

29. Aaronson NK, Ahmedzai S, Bergman B, et al. The European Organization for Research and Treatment of Cancer QLQ-C30: a quality of life instrument for use in international clinical trials in oncology. *J Natl Cancer Inst* 1993; 85:365–376.

30. Greisinger AJ, Lorimor RJ, Aday LA, et al. Development of a quality of life module for end-stage cancer patients. Proceedings of the Third World Congress of Psycho-Oncology. *Psycho-Oncology* 5: Abstract 45, 1996.

31. Greisinger AJ, Lorimor RJ, Aday LA, et al. Terminally ill cancer patients. Their most important concerns. *Cancer Practice* 1997; 5:147–154.

32. Kaasa S, Ahlner-Elmquist M. European Organization for Research and Treatment of Cancer (EORTC)—Social support and spiritual well-being domains. *J Palliat Care* 1998; 14:111–112.

33. Waldron D, O'Boyle CA, Kearney M, et al. Use of an individualised measure of quality of life; SEIQoL in palliative care: results of a pilot study. *Palliat Med* 1996; 10:57.

34. Waldron D, O'Boyle CA, Kearney M, Moriarty M, Carney D. Quality of life measurement in advanced cancer: Assessing the individual. *J Clin Oncol* 1999; 17:3603–3611.

35. Cohen SR, Mount BM, Strobel MG, Bui F. The McGill Quality of Life Questionnaire: a measure of quality of life appropriate for people with advanced disease. A preliminary study of validity and acceptability. *Palliat Med* 1995; 9:207–219.
36. Cohen SR, Hassan SA, Lapointe BJ, Mount BM. Quality of life in HIV disease as measured by the McGill Quality of Life Questionnaire. *AIDS* 1996; 10:1421–1427.
37. Cohen SR, Mount BM, Tomas J, Mount L. Existential well-being is an important determinant of quality of life: evidence from the McGill Quality of Life Questionnaire. *Cancer* 1996; 77:576–586.
38. Cohen SR, Mount BM, Bruera E, et al. Validity of the McGill Quality of Life Questionnaire in the palliative care setting: a multi-centre Canadian study demonstrating the importance of the existential domain. *Palliat Med* 1997; 11:3–20.
39. Leis A, Cohen SR. Determinants of the quality of life of palliative care patients with cancer and that of their family caregivers. Presentation at the 9th Annual Palliative Care Conference, Humber College, Toronto, Ontario, Canada, 1999.
40. Skevington SM. Investigating the relationship between pain and discomfort and quality of life, using the WHOQOL. *Pain* 1998; 76:395–406.
41. Ganz PA, Coscarelli Schag CA, Kahn B, et al. Describing the health-related quality of life impact of HIV infection: findings from a study using the HIV Overview of Problems—Evaluation System (HOPES). *Qual Life Res* 1993; 2:109–119.
42. Nokes KM, Wheeler K, Kendrew J. Development of an HIV assessment tool. *Image* 1994; 25:355–359.
43. Wu AW, Rubin HR, Mathews WC, et al. A health status questionnaire using 30 items from the Medical Outcomes Study. *Med Care* 1991; 29:786–798.
44. McGee HM, O'Boyle CA, Hickey A, et al. Assessing the quality of life of the individual: the SEIQoL with a healthy and gastroenterology unit population. *Psychol Med* 1991; 21:749–759.
45. Hickey AM, Bury G, O'Boyle CA, et al. A new short form individual quality of life measure (SEIQoL-DW): application in a cohort of individuals with HIV/AIDS. *Brit Med J* 1996; 313:29–33.
46. Rathbone GV, Horsley S, Goacher J. A self-evaluated assessment suitable for seriously ill hospice patients. *Palliat Med* 1994; 8:29–34.
47. Waldron D. *Measurement of Individualised Quality of Life Within a Palliative Care Population.* Thesis for the degree of Doctor of Medicine, University College Galway, Ireland, 1997.
48. Kaasa S, Maastekaasa A, Stokke I, Naess S. Validation of a quality of life questionnaire for use in clinical trials for treatment of patients with inoperable lung cancer. *Euro J Cancer Clin Oncol* 1988; 24:691–701.
49. MacAdam DB, Smith M. An initial assessment of suffering in terminal illness. *Palliat Med* 1987; 1:37–47.
50. Ferrans CE. Development of a quality of life index for patients with cancer. *Oncol Nurs Forum* 1990; 17(3):15–21.
51. Ferrell BR, Ferrell BA, Ahn C, Tran K. Pain management for elderly patients with cancer at home. *Cancer Supplement* 1994; 74(7):2139–2146.
52. Ferrell B, Grant M, Padilla G, et al. The experience of pain and perceptions of quality of life: Validation of a conceptual model. *The Hospice Journal* 1991; 7:9–24.
53. McMillan SC, Mahon M. A study of quality of life of hospice patients on admission and at week 3. *Cancer Nurs* 1994; 17:52–60.

54. Skevington SM, MacArthur P, Somerset M. Developing items for the WHOQOL: An investigation of contemporary beliefs about quality of life related to health in Britain. *Brit J Health Psychol* 1997; 2:55–72.
55. Spitzer WO, Dobson AJ, Hall J, et al. Measuring the quality of life of cancer patients. *J Chronic Dis* 1981; 34:585–597.
56. Cohen SR, Mount BM. Good days, bad days: Quantitative and qualitative differences for oncology patients. *J Palliat Care* 1996; 12:62.
57. Cohen SR, Mount BM. Living with cancer: "Good Days" and "Bad Days"—What produces them? Can the McGill Quality of Life Questionnaire distinguish between them? *Cancer* 2000; 89:1854–1865.
58. Sterkenburg CA. A reliability and validity study of the McMaster Quality of Life Scale (MQLS) for a palliative population. *J Palliat Care* 1996; 12(1):18–25.
59. Higginson IJ, McCarthy M. A comparison of two measures of quality of life: their sensitivity and validity for patients with advanced cancer. *Palliat Med* 1994; 8:282–290.
60. McMillan SC. The quality of life of patients with cancer receiving hospice care. *Oncol Nurs Forum* 1996; 23:1221–1228.
61. McMillan SC, Mahon M. Measuring quality of life in hospice patients using a newly developed Hospice Quality of Life Index. *Qual Life Res* 1994; 3:437–447.
62. Weitzner MA, Jacobsen PB, Wagner H Jr., et al. The Caregiver Quality of Life Index—Cancer (CQOLC) scale: development and validation of an instrument to measure quality of life of the family caregiver of patients with cancer. *Qual Life Res* 1999; 8:55–63.
63. Weitzner M, Stein K, Jacobsen P, Gearing-Small M. Development of a family caregiver quality of life instrument: Psychometric properties and preliminary factorial structure. *Qual Life Res* 1998; 7:673–674.
64. Weitzner MA, McMillan SC, Jacobsen PB. Family caregiver quality of life: Differences between curative and palliative cancer treatment settings. *J Pain Symptom Manage* 1999; 17:418–428.
65. Cohen SR, Leis A. Determinants of the quality of life of family caregivers of palliative care patients with cancer. Presentation at the Annual Meeting of The Canadian Association of Psychosocial Oncology, Edmonton, Alberta, Canada, 1999.
66. Kristjanson LJ, Sloan JA, Dudgeon D, Adaskin E. Family members' perceptions of palliative cancer care: predictors of family functioning and family members' health. *J Palliat Care* 1996; 12:10–20.
67. Cassileth BR, Lusk EJ, Strouse TB, et al. A psychological analysis of cancer patients and their next-of-kin. *Cancer* 1985; 55:72–76.
68. Hull, MM. Family need and supportive nursing behaviors during terminal care: a review. *Oncol Nurs Forum* 1990; 16:787–792.
69. Zacharias DR, Gilg CA, Foxall MJ. Quality of life and coping in patients with gynecologic cancer and their spouses. *Oncol Nurs Forum* 1994; 21:1699–1706.
70. Given CW, Given B, Stommel M, Collins C, et al. The Caregiver Reaction Assessment (CRA) for caregivers to persons with chronic physical and mental impairments. *Res Nurs Health* 1992; 15:271–283.
71. Stetz KM. The relationship among background characteristics, purpose in life, and caregiving demands on perceived health of spouse caregivers. *Sch Inq Nurs Pract* 1989; 3:133–153.

72. Leis AM, Kristjanson L, Koop PM, Laizner A. (1997). Family health and the palliative care trajectory: a cancer research agenda. *Cancer Prevention & Control* 1997; 1:352–360.

73. Kurtz ME, Given B, Kurtz JC, Given CW. The interaction of age, symptoms, and survival status on physical and mental health of patients with cancer and their families. *Cancer Supplement* 1994; 74:2071–2078.

74. Holing EV. The primary caregiver's perception of the dying trajectory. *Cancer Nurs* 1986; 9(1):29–27.

75. Hinton J. Can home care maintain an acceptable quality of life for patients with terminal cancer and their relatives? *Palliat Med* 1994; 8:183–196.

76. Kinney JM, Stephens MA. Caregiving Hassles Scale: Assessing the daily hassles of caring for a family member with dementia. *The Gerontologist* 1989; 29(3):328–332.

77. Robinson B. Validation of a caregiver strain index. *J Gerontology* 1983; 38:344–348.

78. Zarit SH, Reever KE, Bach-Peterson J. Relatives of the impaired elderly: Correlates of feelings of burden. *The Gerontologist* 1980; 20:649–655.

79. Grobe ME, Ahmann DL, Ilstrup DM. Needs assessment for advanced cancer patients and their families. *Oncol Nurs Forum* 1982; 9:26–30.

80. Harrington V, Lackey NR, Gates MF. Needs of caregivers of clinic and hospice cancer patients. *Cancer Nurs* 1996; 19:118–125.

81. Kristjanson LJ, Atwood J, Degner LF. Validity and reliability of the family inventory of needs (FIN): measuring the care needs of families of advanced cancer patients. *J Nurs Measurement* 1995; 3:109–126.

82. Steele RG, Fitch MI. Needs of family caregivers of patients receiving home hospice care for cancer. *Oncol Nurs Forum* 1996; 25:823–828.

83. Fakhoury W, McCarthy M, Addington-Hall J. Determinants of informal caregivers' satisfaction with services for dying cancer patients. *Soc Sci Med* 1996; 42:721–731.

84. Kristjanson LJ. Validity and reliability testing of the FAMCARE Scale: Measuring family satisfaction with advanced cancer care. *Soc Sci Med* 1993; 36:693–701.

85. Higginson IJ, McCarthy M. Validity of the support team assessment schedule: do staffs' ratings reflect those made by patients or their families? *Palliat Med* 1993; 7:219–228.

86. Kornblith AB, Herr HW, Ofman US, et al. Quality of life of patients with prostate cancer and their spouses. *Cancer* 1994; 73:2791–2802.

87. Reele BL. Effect of counseling on quality of life for individuals with cancer and their families. *Cancer Nurs* 1994; 17:101–112.

88. Mohide EA, Torrance GW, Streiner DL, Pringle DM, Gilbert R. Measuring the well-being of family caregivers using the time trade-off technique. *J Clin Epidemiol* 1988; 41:475–482.

89. McMillan SC, Mahon M. The impact of hospice services on the quality of life of primary caregivers. *Oncol Nurs Forum* 1994; 21:1189–1195.

90. McMillan SC. Quality of life of primary caregivers of hospice patients with cancer. *Cancer Practice* 1996; 4:191–198.

91. Davies B, Reimer JC, Martens N. Families in supportive care.—Part I: The transition of fading away: The nature of the transition. *J Palliat Care* 1990; 6:12–20.

92. Davies B, Chekryn Reimer J, Brown P, Martens N. *Fading Away: The Experience of Transition in Families with Terminal Illness*. Amityville, NY: Baywood Publishing Company, Inc., 1995.

93. Kristjanson LJ, Leis A, Koop PM, et al. Family members' care expectations, care perceptions, and satisfaction with advanced cancer care: Results of a multi-site pilot study. *J Palliat Care* 1997; 13:5–13.

94. Sawyer MG, Sarris A, Baghurst PA, Cross DG, Kalucy RS. Family assessment device: Reports from mothers, fathers, and adolescents in community and clinic families. *J Marital Family Therapy* 1988; 14:287–296.

95. Hampson RB, Beavers WR. *Successful Families: Assessment and Intervention.* New York: W.W. Norton, 1990.

96. Epstein NB, Baldwin LM, Bishop DS. The McMaster Family Assessment Device. *J Marital Family Therapy* 1983; 9:171–180.

97. Guyatt GH, Cook DJC. Health status, quality of life, and the individual. *JAMA* 1994; 272:630–631.

98. Mount BM, Cohen SR. Quality of life in the face of life-threatening illness: what should we be measuring? *Curr Oncol* 1995; 2:121–125.

99. Cella D. The Functional Assessment of Cancer Therapy-Anemia (FACT-An) Scale: A new tool for the assessment of outcomes in cancer anemia and fatigue. *Sem Hematol* 1997; 34(Suppl 2):13–19.

11

Economic Outcomes and Palliative Care

THOMAS J. SMITH AND LAURIE LYCKHOLM

The cost of cancer care is rising because of increasing age, more cancer cases, increased demand for treatment, and new expensive technologies. Our limited resources must be rationed wisely so that we can provide both curative and palliative care. The ethical implications of using economic and management outcomes rather than traditional health outcomes include shifting emphasis from helping at all cost to helping at a cost society can afford, how much society is willing to pay, the value of care to the dying versus those with curable illnesses, and tolerance of suboptimal care.

The outcomes of palliative care do not differ from other cancer treatment, from the perspective of economics or health service research. For treatment to be justified, there must be some demonstrable improvement in disease-free or overall survival, toxicity, quality of life, or cost effectiveness. Palliative care usually does not change survival, and it does not have a measurable cost-effectiveness ratio since palliative therapy does not gain years of life. There may be little change in quality-adjusted life years because the improvements in health state are too small to measure with current instruments, or are lost in the impact of the disease.

Only a few studies have assessed the economic outcomes of palliative therapy. The major areas of interest include the following: (1) palliative chemotherapy versus best supportive care; (2) supportive care for cancer symptoms; (3) the process and structure of care; (4) follow up; and (5) hospice care. Palliative first line chemotherapy for Stage III and IV non-small cell lung cancer, mitoxantrone for prostate cancer, and fluorouracil-based chemotherapy for gastrointestinal cancer all have acceptable cost-effectiveness ratios. Supportive care effectiveness and cost for infections, nausea, and pain can be improved. Hospice care saves at best 3% of total care cost, but gives care equal to non-hospice care. Coordination of palliative care will save 40% of costs but will not improve the clinical outcomes of dying patients.

Whether half full or half empty, it *will* be a smaller glass.

Detmer, 1997[1]

Why Are Economic Outcomes Important?

Health care spending and health care quality are major problems in the United States. Cancer care costs have risen from \$35 billion in 1990[2] to \$40 billion in 1994[3] to one estimate of \$50 billion by 1996.[4] We are spending a significant amount on high technology care for the elderly, since nearly one-third of all Medicare spending is on patients in their last year of life,[5,6] and those funds cannot be spent on preventive services or chronic disease conditions for the same population.[7] In the largest Virginia insurance plan, the top 1% of the population consumes 30% of the resources. The pressure on health care funds will increase due to increased demands for care from an educated elderly population, more elderly long term survivors, new and expensive technologies, new diseases, and demands for cost cutting.

It is clear that the process of care may not be optimal for all patients, and that quality of palliative care could improve. The SUPPORT study showed that half of all dying patients had unnecessary pain and suffering in their final days of life while in the hospital.[8] Nearly half of patients suffer unnecessary pain even when cared for by oncologists or academic oncologists.[9] The care given to cancer patients in general can be improved.[10–12] For breast cancer as an example: (1) some states have five times the number of mastectomies versus the preferred method of breast conserving lumpectomy and radiation;[13,14] (2) there is substantial under use of adjuvant therapy;[15] and (3) there is underuse of surveillance mammography in patients after breast cancer treatment, with about 20% having no follow up mammogram within 2 years.[16] For other illnesses, we have documented substantial underuse of thoracotomy in the elderly with lung cancer compared to younger patients,[17] and similar patterns in prostate cancer.[18]

The whole neglected issue of cancer care quality is now under discussion, with active efforts to improve it.[19] The relationship of volume to quality is striking: (1) a significant (5%–10%) overall survival advantage at a cancer specialty center for breast cancer, rather than at community hospitals;[20,21] (2) better survival for testicular cancer patients treated at specialist centers;[22] (3) better survival and fewer complications for ovarian cancer surgery performed by specialist gynecologic oncologists rather than general surgeons or gynecologists,[23] and (4) better survival for prostate cancer patients at high-volume centers.[10]

We have identified some important questions about economic outcomes and palliative care (Table 11.1). We reviewed Medline from 1970 to 1998 for relevant articles, and did selected searches within bibliographies.

Table 11.1. Types of studies of health and service research

Type of study	Question posed
Policy analysis	What outcomes justify treatment? Who should make those decisions?
Type of care: chemotherapy versus best or other types of supportive care chemotherapy	Does chemotherapy save money compared to best supportive care, when all costs are considered?
The site of service	Is home versus hospitals more effective and less costly?
Structural and process changes in care	Can costs of care be reduced by changes in how it is delivered? For example, by coordination or at home?
Hospice versus non-hospice	Does hospice improve quality of life or reduce costs of care?
Advanced directives and do not resuscitate orders	Do advanced directives influence medical treatment decisions or change costs?

The Ethics of Adding Economic Outcomes

In the modern arena of health care, non-medical concerns such as cost control, oversight and audit, utilization review and decreasing liability risk have assumed a significant role. Some authorities have argued that such management tools are not inherently unethical.[24] Cost control is certainly not inherently unethical, but should be considered secondary to the goal of quality care. The goals of medicine are grounded in a tradition of promoting health and providing comfort and relief of suffering in a just manner. Cost control through aggressive disease management may actually promote these goals in making more or better care available.

Cost control must be differentiated from profit motivation and entrepreneurship, which have never been considered the goals of medicine. These activities in the context of medical care are unethical in that they may make medical care more expensive and difficult to access, especially for those who are socially disadvantaged. They may also create further conflicts of interest in already precarious fiduciary relationships between physicians and their patients. A code of ethics that covered everyone, rather than just one group, might be useful.[25]

Tolerance of sub-optimal care is an equally important ethical issue, and one that is rarely mentioned in either ethical or management studies. Studies such as the SUPPORT study have revealed that many aspects of end of life care are still suboptimal. The national dialogue about physician assisted suicide might also indicate that end of life care has not been optimized, thus resulting in despair and frustration so significant as to urge dying persons to consider suicide to end their suffering. If palliative care can be improved, or made less costly, or both without sacrificing quality of care, it must be done in the service of promoting the values of beneficence, compassion, and respect for autonomy.

This movement is occurring on a national level, with the advent of several important/ national/international/large initiatives [Project on Death in America (PDIA), Education of Physicians on End of Life Care (EPEC), etc.]. HCFA's approval of an ICD-9 code for palliative care was hoped by some to indicate its significance in the health care system.[26] The economic outcomes are not known, and may be difficult to measure, but regardless, the ethical impetus to correct the deficiency is critical.

Another serious ethical question is the ownership of disease management models. Should management tools that improve care be protected, or be available to the general public? If one developed a tool that improved care at markedly lower cost, one could argue that it should be made available for widespread distribution, much like polio vaccine.

Some have argued that budgets should not be balanced with penalty to one group such as the elderly or those on Medicare.[27,28] Many health care goods are rationed justly according to age, such as transplants, coronary bypass, and hemodialysis, based on the theory of equality of opportunity according to ability to benefit from such procedures.[29] However, palliative care is different in that age does not determine whether a person stands to benefit. In this circumstance, the ethic of distributive justice supports the concept that medical and social needs dictate whom stands to benefit most from palliative care.

Downie reported:

> It does not seem reasonable to postulate that the medical needs of the elderly terminally ill are any less than those of younger patients, and indeed they may be greater because of multiple additional pathologies associated with aging.[30]

Sidgwick's argument that each moment of life is equally valuable no matter when it occurs[31] is most poignant in the instance of palliative care.

Patients may view benefit and toxicity in ways very different from their health care providers, and from those who are well. Dying patients would undergo almost any treatment toxicity for a 1% chance of short-term survival, while their doctors and nurses would not, and these decisions were not changed after patients experienced the toxicity of treatment.[32] A study of palliative radiotherapy for brain tumor patients showed little survival and modest functional benefit, and a substantial decrement in intellectual function, but most patients and families would still want it.[33,34]

What is the Right Amount to Spend on Health Care?

This question cannot be answered without knowing the economic and cultural particulars of a country or even health system. Blanket statements about a percentage of the Gross National Product (GNP) may be misleading if a comparison country spends a higher percentage on social net programs but less on direct medical care costs. Comments about health care spending as a percent of the GNP may also reflect opinions about alternative uses, for example, "We should stop spending money on defense and spend it on health care." In the United States, the amount spent on education has declined from 6% to 5% of GNP, while the amount spent on health care (especially for the elderly) has risen from 6% to about 14%.[35]

Should There Be Special Economic or Policy Considerations for Palliative Care?

No, in general. Most health care policy analysts and economists would argue that all care should be evaluated equally. For example, a therapy that gains 1 week for 52 patients should be valued as much as an equivalent cost therapy that gains 52 weeks for 1 patient.[36] Recently, some health economists have argued that time given to those who are most at risk should be valued more (e.g., time added in the last 6 months of life should be given triple value).[37] The analogy was made to food and hunger: a sandwich given to a starving person would be of more intrinsic value than one given to a person who already had many sandwiches. Such discussions, while interesting, are outside the scope of this chapter.

The World Health Organization has made lists of priorities for health care. In cancer, palliative care has always been included in the same category as curative therapy for Hodgkins's disease. In part, this was done because most palliative care is so inexpensive.[38]

What are Important Economic Outcomes?

Economic outcomes are not different from clinical outcomes, except that cost must be considered along with clinical benefit. Only one medical group, the American Society of Clinical Oncology, has published recommendations on what benefit is justified to recommend a medical intervention, listed in Table 11.2.[39] Of note, ASCO could not define the lowest amount of benefit

Table 11.2. Outcomes that justify a medical intervention

Justify	Do not justify
Improved overall survival	False hope that survival will be improved
Improved disease free survival	
Improved formal quality of life	
Less toxicity	
Improved cost effectiveness	Cost alone

Table 11.3. Standard definitions for economic outcome analysis

Term	Definition	Comment
Resource utilization	Number of units used, e.g., 9 hospital days	Best collected prospectively, using a combination of clinical research forms, hospital bills, and patient diaries for outpatient or off-site events.
Charge	What is billed to the patient	May be fair representation of the cost of service. Can be accurately converted to costs using ratio of charges to cost.[41]
Cost	What it costs society to provide the service	
Direct medical cost	Cost of standard medical interventions	Usual cost-drivers include: hospital days, professional fees, diagnostic tests, pharmacy fees, and other (blood products, operating room, or emergency services, etc.)
Direct nonmedical cost	Costs of medical interventions not captured, but directly caused	Includes: transportation, time lost from work, caregiver costs, etc. most are not covered by insurance and may be out-of-pocket costs.
Perspective	The viewpoint of the analysis	Should be explicitly stated. Most analyses are done from the perspective of society (valuing this intervention versus other uses of the same money) or a health care system (valuing this intervention against other local health care needs.) The perspective of the individual patient or provider may give less attention to the needs of others.[42,43]
Discounting	Adjusts value of intervention for future benefit to present time amount	Health effects and costs should normally be discounted at 3%/year.

Source: Modified from Smith et al.[36]

that justified an intervention, for example, 2 weeks of quality survival, but recommended that the benefit be weighed against the toxicity and costs. If cost effectiveness data are not available, then cost consciousness with attention to lowest costs for comparable results would be appropriate; cost alone is not sufficient, since more expensive treatments such as bone marrow transplantation for relapsed leukemia may give better survival at reasonable cost effectiveness.[36]

The economic data necessary to make decisions about treatment may be collected in much the same way as clinical information, and standard formats for collection and analysis are now available.[40] Some standard definitions are listed in Table 11.3.

Table 11.4. Ways to balance clinical and cost studies

Type of study	*Advantages and disadvantages*
Clinical outcomes only	Ignores costs. e.g., Easy to choose among clearly superior therapies such as cisplatin for testicular cancer; harder among all others that give lesser benefits at high costs.
Cost only, e.g., costs of treating febrile neutropenia	Ignores clinical outcomes. Does not help choose among clinical strategies. e.g., The cost of CSF mobilization of stem cells may be higher than that of bone marrow collection, but it saves money later by reducing hospital stay.[45]
Costs and clinical outcomes together	
Cost-minimization	Assumes that two strategies are equal; lowest cost strategy is preferred
Cost-effectiveness	Compares two strategies; assigns $ per additional LY saved by strategy. Example: at present, CSFs have not improved survival, so cost must be lower for therapy to be cost-effective.
Cost-utility	Compares two strategies; assigns $ per additional LY saved by strategy, then estimates the quality of that benefit in $/QALY. e.g., No data show significant improvement in quality of life or utilities in patients who have received CSFs, so unlikely to have major impact.
Cost-benefit	Compares two strategies but converts the clinical benefits to money, e.g., a year of life is worth $100,000. Possible but rarely done due to difficulty in assigning $ value to benefit; requires assigning a $ value to human life.

CSF, colony stimulating factor; LY, year of life; QALY, quality-adjusted year of life.

Cost Effectiveness as an Outcome

One approach to funding treatments has been based on cost-effectiveness ratios.[36] Laupacis and colleagues in Canada proposed explicit funding criteria: (1) treatments that worked better and are less expensive be adopted; (2) treatments with cost-effectiveness ratios <$20,000 per additional year of life (LY) gained be accepted, with the recognition that they cost additional resources; (3) treatments with cost effectiveness ratios $20,000–$100,000/LY be examined on a case by case basis with caution; (4) and treatments with cost effectiveness ratios of >$100,000/LY be rejected.[44] This approach is valid in a system where all resources are shared equally; it is not clear how this system applies to other health care systems where resources may not be shared.[43] Alternatively, patients might be allowed to purchase additional insurance for expensive treatments, or pay for them out of pocket. In the United States, there has been no accepted answer but most authorities have agreed on an implicitly defined benchmark of $35,000–$50,000 per year of life saved.[36]

It is important to organize data in a way that balances clinical and cost information side by side as shown in Table 11.4.

Table 11.5. Chemotherapy versus best supportive care or alternative treatments

Topic	Conclusion
Lung cancer	
Chemotherapy versus best supportive care in non-small cell lung cancer[52]	Chemotherapy gained 8–13 weeks compared to best supportive care. Chemotherapy generally saved money for the province of Ontario, from a savings of CAN$8000 to additional cost of CAN$20,000 depending on assumptions. Similar results found for vinorelbine and cisplatin.[54]
Combined modality including chemotherapy versus radiation or surgery for Stage III non-small cell lung cancer[55–57]	Chemotherapy in combination with radiation or surgery adds clinical benefit; for chemotherapy plus radiation 1- and 5-year survival is increased from 40% to 54% and 6% to 17%, for instance. The addition of chemotherapy for IIIA patients added cost of CAN$15,866, and addition of chemotherapy to IIIB patients added CAN$8912. The cost year of life gained was well within accepted bounds at CAN$3348 to CAN$14,958.
Alternating chemotherapy for small cell lung cancer[67]	The alternating chemotherapy arm cost more, but because it was more effective, the marginal cost effectiveness was only $4560/LY.
Gastrointestinal cancer	
Chemotherapy versus best supportive care followed by chemotherapy for GI cancer patients[58]	Chemotherapy added 5 months median survival if given early rather than late, with symptom palliation for 4 months. The additional cost of about CAN$20,000/life year was within accepted bounds.
Prostate cancer	
Palliative chemotherapy with mitoxantrone plus prednisone versus prednisone[59,60]	Mitoxantrone did not improve survival, but improved quality of life as measured by several indices, and the mitoxantrone strategy cost less than prednisone supportive care.
Breast cancer	
High dose chemotherapy for limited metastatic disease versus standard chemotherapy[64]	High dose chemotherapy added 6 months at a cost of CAN$58,000, or CAN$116,000/LY; this is palliative care as this treatment has not been shown to be curative.
Other	
Acute myelogenous leukemia[66]	Chemotherapy, compared to supportive care, added additional cost but the cost effectiveness was CAN$18,000/LY, within acceptable limits.

LY, year of life.
Source: Modified from Smith et al.[36]

164

Chemotherapy is one of several types of palliative care and may be helpful for symptom relief or to prolong survival, as long as the switch to supportive care is made while resources and good quality time are still available.[46]

It is possible to give chemotherapy and either save money, or have a cost effectiveness within accepted limits as shown in Table 11.5. Patient treated with chemotherapy for non-small cell lung cancer have a small benefit, estimated at 2–4 months in most series,[47,48] and symptom relief in up to 60%.[49] Both the American Society of Clinical Oncology[50] and Ontario government[51] recommend consideration of chemotherapy for suitable patients. Jaakimainen et al. found that chemotherapy actually saved disease management costs compared to best supportive care by preventing hospitalizations late in the disease course. The cost effectiveness ratios ranged from $–8000 (cost saving) to $+20,000 Canadian for each additional year of life.[52] Smith and colleagues found that chemotherapy with cisplatin and vinorelbine, compared to vinorelbine alone or cisplatin and vindesine, added substantial clinical benefit[53] at a reasonable cost effectiveness of $15,000–$17,000 per year of life.[54] Given the benefit and low cost of the drugs, vinorelbine and cisplatin compared to best supportive care would give results similar to those of Jaakimainen and colleagues.[52] Evans and colleagues used decision analysis to show that chemotherapy in combination with radiation and/or surgery for Stage IIIA or IIIB disease, in comparison to treatment without chemotherapy would improve survival at a cost of $3348 to $14,958 Canadian per year of life saved.[55] The model showed benefit at a reasonable cost under all situations of reasonable clinical efficacy. The chemotherapy treatments fit existing monetary guidelines for use.[56,57]

A trial of fluorouracil-based chemotherapy for gastrointestinal cancer patients randomized to first-line chemotherapy versus best supportive care that could include later chemotherapy for symptom control showed benefit at acceptable cost-effectiveness ratios.[58] For the whole group, chemotherapy enhanced survival by about 5 months at a cost of about $20,000 per year of life gained, within accepted bounds.[36] For subsets of types of cancer, such as gastric cancer, the treatment was effective at a reasonable cost. For most other subsets, the patient numbers were too small to draw meaningful conclusions about either clinical effect or cost-effectiveness.

For patients with metastatic prostate cancer mitoxantrone added a small clinical benefit in terms of pain relief and symptom control in 23 of 80 patients, lasting for 6 more months than prednisone alone, but did not alter survival when compared to prednisone alone.[59] Although initial drug costs were higher, total disease costs were lower in the group that received mitoxantrone as initial treatment,[60] so good chemotherapy palliation could be accomplished at no additional cost to society. Total androgen blockade produced small clinical benefit at an acceptable cost to society, compared to single androgen blockade.[61]

There have been no studies on the effectiveness or cost effectiveness of chemotherapy for metastatic breast cancer compared to best supportive care. Hospitalization accounts for the majority of costs, while chemotherapy has been

Table 11.6. Site of service

Topic	Conclusion
Narcotics	Narcotics at home per diem costs were higher for home patients, but total costs were lower with equivalent palliation.[68]
Inpatient or outpatient chemotherapy	Outpatient administration was less expensive, US$184 versus US$223 in.[69]
Home or inpatient/clinic chemotherapy	Home chemotherapy was safe, well accepted, and cost less per treatment.[70]

a relatively trivial cost in the United Kingdom.[62] High-dose chemotherapy is commonly used for incurable metastatic disease, and in the one randomized controlled trial, it doubled overall survival from 10.4 to 20.8 months but did not produce a long-term survival plateau.[63] In the only available study of comparative treatment, Hillner et al.[64] compared best standard chemotherapy to high-dose chemotherapy with a stem cell transplant. High-dose chemotherapy (HDC) added about 6 months at a cost-effectiveness ratio of $116,000 per year of life gained, outside the bounds of accepted treatments. Of interest, drug costs for most breast cancer patients amount to less than 10% of the total cost.[65]

Acute myelogenous leukemia chemotherapy cost more than supportive care and certain death, and allogeneic transplant was even more effective. The transplant survival benefit 48% versus 21% at 5 years was sufficient to offset higher costs of treatment and make the cost-effectiveness ratio about $18,000/LY.[66]

The less expensive a setting, the less costly the intervention, as shown in Table 11.6. Home narcotic infusions had lower total costs due to less hospital costs despite higher drug equipment and nursing costs.[68] Outpatient administration of chemotherapy was less expensive than inpatient administration.[69] Home chemotherapy compared to outpatient chemotherapy was well-accepted with only two of 424 patients electing to discontinue home treatment, safe, and no more costly with an average cost $50 compared to $116 in hospital, with equal total costs.[70]

Disease management strategies have shown some modest improvements, with better quality of care, less cost, and high patient satisfaction. The available studies are shown in Table 11.7.

Coordinated care may be one of the most successful disease management strategies. The Medicare Hospice Benefit requires nurse coordination, team management, easy access to low per diem hospital beds for respite or temporary care, and expanded drug coverage.[71,72] Adding a nurse coordinator for terminally ill patients in England did not change any disease outcomes; patients still died, and most still had some unrelieved symptoms, but patient and family satisfaction was helped slightly.[73] The total costs were reduced from £8814 to £4414 (US$12,870 to $6444) from decreased hospital days for a cost savings of 41% in almost all conditions.[74]

Home nursing care was associated with more patients dying at home.[75]

Table 11.7. Process or structural changes in care

Topic	Conclusion
Reducing uncontrolled pain admissions	A system wide intervention of focus on pain management, a supportive care consultation team, and making a pain resource center. This was associated with a reduction in admissions from 255/5772 (4.4%) to 121/4076 (3.0%), at a projected cost savings of US$2,719,245.[76]
Presence of nursing care for end of life	Nursing care availability allowed more patients to die at home consistent with the wishes of most patients.[75]
Clinical practice guidelines for supportive care: antiemetics, treatment of febrile neutropenia, treatment of pain	A division changed practice to standardized oral antiemetics, and once-daily ceftriaxone and gentamicin. Cost savings were estimated at US$250,000 for each intervention, yearly.[72,79,80]

One center did a pain management intervention with enhanced institutional education programs, a highly visible respected consultative team, and a pain resource center for nurses and families. This was associated with a decrease in admissions and re-admissions for pain control with marked cost savings.[76] The study was not randomized, and could not account for other significant changes such as the growth of managed care with restricted admission policies. However, the conclusion must be that this is better pain management, better medical care, and probably saves money.

Teaching medical staff about choices for intensive care unit use can improve economic outcomes. An ethicist in the surgical intensive care unit (SICU) addressed the issues of patient choice about dying and the ethics of futile care. This was associated with a decrease in length of stay from 28 to 16 days, and a decrease in SICU days from 2028 to 1003 days, far greater than observed in other parts of the hospital. Cost savings were estimated at $1.8 million.[77] Dowdy and colleagues did pro-active ethics consultations for all mechanically ventilated patients beyond 4 days, and showed improved length of stay (less use of the intensive care unit, either by discontinuing futile care or transferring the patient to lesser intensity units) and a decrease in costs.[78]

Clinical practice guidelines for supportive care may decrease costs, but formal data have not been published (reviewed by Smith[72]). Standardization of care can improve the process of care even if not the outcomes, for most areas studied.[11,12]

The available data do not show that hospice improves care or saves money, as shown in Table 11.8.[72,81,82]

A large randomized controlled trial of hospice versus standard care showed that hospice did not improve quality of care by any measured benchmark (pain, ability to perform activities of daily living). Patients still used many hospital days, 48 for control, 51 for hospice, but more of the hospice patients were hospitalized on the hospice unit. There was no difference in diagnostic procedures, or total costs of about $15,000 per patient.

Table 11.8. Hospice versus non-hospice care

Topic	Conclusion
Randomized controlled trial of hospice versus non-hospice care in Veterans Hospital	Hospice did not improve or worsen quality of care by any measured benchmark (pain, ability to perform activities of daily living.). There was no difference in diagnostic procedures. Total costs were $15,000 per patient, with no difference in the arms.[86]
Hospice election versus standard care, Medicare beneficiaries, 1992	Medicare saved $1.65 for each $1 spent on hospice programs; most of the savings occur during the last month of life[83]
Hospice election versus standard care, Medicare beneficiaries, 1988	Medicare saved $1.26 for each $1 spent on hospice programs; most of the savings occur during the last month of life[84]
Total costs from data bases	No significant difference in total costs from diagnosis to death, but significant cost savings of 39% for hospice patients who were in hospice over 2 weeks.[87]
Total disease management costs comparing those who elected hospice to those who did not	No difference or slightly higher costs among Medicare beneficiaries who elected hospice. Within the hospice period, average 27 days, costs were slightly lower for those who elected hospice.[72]
Home care	Home care provided by relatives is not much different ($4563 for each 3-month period) than costs in a nursing home or similar setting. The sicker the patient became, the more the cost to the family regardless of diagnosis. Costs were lowest when the patient and care giver lived in the same household.[88,89]
Matching resource use to the dying patient	Hospice patients more likely to receive more home nursing care, and spend less time in the hospital than conventional care patients. Conventional care was the least expensive when overall disease management costs were calculated, but hospital-based hospice ($2270) and home care hospice ($2657) were less expensive than conventional care ($6100) in the last month of life.[85]

All amounts in US dollars.

More recent data suggest that hospice care can be cost-saving.[83] In the 1992 Medicare files those who elected hospice cost less than cancer patients who did not elect hospice. For those who enrolled in the last month of life, typically over half of Medicare patients, Medicare saved $1.65 for each $1 spent. Those who elected hospice tended to use more resources in the months from diagnosis until about 3 months before death, so the total disease management savings were close to zero. Similar findings were reported previously.[84]

Hospice may actually not be saving total disease management costs, but just shifting them to costs not captured by our current accounting systems. In our own study of Medicare hospice use in Virginia, total disease management costs were actually higher for those who eventually elected hospice. Those who elect hospice tend to be patients with resources to absorb more home care costs, more out-of-pocket drug costs, etc. The data are consistent with an affluent group of patients

Table 11.9. Use of advanced directives, do not resuscitate orders

Study	Conclusion
California Durable Power of Attorney for Health Care placed on chart[92]	No effect on treatment charges, types of treatment, or health status.
DNR[93]	Average of $57,334 for those without DNR orders, to $62,594 with those with DNR orders.
Advanced directives in SUPPORT hospitals[91]	No cost savings with advance directives. For patients prior to the SUPPORT intervention, there was a 23% reduction in cost associated with presence of advance directives, $21,284 with compared to $26,127 without. The intervention patients were more likely to have advance directives documented. Average cost was $24,178 for those without advanced directives, $28,017 for those with advanced directives on the intervention arm.

DNR, do not resuscitate.
All amounts in US dollars.

using all the resources needed for treatment, then using hospice resources in addition. There are no published data on whether the medically undeserved use hospice, will accept its philosophy, or how much those patients will cost the system.[72]

Database studies have shown similar results. In a retrospective study of 12,000 patients at 40 centers, Aiken et al. found that hospice patients were more likely to receive home nursing care, and spend less time in the hospital than conventional care patients.[85] Of the three models of care evaluated, conventional care was the least expensive when overall disease management costs were calculated, but hospital-based hospice ($2270) and home care hospice ($2657) were less expensive than conventional care ($6100) in the last month of life.

Advanced directives, such as do not resuscitate (DNR) orders, have been advocated to allow patients to make autonomous choices about their care at the end of life and possibly reduce costs by preventing futile care. However, as reviewed by Emanuel and Emanuel, there has been no cost savings associated either with the use of advanced directives or DNR orders[81,90] (Table 11.9). These findings have been confirmed in the more recent SUPPORT study.[91]

Advanced medical planning is clearly a part of palliative care and care of the dying. Norman Levinsky has questioned whether advanced medical planning has become an economic strategy as much as a way to respect a patient's wishes. He says,

> Confusion between advance planning as a method to find out what the patient wants and advance planning as a mechanism to reduce medical care and thereby contain costs represents a clear danger to the goals of informed consent and autonomy for patients.[27]

In one randomized study of 204 patients with life threatening diseases, it was found those who executed an advance directive had no significant positive or negative effect on a patient's well-being, health status, medical treatments, or medical treatment charges.[92]

Conclusion

Economic outcomes will become increasingly important for all types of health care, including palliative care. The few studies show substantial opportunities for improvement by using disease management strategies. Chemotherapy for some cancers (non-small cell lung cancer, prostate cancer, and gastrointestinal cancer) is reasonably effective and has acceptable cost-effectiveness ratios; this does not apply to any regimen that has not been formally evaluated. Coordination of palliative care shows no major clinical benefit but major cost savings. Directed ethical interventions about futile care appear to produce significant cost-savings. The use of advanced directives or hospice care may be good medical care but are do not produce major economic benefit.

References

1. Detmer DE. Half empty or half full, it will be a smaller glass. *Inquiry* 1997; 34:8–10.
2. Brown ML. The national economic burden of cancer. *JNCI* 1990; 82:1811–1814.
3. Brown ML, Hodgson TA, Rice DP. Economic impact of cancer in the U.S. In: Schottenfeld D, Fraumeni J, eds. *Cancer, Epidemiology, and Prevention.* London: Oxford University Press, 1996.
4. Rundle RL. Salick Pioneers Selling Cancer Care to HMOs. *The Wall Street Journal,* Monday, August 12, 1996, B1–B2.
5. Lubitz JD, Riley GF. Trends in Medicare payments in the last year of life. *N Engl J Med* 1993; 328:1092–1096.
6. Lubitz J, Beebe J, Baker C. Longevity and Medicare expenditures. *N Engl J Med* 1995; 332:999–1003.
7. Welch HG, Wennberg DE, Welch WP. The use of Medicare home health care services. *N Engl J Med* 1996; 335:324–329.
8. The SUPPORT Principal Investigators. A controlled trial to improve care for seriously ill hospitalized patients. The study to understand prognoses and preferences for outcomes and risks of treatments (SUPPORT). *JAMA* 1995; 274:1591–1598.
9. Cleeland CS, Gonin R, Hatfield AK, et al. Pain and its treatment in outpatients with metastatic cancer. *N Engl J Med* 1994; 330:592–596.
10. Hillner BE, Smith TJ. Assessing the quality of cancer care in the United States. A report to the Institute of Medicine and National Cancer Advisory Board. Part I: The quality of cancer care. Does the literature support the rhetoric? *J Clin Oncol* 2000; 18:2327–2340.
11. Smith TJ, Hillner BE. Assessing the quality of cancer care in the United States. A report to the Institute of Medicine and National Cancer Advisory Board. Part II: Clinical practice guidelines, critical pathways, and care maps. *J Clin Oncol* 2000; 18:2327–2340.

12. Hillner BE, Smith TJ. Assessing the quality of cancer care in the United States. A report to the Institute of Medicine and National Cancer Advisory Board. Part III: Models of excellence. *J Clin Oncol* 2000; 18:2327–2340.

13. Farrow DC, Hunt WC, Samet JM. Geographic variation in the treatment of localized breast cancer. *N Engl J Med* 1992; 326:1097–1101.

14. Nattinger AB, Gottlieb MS, Veum J, Yahnke D, Goodwin JS. Geographic variation in the use of breast-conserving treatment for breast cancer. *N Engl J Med* 1992; 326:1102–1107.

15. Hillner BE, Penberthy L, Desch CE, McDonald K, Smith TJ, Retchin SR. Variation in staging and treatment of local and regional breast cancer in the elderly. *Breast Cancer Res Treat* 1996; 40:75–86.

16. Hillner BE, MacDonald MK, Penberthy L, et al. Measuring standards of care for early breast cancer in an insured population. *J Clin Oncol* 1997; 15(4):1401–1408.

17. Smith TJ, Penberthy L, Desch CE, et al. Differences in initial treatment patterns and outcomes of lung cancer in the elderly. *Lung Cancer* 1995; 13:235–252.

18. Desch CE, Penberthy L, Newschaffer C, et al. Factors that determine the treatment of local and regional prostate cancer. *Med Care* 1996; 34(2):152–162.

19. Hillner BE, Smith TJ. Hospital volume and patient outcomes in major cancer surgery: a catalyst for quality assessment and concentration of cancer services. *JAMA* 1998; 280(20):1783–1784.

20. Gillis CR, Hole DJ. Survival outcome of care by specialist surgeons in breast cancer: a study of 3786 patients in the west of Scotland. *BMJ* 1996; 312:145–148.

21. Sainsbury R, Haward R, Rider L, Johnstone C, Round C. Influence of clinician workload and patterns of treatment on survival from breast cancer. *Lancet* 1995; 345:1265–1270.

22. Feuer EJ, Frey CM, Brawley OW, et al. After a treatment breakthrough: a comparison of trial and population-based data for advanced testicular cancer. *J Clin Oncol* 1994; 12:368–377.

23. Nguyen HN, Averette HE, Hoskins W, Penalver M, Sevin B, Steren A. National survey of ovarian carcinoma Part V. The impact of physician's specialty on patient's survival. *Cancer* 1993; 72:3663–3670.

24. Berger JT, Rosner F. The ethics of practice guidelines. *Arch Intern Med* 1996; 156:2051–2056.

25. Smith R. An ethical code for everybody in health care: A code that covered all rather than single groups might be useful. *BMJ* 1997; 315(7123):1633–1634.

26. Cassel CK, Vladeck BC. ICD-9 Code for palliative or terminal care. *N Engl J Med* 1996; 335:1232–1234.

27. Levinsky NG. The purpose of advance medical planning—autonomy for patients or limitation of care? *N Engl J Med* 1996; 335:741–743.

28. Callahan D. Controlling the costs of health care for the elderly—fair means and foul. *N Engl J Med* 1996; 335:744–746.

29. Daniels N. *Just Health Care.* New York: Cambridge University Press, 1985.

30. Randall F. *Palliative Care Ethics: A Good Companion.* New York: Oxford University Press; 1996.

31. Sidgwick H. *The Methods of Ethics.* London: McMillan, 1907.

32. Slevin ML, Stubbs L, Plant HJ, et al. Attitudes to chemotherapy: comparing views of patients with cancer with those of doctors, nurses, and general public. *BMJ* 1990; 300:1458–1460.

33. Davies E, Clarke C, Hopkins A. Malignant cerebral glioma—I: Survival, disability, and morbidity after radiotherapy. *BMJ* 1996; 313:1507–1512.

34. Davies E, Clarke C, Hopkins A. Malignant cerebral glioma—II: Perspectives of patients and relatives on the value of radiotherapy. *BMJ* 1996; 313:1512–1516.

35. Lamm RD. The ghost of health care future. *Inquiry* 1994; 31:365–367.

36. Smith TJ, Hillner BE, Desch CE. Efficacy and cost-effectiveness of cancer treatment: rational allocation of resources based on decision analysis. *JNCI* 1993; 85:1460–1474.

37. Waugh N, Scott D. How should different life expectancies be valued? *BMJ* 1998; 316(7140):1316.

38. Olweny CL. Ethics of palliative care medicine: palliative care for the rich nations only! *J Palliat Care* 1994; 10(3):17–22.

39. American Society of Clinical Oncology Outcomes Working Group (core members). Outcomes of cancer treatment for technology assessment and cancer treatment guidelines. *J Clin Oncol* 1995; 14:671–679.

40. Brown ML, Glick HA, Harrell FE, et al. *Integrating Economic Analysis Into Cancer Clinical Trials: The National Cancer Institute American Society of Clinical Oncology Economics Workbook*, 1998:1.

41. Shwartz M, Young DW, Siegrist R. The ratio of costs to charges: how good a basis for estimating costs? *Inquiry* 1995; 32:476–481.

42. Smith TJ, Bodurtha JN. Ethical considerations in oncology: balancing the interests of patients, oncologists, and society. *J Clin Oncol* 1995; 13:2464–2470.

43. Smith TJ. Which hat do I wear? *JAMA* 1993; 270:1657–1659.

44. Laupacis A, Feeny D, Detsky AS, Tugwell PX. How attractive does a new technology have to be to warrant adoption and utilization? Tentative guidelines for using clinical and economic evaluation. *Can Med Assoc J* 1992; 146:473–481.

45. Smith TJ, Hillner BE, Schmitz N, et al. Economic analysis of a randomized clinical trial to compare filgrastim-mobilized peripheral blood progenitor cell transplantation and autologous bone marrow transplantation in patients with Hodgkin and non-Hodgkin lymphoma. *J Clin Oncol* 1997; 15:5–10.

46. Smith TJ, Desch CE, Hillner BE. Ways to reduce the cost of oncology care without compromising the quality. *Cancer Invest* 1994; 12:257–265.

47. Blair SN, Kohl HWI, Barlow CE, Paffenbarger RS, Jr, Gibbons LW, Macera CA. Changes in physical fitness and all-cause mortality. A prospective study of healthy and unhealthy men. *JAMA* 1995; 273:1093–1098.

48. Souquet PJ, Chauvin F, Boissel JP, et al. Polychemotherapy in advanced non-small cell lung cancer: a meta-analysis. *Lancet* 1993; 342:19–21.

49. Adelstein DJ. Palliative chemotherapy for non-small cell lung cancer. *Semin Oncol* 1995; 22:35–39.

50. American Society of Clinical Oncology. Clinical practice guidelines for the treatment of unresectable non-small-cell lung cancer. *J Clin Oncol* 1997; 15(8):2996–3018.

51. Evans WK, Newman T, Graham I, et al. Lung cancer practice guidelines: lessons learned and issues addressed by the Ontario Lung Cancer Disease Site Group. *J Clin Oncol* 1997; 15(9):3049–3059.

52. Jaakimainen L, Goodwin PJ, Pater J, Warde P, Murray N, Rapp E. Counting the costs of chemotherapy in a National Cancer Institute of Canada randomized trial in non-small cell lung cancer. *J Clin Oncol* 1990; 8:1301–1309.

53. Le Chevalier T, Brisgand D, Douillard JY, et al. Randomized study of vinorelbine and cisplatin versus vindesine and cisplatin versus vinorelbine alone in advanced non-small cell lung cancer: results of a European multicenter trial including 612 patients. *J Clin Oncol* 1994; 12:360–367.

54. Smith TJ, Hillner BE, Neighbors DM, McSorley PA, Le Chevalier T. An economic evaluation of a randomized clinical trial comparing vinorelbine, vinorelbine plus cisplatin and vindesine plus cisplatin for non-small cell lung cancer. *J Clin Oncol* 1995; 13:2166–2173.

55. Evans WK, Will BP, Berthelot JM, Earle CC. Cost of combined modality interventions for stage iii non-small-cell lung cancer. *J Clin Oncol* 1997; 15(9):3038–3048.

56. Evans WK, Will BP. The cost of managing lung cancer in Canada. *Oncol Hunting* 1995; 9(suppl 11):147–153.

57. Evans WK, Will BP, Berthelot JM, Wolfson MC. The economics of lung cancer management in Canada. *Lung Cancer* 1996; 14(1):13–17.

58. Glimelius B, Hoffman K, Graf W, et al. Cost-effectiveness of palliative chemotherapy in advanced gastrointestinal cancer. *Ann Oncol* 1995; 6(3):267–274.

59. Tannock IF, Osoba D, Stockler MR, et al. Chemotherapy with mitoxantrone plus prednisone or prednisone alone for symptomatic hormone-resistant prostate cancer: a Canadian randomized trial with palliative end points. *J Clin Oncol* 1996; 14(6):1756–1764.

60. Bloomfield DJ, Krahn MD, Tannock IF, Smith TJ. Economic evaluation of chemotherapy with mitoxantrone plus prednisone for symptomatic hormone resistant prostate cancer (HRPC) based on a Canadian randomized trial (RCT) with palliative endpoints. Proceedings of ASCO 17, 1997.

61. Hillner BE, McLeod DG, Crawford ED, Bennett CL. Estimating the cost effectiveness of total androgen blockade with flutamide in M1 prostate cancer. *Urology* 1995; 45(4):633–640.

62. Richards MA, Braysher S, Gregory WM, Rubens RD. Advanced breast cancer: use of resources and cost implications. *Br J Cancer* 1993; 67:856–860.

63. Bezwoda WR, Seymour L, Dansey RD. High-dose chemotherapy with hematopoietic rescue as primary treatment for metastatic breast cancer: a randomized trial. *J Clin Oncol* 1995; 13:2483–2489.

64. Hillner BE, Smith TJ, Desch CE. Efficacy and cost-effectiveness of autologous bone marrow transplantation in metastatic breast cancer. Estimates using decision-analysis while awaiting clinical trial results. *JAMA* 1992; 267:2055–2061.

65. Holli K, Hakama M. Treatment of the terminal stages of breast cancer. *BMJ* 1989; 298:13–14.

66. Welch HG, Larson EB. Cost-effectiveness of bone marrow transplantation in acute nonlymphocytic leukemia. *N Engl J Med* 1989; 321:807–812.

67. Goodwin PJ, Feld R, Evans WK, Pater J. Cost-effectiveness of cancer chemotherapy: an economic evaluation of a randomized trial in small-cell lung cancer. *J Clin Oncol* 1988; 6:1537–1547.

68. Ferris FD, Wodinsky HB, Kerr IG, Sone M, Hume S, Coons C. A cost-minimization study of cancer patients requiring a narcotic infusion in hospital and at home. *J Clin Epidemiol* 1991; 44:313–327.

69. Wodinsky HB, DeAngelis C, Rusthoven JJ, et al. Re-evaluating the cost of outpatient cancer chemotherapy. *Can Med Assoc J* 1987; 137:903–906.

70. Lowenthal RM, Piaszczyk A, Arthur GE, O'Malley S. Home chemotherapy for cancer patients: Cost analysis and safety. *Med J Aust* 1996; 165(4):184–187.
71. Harris NJ, Dunmore R, Tscheu MJ. The Medicare hospice benefit: fiscal implications for hospice program management. *Cancer Management* 1996; May/June:6–11.
72. Smith TJ. *End of Life Care: Preserving Quality and Quantity of Life in Managed Care.* ASCO Educ Book, 33rd Annual Meeting, 1997:303–307.
73. Addington-Hall JM, MacDonald LD, Anderson HR, et al. Randomized controlled trial of effects of coordinating care for terminally ill cancer patients. *BMJ* 1992; 305:1317–1322.
74. Raftery JP, Addington-Hall JM, MacDonald LD, et al. A randomized controlled trial of the cost-effectiveness of a district co-ordinating service for terminally ill cancer patients. *Palliat Med* 1996; 10:151–161.
75. McWhinney IR, Bass MJ, Orr V. Factors associated with location of death (home or hospital) or patients referred to a palliative care team. *Can Med Assoc J* 1995; 152(3):361–370.
76. Grant M, Ferrell BR, Rivera LM, Lee J. Unscheduled readmissions for uncontrolled symptoms. *Nurs Clin North Am* 1995; 30(4):673–682.
77. Holloran SD, Starkey GW, Burke PA, Steele G Jr, Forse RA. An educational intervention in the surgical intensive care unit to improve ethical decisions. *Surgery* 1995; 118(2):294–298.
78. Dowdy MD, Robertson C, Bander JA. A study of proactive ethics consultation for critically and terminally ill patients with extended lengths of stay. *Crit Care Med* 1998; 26(2):252–259.
79. Smith TJ. Reducing the cost of supportive care, Part I: Antibiotics for febrile neutropenia. *Clin Oncol Alert* 1996; 11:46–47.
80. Smith TJ. Reducing the cost of supportive care II: Anti-emetics. *Clin Oncol Alert* 1996; 11:62–64.
81. Emanuel EJ. Cost savings at the end of life. What do the data show? *JAMA* 1996; 275:1907–1914.
82. Emanuel EJ, Emanuel LL. The economics of dying. The illusion of cost savings at the end of life. *N Engl J Med* 1994; 330:540–544.
83. National Hospice Organization. *An Analysis of the Cost Savings of the Medicare Hospice Benefit.* Miami, FL: Lewin-VHI Inc, 1997.
84. Kidder D. The effects of hospice coverage on Medicare expenditures. *Health Serv Res* 1992; 27:195–217.
85. Aiken LH. Evaluation and research and public policy: lessons learned from the National Hospice study. *J Chronic Dis* 1986; 39:1–4.
86. Kane RL, Berstein L, Whales J, Leibowitz A, Kaplan S. A randomized control trial of hospice care. *Lancet* 1984; 1:890–894.
87. Brooks CH, Smyth-Staruch K. Hospice home care cost savings to third party insurers. *Med Care* 1984; 22:691–703.
88. Stommel M, Given CW, Given BA. The cost of cancer home care to families. *Cancer* 1993; 71:1867–1874.
89. Given BA, Given CW, Stommel M. Family and out-of-pocket costs for women with breast cancer. *Cancer Pract* 1994; 2:187–193.
90. Emanuel EJ, Emanuel LL. The economics of dying: The illusion of cost savings at the end of life. *N Engl J Med* 1994; 330(8):540–544.

91. Teno J, Lynn J, Connors AF Jr, et al. The illusion of end-of-life resource savings with advance directives. SUPPORT Investigators. Study to Understand Prognoses and Preferences for Outcomes and Risks of Treatment. *J Am Geriatr Soc* 1997; 45(4):513–518.
92. Schneiderman LJ, Kronick R, Kaplan RM, Anderson JP, Langer RD. Effects of offering advance directives on medical treatments and costs. *Ann Intern Med* 1992; 117(7):599–606.
93. Maksoud A, Jahnigen DW, Skibinski CI. Do not resuscitate orders and the cost of death. *Arch Intern Med* 1993; 153(10):1249–1253.

12

Symptom Assessment Outcomes in Home-Based Palliative Care

FRANCO DE CONNO AND CINZIA MARTINI

In view of the fact that 90% of patients assisted by palliative care centers suffer from advanced cancer,[1] the purpose of this chapter is to analyze the use of symptom assessment as outcome of home-based palliative care strategies for advanced cancer patients.

Indeed, it is necessary to define the population of patients on which palliative care is focused as consisting of terminal patients who, with the exception of very rare cases, are not intended to be treated with specific cancer therapies and for whom the therapeutic goal exclusively consists of symptom control intended as subjective well-being.

Home care for advanced cancer patients requiring palliative care first established and has developed for various reasons. Today, palliative care is given in different settings: in palliative care units (PCU) in general hospitals or cancer hospitals, in hospices, and in home care units. These models are not alternatives, but rather integrate each other. Their availability is aimed at guaranteeing adequate response to the various problems emerging in the care of advanced cancer patients.

Among the various reasons that have determined the development of home-based palliative care, there is primarily the acknowledgement of the wish, expressed by healthy as well as ill individuals, to die in their own homes, surrounded by the affection of their loved ones. There is, however, an equally significant resource allocation problem of the various States' health policies. In fact, although common ethics assigns extreme importance to the life of the dying individual, in practice there are always many obstacles in the way of planning adequate global health and assistance services for patients in the terminal phase of the disease.

When there is the possibility of choice, individual preferences range from home care to hospitalization. It should therefore not be a question of choosing between good home care and good hospital or hospice care, but the different options are both needed. Home assistance first of all assumes compliance with the patient's preference as to home or hospital, often a much more complex and personal issue when compared to any external evaluation.[2]

This century has witnessed a progressive trend toward terminal status hospitalization, since the hospital is viewed as the place where it is possible to perform diagnostic examinations and treatments from the most simple to the most sophisticated, and where medical and nursing personnel is present around the clock. In the public's opinion, all this is equivalent to the best care possible. Furthermore, especially in large cities, family and community life is conditioned by small living quarters and long working hours that do not leave much time for the care of a dying patient who instead needs adequate space and continuous assistance. Conversely, hospitals have developed into places specialized in the care of acute pathologies and provide high-tech diagnostics and therapies, but precisely because of their structure are poorly equipped for the care of terminal patients.

Certainly in the last 20 years, palliative care programs for cancer patients have attempted to invert this tendency to hospitalize death. An epidemiological study performed in Genoa, Italy demonstrated that the trend of home cancer-related death rate can be influenced by offering home care services. Indeed, between 1985 and 1990 it increased from 28% to 33% in association with the development of palliative home care services for patients with advanced cancer.[3]

In industrialized countries today, over 80% of cancer-related deaths occur in hospitals. The experience of many palliative home care teams has shown that the percentage of patients who underwent home care services died in their own homes in significantly higher percentages. To date it is impossible to prove that the offer of home assistance has any effect on the will or capability of our society in assisting terminal patients at home up to their death, whereas there is certainly a significant population of terminal patients receiving palliative home care, no matter whether they die at home or in a hospital or hospice. A study conducted by Parkes shows that in the case of palliative home care, the period spent by terminal patients at home is longer even when they then die in hospice. It is therefore necessary to verify the palliative home care methods, the resources dedicated to them, and their effectiveness in achieving the expected therapeutic results.

Symptom Outcome

The first goal of palliative care is to improve the quality of life in the advanced stages of incurable diseases. There is global consensus in deeming the control of the physical and psychological symptoms an element of primary importance in the terminal patient's quality of life.[4]

Measuring and documenting the outcomes of symptom assessment is, therefore, meaningful from a clinical perspective for individual patient monitoring and therapeutic decision making, from a quality insurance perspective for auditing the care provided by different services and setting of care and from a research perspective to determine significant end-points for clinical research.[5]

Pain and symptom management in the home presents a challenge to health care professionals. A peculiarity of palliative home care is the fundamental role played by the family, even more important than in the hospice setting, and the initial assessment of the patient and family are the key to making an appropriate care plan. Most of the nursing provided at home is given by the patient's family, and the emotional involvement with the lack of specific knowledge may be source of great anxiety. These factors clearly affect symptom evaluation, too.

Explanation of the causes of the symptomatology and of the therapeutic options to the patient and his or her family is mandatory when planning a therapeutic strategy that will focus on symptom prevention, anticipation of acute events, and preparing the family for eventual problems. Patient and family counseling is therefore indispensable.

Symptom evaluation appears to be crucial in that it is the only parameter guiding care planning. Although other clinical evaluations obviously are also important, they take on secondary importance with respect to the main objective. The symptom must, therefore, be seen as a multidimensional concept (physical, psychological, existential), and the subjective aspect must be stressed in the clinical relationship with the patient and with his family, in assessing the outcomes and in scientific research.

Based on our experience over the last 18 years, we can state that pain and other symptom management, and psychosocial support can be efficaciously delivered at home.[6]

Symptom Prevalence

It is not easy to compare symptom prevalence tables in advanced cancer patients because the checklists differ, the data collection methods differ, the taxonomy sometimes used differs, especially as regards psychological symptoms, and the studied population's survival differs, ranging from several months to a few weeks.

Physical symptoms

Numerous surveys have documented the high prevalence of symptoms in patients with advanced cancer. Several studies confirmed that most patients experience multiple symptoms. Advanced cancer patients' symptom prevalence data unanimously show asthenia, anorexia and pain as being the most frequent symptoms, followed by dyspnea, confusion, and vomiting[7–13] whereas the most distressing symptoms are pain and dyspnea.[14] Pain is experienced by approximately 70%–90%

of patients with advanced cancer.[15] Fatigue or asthenia are reported by 75% of cancer patients[16,17] and in almost half of the patients admitted to St Christopher's Hospice,[18] the prevalence of anorexia is in the range of 30%–80%.[9,10]

It is possible to outline a model—almost a final common path—characterizing the clinical approach to the terminal phases of advanced cancer, independently from the type of primary tumor, and that includes, as regards physical symptoms: pain, appetite deterioration, cognitive disorders, gastrointestinal disorders, and respiratory distress.[19]

Psychological symptoms

Physical symptoms are reported as more common than psychological symptoms but when specific psychological measures are applied, the latter have high prevalence rates. The prevalence of major psychiatric disorders in cancer patients has been reported to be 2%–6%[20] but the prevalence of psychological symptoms is higher.[21] In fact, depressive or anxious symptoms are quite frequent in cancer patients with adjustment disorders, reported as high as 47%.[20]

Symptom Assessment

Symptom evaluation is a complicated matter and includes various aspects beyond simple prevalence. Evaluation is a process that can go from simple and immediate to extremely complex. There are various aspects to be considered:

- the multiplicity of cancer patient symptoms
- the multidimensionality of the symptoms—it is, in fact, possible to discern a symptom's intensity, duration, frequency, as well as the degree of distress it causes in the individual patient
- the possible interaction between different symptoms (e.g., anorexia and pain)[22]
- the interaction between symptoms and the subject's functionality/ autonomy[10]
- the possible interaction between the symptoms and the patient's awareness of the disease, of its terminal nature, or both
- the interaction between symptoms and quality of life.[14]

Only an accurate evaluation allows for the identification of the cause(s) of a symptom, and especially for the understanding of the interrelationship between the various causes and the various manifestations of the symptom.

The need to implement an objective evaluation of symptoms has boosted the search for standard assessment methods through the use of specific instruments capable of providing valid and repeatable quantification.

If symptom evaluation is useful, this raises the question. Is there a practical approach for symptom evaluation in far–advanced cancer patients receiving home care?

Symptoms are by definition perceptions, and, therefore, subjective. For this reason, the assessment of symptoms is a particularly difficult task. Moreover, the same semantic and terminology-related definition may vary for given symptoms in different individuals. Finally, linguistic translations do not always succeed in defining the same content for a given word. For example, most surveys report that fatigue is the most common symptom in the population with advanced cancer but the complaint of fatigue may actually reflect the presence of several other related symptoms. Patients use fatigue to describe lack of energy or vitality, muscle weakness, tiredness, or sleepiness. This indicates that symptom assessment not only must be conducted using specifically designed instruments, but also that said instruments must be validated along with their versions in languages different from the original.

Symptoms are multidimensional. It is possible to measure these various dimensions: intensity, frequency, duration, characteristics, as it is also possible to measure their degree of psychological (global distress) and physical impact on the patient's daily functions and in general on his or her quality of life.

The fact that symptoms are subjective leads to the conclusion that the best source of information is the patient himself. Unfortunately, in the terminal phases of the disease, the patient may be incapable of providing this information due to excessively deteriorated physical and cognitive conditions.

When the symptom is accompanied by an objective sign, it is possible to monitor the latter, as is the case with vomiting, for example, but objective assessment cannot replace subjective assessment tout court. The difficulties in assessing symptoms in patients who are dying have led to the use of data from observers, despite concerns about the validity of this methodology. Observer ratings of symptom severity correlate poorly with patient ratings and are generally an inadequate substitute for patient reporting.[23–25]

Peruselli found a congruence in 63% of reported instances when the patients' own descriptions of their symptoms were compared with their symptoms as identified by nursing staff. Agreement was more frequently found with somatic symptoms than with psychological ones.[26] Some observations make this topic intriguing: a survey of 154 inpatients and home care cancer deaths found that approximately 33% of patients were able to interact 24 hours before death, 5% could interact 12 hours before, and 8% were able to communicate in the last hour of life.[27]

One may debate at this point whether or not symptom assessment finds its natural and final limitation in when the patient can no longer be the source of information. Conversely, is it feasible to find a compromise and identify other sources of information? Could this source be the family? Or the team of carers? Is the situation different for the patient living the last phase of the disease in a hospice or at home? Great efforts are being made to collect data on the last stage of life, allowing for the limitations of these assessments in regard to symptoms.

Validated Symptom Assessment Instruments

There are instruments that measure multiple symptoms and instruments that measure one specific symptom. These instruments should be simple and not excessively time-consuming aiming at a good compliance over time, enable self-assessment, validity, reliability, and multidimensionality.

They should be inserted as far as possible within a patient-operator relationship context. One common difficulty resides in scarce compliance, not on the part of the patient but of the operator who views the giving out of a questionnaire as a cold, detached, and useless gesture in clinical practice.

Instruments for assessing single symptoms

The measurement of subjective variables and in particular of symptoms suffers from the absence of an external golden standard to establish the validity of a given measurement instrument. An operational solution of this problem is the use of visual analogue scales (VAS), and the numerical and verbal rating scales (NRS, VRS). All these scales share the characteristic of forcing the subject experiencing a given sensation or symptom to rate the magnitude of his or her subjective feeling from minimum to maximum. The intensity rating is expressed on an abstract continuum (as in the VAS) or by numbers (NRS) or words (VRS) representing different grading of intensity distributed between the minimum and maximum intensities. These methods although apparently simple should be carefully understood considering the complex psychophysical, and statistical issues implicated. It is however useful to recognize that many different clinical variables can be measured by VAS, NRS, and VRS provided the validity of the method and its measurement properties have been established and its clinical meaning clarified.

Pain

Pain is certainly the most studied symptom from a measurement perspective. Pain-related items are present in all symptom checklists for cancer patients. There are, however, various specific instruments for pain assessment, which can be distinguished into monodimensional and multidimensional. The former assess pain intensity and relief and include visual analogue, numeric, and categoric (verbal) scales. Among the multidimensional instruments, the most renowned are the Brief Pain Inventory and the McGill Pain Questionnaire.

The Brief Pain Inventory is self-administered. Numeric scales, ranging from 0 to 10, indicate the intensity of pain in general, at its worst, at its least, and right now. Seven questions indicate the degree to which pain interferes with function, mood, sleep, and enjoyment of life. It has been translated and validated into several languages.[28]

The McGill Pain Questionnaire is a self-administered questionnaire that provides global scores and subscale scores that reflect the sensory, affective, and evaluative dimensions of pain.[29,30] A short form of the questionnaire is available.[31]

Dyspnea

Dyspnea occurs in 21%–70% of patients with advanced cancer. There are several methods to assess dyspnea but only few have been used in cancer patients. Different tests have been used in cardiopulmonary diseases: a five-points scale developed by Fletcher,[32] the Chronic Respiratory Questionnaire,[33–35] the Borg Scale (Ratio of Perceived Exertion),[36] the Oxygen Cost Diagram,[37] and the Dyspnea Index.[38] They have been recently reviewed.[39]

Fatigue/asthenia

Fatigue/asthenia is a complex symptom difficult to assess. The following tools have been proposed:

The Piper Fatigue Self-Report Scale. This is a 41-item scale to evaluate the multidimensionality of fatigue—that is, intensity, distress, and impact on patients during radiotherapy. It has excellent reliability and moderate construct validity in this population.[40]

The VAS-F (Visual Analogue Scale-Fatigue). This 18-item scale evaluates the multidimensionality of fatigue in patients with sleep disorders. It has high internal consistency and correlates significantly with the fatigue subscale of POMS.[41]

The Edmonton Functional Assessment Tool (EFAT). The EFAT is a validated instrument to assess asthenia in the context of the functional and performance status of terminally ill patients. Ten items are rated according to predetermined standards of performance, which are described in behavioral terms. These descriptors are ranked from 0 to 3, 0 being independent and 3 being totally dependent. Numerical ratings of the EFAT allow a visual display of performance status, facilitating communication of performance status to the multidisciplinary team. It has been found to have good values for validity and reliability and it seems to change appropriately according to the changes in the patients' clinical status.[42]

Nausea and vomiting

Nausea and vomiting in advanced cancer occur as a manifestation of the disease process or as a complication of drugs used for symptom control. Reuben and Mor, using the data of the National Hospice Study, found that nausea and vomiting developed in 62% of terminal cancer patients in the last 6 months of life, with prevalence rates of at least 40% during the last 6 weeks.[43]

Morrow Test. This self-assessment method includes 17 items. Nausea and vomiting frequency and intensity are evaluated with Likert scales; duration is also recorded. It has been specifically designed for chemotherapy-induced emesis.[44]

Overall Nausea Index. This instrument is based on three indices—nausea evaluation index, nausea global intensity, and nausea intensity visual analogue scale. It is a modified version of the McGill Pain Questionnaire with the term nausea substituted for the term pain.[45]

Cognitive impairment

Symptoms of cognitive impairment can be screened and assessed with many different methods among which the most commonly used are the MiniMental Status Exam[46] and the Blessed Orientation-Memory-Concentration Test.[47] In terminally ill cancer patients, symptoms of cognitive impairment are often associated with the diagnosis of delirium. The diagnosis of delirium is based on criteria outlined by the American Psychiatric Association in the DSM-IV, and several tools have been developed and validated to facilitate this diagnosis, for example, the Confusion Assessment Method,[48] the Delirium Rating Scale,[49] and the Delirium Symptom Interview.[50]

Instruments for assessing multiple symptoms

Edmonton Symptom Assessment System

This instrument is based on nine visual analogue scales measuring pain, activity, nausea, depression, anxiety, drowsiness, appetite, wellbeing, and shortness of breath, which are completed twice a day in the palliative care unit. Its validity and reliability have not been completely studied.[51]

Symptom distress scale

This scale is used to evaluate the subjective perception of symptoms. It is self-administered and has 13 items with responses rated on a 5-point Likert scale ranging from 1 (no distress) to 5 (extreme distress). It evaluates the frequency and intensity of pain, frequency and intensity of nausea, appetite, bowel pattern, breathing, coughing, fatigue, insomnia, concentration, and two psychological symptoms, appearance and mood.[52]

Rotterdam Symptom Checklist

It was developed as a tool to measure the symptoms reported by cancer patients; this questionnaire uses a 4-point Likert scale to evaluate 34 physical and psychological symptoms plus 8 items defining the impact of symptoms on the activities of daily living. It gives information about symptom distress but not about the intensity and the frequency.[53]

The European Organization for Research and Treatment in Cancer QLQ-C30

This is a self-reporting questionnaire of quality of life that incorporates 9 multi-item scales, 5 functional scales (physical, role, cognitive, emotional, and social), 3 symptom scales (fatigue, pain, nausea, and vomiting) and a global health and quality of life scale. Several single-item symptom measures are also included.[54]

Memorial symptom assessment scale (MSAS)
It is self-administered and provides multidimensional information about 32 physical and psychological symptoms. Severity, frequency, and distress are evaluated. Its reliability and validity has been proven in the cancer population.[55]

Therapy impact questionnaire
It has been validated for quality of life assessment in advanced cancer patients and is composed of 36 items that assess physical symptoms (24 items), functional status (3 items), concomitant emotional and cognitive factors (6 items), and social interaction (2 items). A global well-being judgement completes the Therapy Impact Questionnaire (TIQ). It uses a 4-point verbal Likert scale from "not at all" to "very much".[56]

Supportive team assessment schedule
Higginson and McCarthy have proposed an assessment method that uses the AUDIT concept, resulting in the most renowned instrument of this type. It contains 17 items assessing gravity with a rating from 0 to 6, including those for the control of pain and of other symptoms (in two separate items). Supportive Team Assessment Schedule (STAS) ratings completed by 2 palliative care teams were compared with patients' ratings and with carer's ratings of 7 out of 17 items. Team ratings were usually closer to those of the patients than those of the carer.[57]

Other instruments validated in palliative care are reviewed by Hearn and Higginson.[5]

Experience of Symptom Assessment in Home Care

The patient receiving home care usually has a short life expectancy, even though the criteria for activating this type of service may vary. Cases reported show that the mean duration of home assistance varies from 29 days[58] to 62 days.[59] These values do not differ much from those of the National Hospice Study where 50% of patients had a survival rate shorter than 35 days.[1]

Higginson reports the evaluation of symptoms in 86 cancer patients referred to a district terminal care support team. The symptoms were rated throughout care using a standardized schedule with a score of seven points corresponding to a progressive worsening of the symptom. The mean length of time in care was 62 days with a mean of 7.2 weekly assessments. Pain was the most common main symptom (41%) at referral, but became less prominent over time. After the first week of care, weakness or dyspnea became main symptoms and in the last week became the most common uncontrolled symptoms (21%). The scores suggest that pain was controlled very early in care, while dyspnea increased with the approach of death.[59]

Mercadante reported the experience of a home palliative care unit with 745 terminal cancer patients in 4 years in Palermo, Sicily. Data about symptoms were recorded but only pain was measured. Pain was assessed using a VAS, considering pain level good when kept at the level of slight or moderate, less than 4 cm using VAS. Pain was controlled according to the criterion in more than 80% of cases.[60]

The home care team of the National Cancer Institute of Milan used the TIQ for symptom and quality of life assessment in 348 terminal cancer patients over 3 years. The duration of the assistance ranged between 1 and 6 weeks for 50% of the patients, but for one third of them it was shorter than 2 weeks. Eight-six percent of patients died at home and 14% died in hospitals. Multivariate analysis showed that only a higher degree of family support was associated with home death. The prevalence of distressing symptoms indicates that severe uncontrolled pain had a major role in patients being referred for symptom control to the service (50% of all cases) and pain was the only symptom showing substantial improvement throughout the home care duration. However, a significant group of patients still complained of severe pain in their last week of life (23.8%). Among the other symptoms, dyspnea showed an increasing trend and poor control, also in agreement with previous observations, and was 15.3% in the last week of life. Psychosocial distress, as evaluated by the TIQ, did not show significant changes from the first to the last week of care.[6]

Peruselli et al. used the symptom distress scale (SDS) developed by McCorkle and Young for the evaluation of the degree of symptom distress in 106 terminal cancer patients cared for at home. The median survival in palliative home care was 29 days. The SDS score demonstrated a reduction in symptom distress after starting home care. The improvement in symptom distress was more pronounced in the group of patients with an initially higher level of distress whose symptom control was essentially good until death. On the contrary, in the group of less severe cases, the trend was quite different, with a gradual, albeit slow, deterioration. Palliative care was effective in mitigating pain and in part stimulating appetite, curbing nausea, and controlling psychological aspects, whereas the outcome for social and functional aspects worsened independent of the home care support.[58]

Recently, symptom prevalence and outcome for inpatients and outpatients referred to a palliative care team were evaluated with E-STAS, an extension of STAS. The most common symptoms at referral were psychological distress 93%, anorexia 73%, pain 59% and mouth discomfort 59%. In all symptoms, except depression, there were statistically significant improvements from first to last assessment.[61]

In conclusion, in a setting of severely debilitated patients in home care or in hospices, it is best to use simple and short assessment instruments that, although they do not give in-depth assessment of the various aspects of symptoms, are nonetheless useful for monitoring the clinical situation and its evolution.

Results of Measuring Symptom Outcome in Comparing Different Settings of Care

One of the major issues debated in palliative care is which setting of care is more appropriate to offer good palliative care. Studies aimed at comparing different settings of care on the basis of their results in symptom control are excessively rare.

Kane et al. reported no significant differences between terminally ill cancer patients randomly assigned to receive hospice or conventional care in measures of pain and other symptoms. Both patients and their family caregivers were more satisfied with the hospice care and significantly less anxious than those without support.[62]

The results of the National Hospice Study comparing hospice care with conventional care indicate that pain and symptom control were better in the inpatient hospice setting than in home care or conventional care.[1] The NHS was conducted on 1754 terminal patients selected in 40 hospices distributed nationally and 14 conventional cancer care settings. Patients had to have cancer, have a primary care person to help care for them, and have a life expectancy of 6 months or less. Patients and their caregivers were interviewed biweekly regarding the patient's condition, symptoms, and services provided. The last interview occurred, on average, 7 days prior to death, the second to last interview occurred about 21 days before death and the third to last interview occurred 35–42 days before death. Patient's experiences of symptoms were measured using a modified set of questions from Melzack.[29] If the patient were unable to respond to the interview, the caregiver was asked whether the symptom had occurred, although not about how severe it was.[63]

In the past, the data from Parkes comparing pain control at home, in hospital and in hospice in a specific area of the city of London had been based on the memories of a patient's surviving relative. Parkes concluded that pain control in the hospital was equivalent to that obtained in hospice in the 1977–1979 period, whereas 10 years prior to that time the same symptom was better controlled in hospice. In both study periods, the symptom of pain as recalled by the relatives was more severe at home than in a care-giving structure. The percentage of relatives reporting very high levels of anxiety was much higher when the patient had been hospital- or home-assisted compared to when the patient died in hospice. This last result was entirely similar in the two studies conducted 10 years apart.[64]

In another study conducted in 1974–1976, 51 patients who had been cared for by the home care team from St. Christopher's hospice were compared with 51 who had spent time at home during the terminal period but had not received help from the hospice. No significant differences in the incidence of physical and emotional distress were found between the two groups. The length of time that each group spent in hospital during the terminal phase was different in the two groups: 2.6 weeks for patients receiving home care from the hospice, and 5.6 for the other group.[65]

A study conducted by Ventafridda et al. compared home assistance and hospital assistance based on clinical, psychosocial, and economic parameters. The results obtained from two populations of 30 patients each did not show any statistically significant difference regarding pain control, the number of symptoms, or the number of sleeping hours.[66]

Dunphy and Amesbury reviewed all patients cared for by St Joseph's Hospice, London, in the hospice or in home care during 6 months. The average length of time from initial involvement to death was 21.75 days for the hospice group and 40.5 days for the home care group. About the clinical symptoms experienced by the two groups at referral, there was a higher than expected prevalence of both dyspnea and anxiety or depression among the home care group, but the proportion of patients experiencing individual symptoms in both groups was similar.[67]

Symptom Assessment in the Last Phases of Life

The last days of life have been often considered a critical period for palliative care and a time when good palliative care is felt to be particularly necessary. In this period, therefore, the need to document the quality of symptom control in different settings of care is particularly acute although difficult as already mentioned above.

The National Hospice Study (NHS) reported that pain was more prevalent in the last weeks of life and the percentage of patients with persistent or severe pain increased within 2 days of death compared to the previous 6 days.[68] Using the same data, Reuben evidenced an increasing prevalence of dyspnea in the last 6 week of life and 64% in the week before death.[69] In the NHS, 50% of patients were incapable of responding 2 weeks before death, whereas this occurred in 80% of cases 1 week before death. In these cases, data were collected by the caregiver.

Ventafridda et al. evaluated the symptoms of 120 terminal cancer patients assisted by a home care team until death for an average of 41 days, with the aim to document how long before death symptoms appear that patients term unendurable. They observed the presence of unendurable symptoms in 52% of patients on an average of 2 days before death, the most common symptoms being dyspnea, pain, delirium, and vomiting. The intensity of symptoms was assessed by an endurable/unendurable dichotomous category as reported by the patients.[70]

Fainsinger et al. demonstrated that patients in a palliative care unit gradually reduced their compliance with twice daily visual analogue score measures for pain, activity, nausea, drowsiness, appetite, sensation of well-being, depression, and anxiety as their disease progressed. On the day of referral 69% of the VAS were completed by the patient and 28% by the nurse, on the day of death only 8% of the VAS were completed by the patient.[12]

Coyle et al. evaluated the prevalence of symptoms during the last 4 weeks of life of 90 patients who had been followed by their Supportive Care Program. At 4 weeks before death, 71% of patients experienced three or more symptoms and fatigue, weakness, sleepiness, and cognitive impairment were the most common. In the last week sleepiness increased from 24% to 57%, and dyspnea increased from 17% to 28%.[11]

Conclusions

Available data indicate that palliative home care is feasible and that the outcome in terms of symptom control is similar to that of in-hospice care and of conventional care. Family anxiety and emotional burden are more pronounced at home and this aspect should receive more attention by home care programs. The savings of state financial resources in promoting palliative home care has to be balanced with the family, financial, and social resources that are used instead. Anyhow, the offer of special home care must strive for an improvement in home care quality and for documenting its outcomes in terms of symptom control, so as to define the indications and limitations of this kind of palliative care.

Another aspect requiring special attention is the choice of assessment methods in research, considering that here evaluations become more complex. This is a very important issue, because only its development can guarantee improvement of the care models, although we know that they are not indicated for terminal patient conditions, especially during the terminal phases of life.

Assessment of the terminal patient for clinical purposes must be very simple and must foresee the possibility of exploiting the leader relative in the home care setting.

It is obviously very difficult to produce instruments useful in this sense, and the current lack of validated assessment instruments is an indication of this situation.

This is where future efforts should be channeled, and represents one of the many challenges for palliative care.

References

1. Greer D, Mor V, Morris J, Sherwood S, Kidder D, Birnbaum H. An alternative in terminal care: results of the National Hospice Study. *J Chron Dis* 1986; 39:9–26.
2. Hinton J. Comparison of places and policies for terminal care. *Lancet* 1979:29–32.
3. Costantini M, Camoirano E, Madeddu L, Bruzzi P, Verganelli E, Henriquet F. Palliative home care and place of death among cancer patients: a population-based study. *Palliat Med* 1993; 7:323–331.
4. Ventafridda V. Continuing care: a major issue in cancer pain management. *Pain* 1989; 36:137–143.

5. Hearn J, Higginson I. Outcome measures in palliative care for advanced cancer patients: a review. *J Public Health Med* 1997; 19:193–199.

6. De Conno F, Caraceni A, Groff L, et al. Effect of home care on the place of death of advanced cancer patients. *Eur J Cancer* 1996; 32A:1142–1147.

7. Doyle D. Symptom relief in terminal illness. Medicine in Practice 1983; 1:694–698.

8. Baines M. Nausea and vomiting in the patient with advanced cancer. *J Pain Symptom Manag* 1988; 3:81–85.

9. Reuben DB, Mor V, Hiris J. Clinical symptoms and length of survival in patients with terminal cancer. *Arch Int Med* 1988; 148:1586–1591.

10. Ventafridda V, DeConno F, Ripamonti C, Gamba A, Tamburini M. Quality of life assessment during a palliative care program. *Ann Oncol* 1990; 1:415–420.

11. Coyle N, Adelhardt J, Foley KM, Portenoy RK. Character of terminal illness in the advanced cancer patient: pain and other symptoms during last four weeks of life. *J Pain and Symp Manage* 1990; 5:83–89.

12. Fainsinger R, Miller MJ, Bruera E, Hanson J, MacEachern T. Symptom control during the last week of life on a palliative care unit. *J Palliat Care* 1991; 7:5–11.

13. Donnelly S, Walsh D. The symptoms of advanced cancer. *Semin Clin Oncol* 1995; 22:67–72.

14. Portenoy R, Thaler H, Kornblith A, et al. Symptom prevalence, characteristics and distress in a cancer population. *Qual Life Res* 1994; 3:183–189.

15. Portenoy RK. Cancer pain: epidemiology and syndromes. *Cancer* 1989; 63:2298–2307.

16. Smets EMA, Garssen B, Schuster-Uitterhoeve ALJ, de Haes JCJM. Fatigue in cancer patients. *Br J Cancer* 1993; 68:220–224.

17. Bruera E, MacDonald R. Asthenia in patient with advanced cancer. *J Pain Symp Manage* 1988; 3:9–14.

18. Walsh T, Saunders C. Hospice care: the treatment of pain in advanced cancer. *Rec Results Cancer Res* 1984; 89:201–211.

19. Maltoni M, Pirovano M, Scarpi E, et al. Prediction of survival in patients terminally ill with cancer. *Cancer* 1995; 75:2613–2623.

20. Derogatis LR, Morrow GR, Fetting J, Penman D, Piasetsky S, Schmale AM. The prevalence of psychiatric disorders among cancer patients. *J AMA* 1983; 249:751–757.

21. Breitbart W, Bruera E, Chochinov H, Lynch M. Neuropsychiatric syndromes and psychological symptoms in patients with advanced cancer. *J Pain Symp Manage* 1995; 10:131–141.

22. Ingham J, Portenoy R. Cachexia in context: the interaction among anorexia, pain, and other symptoms. In: Bruera E, Higginson I, eds. *Cachexia-Anorexia in Cancer Patients*. New York: Oxford University Press, 1996:158–171.

23. Grossman SA, Sheidler VR, Swedeen K, Mucenski J, Piantadosi S. Correlation of patient and caregiver ratings of cancer pain. *J Pain Symp Manage* 1991; 6:53–57.

24. Clipp EC, George LK. Patients with cancer and their spouse caregivers. Perceptions of the illness experience. *Cancer* 1992; 69:1074–1079.

25. Higginson I, Priest P, McCarthy M. Are bereaved family members a valid proxy for a patient's assessment of dying? *Soc Sci Med* 1994; 38:553–557.

26. Peruselli C, Camporesi E, Colombo AM, et al. Nursing care planning for terminally ill cancer patients receiving home care. *J Palliat Care* 1992; 8:4–7.

27. Ingham J, Portenoy R. The measurement of pain and other symptoms. In: Doyle D, Hanks GWC, MacDonald N, eds. *Oxford Textbook of Palliative Medicine*. 2nd Edition. Oxford: Oxford University Press, 1998:203–219.

28. Daut RL, Cleeland CS, Flanery RC. Development of the Wisconsin Brief Pain Questionnaire to assess pain in cancer and other diseases. *Pain* 1983; 17:197–210.

29. Melzack R. The McGill pain questionnaire: Major properties and scoring methods. *Pain* 1975; 1:277–299.

30. Graham C, Bond S, Gerkovich M, et al. Use of the McGill Pain Questionnaire in the assessment of cancer pain: replicability and consistency. *Pain* 1980; 8:377–387.

31. Melzack R. The short-form McGill Pain Questionnaire. *Pain* 1987; 30:191–197.

32. Fletcher C, Elmes P, Fairbairn A, Wood C. The significance of respiratory symptoms and the diagnosis of chronic bronchitis in a working population. *BMJ* 1959; 2:257–266.

33. Guyatt G, Thompson P, Berman L, et al. How should we measure function in patients with chronic lung disease? *J Chronic Dis* 1985; 38:517–524.

34. Guyatt G, Berman L, Townsend M, et al. A measure of quality of life for clinical trials in chronic lung disease. *Thorax* 1987; 42:773–778.

35. Wijkstra P, Ten Vergert E, Van Altena R, et al. Reliability and validity of the chronic respiratory questionnaire. *Thorax* 1994; 49:465–467.

36. Borg G. Perceived exertion as an indicator of somatic stress. *Scand J Rehabil Med* 1970; 2:92–98.

37. McGavin C, Artvinli M, Naoe H, McHardy G. Dyspnea, disability, and distance walked: comparison of estimates of exercise performance in respiratory disease. *BMJ* 1978; 2:241–243.

38. Mahler D, Weinberg D, Wells C, et al. The measurement of dyspnea: contents, inter-observer agreement, and physiologic correlates of two new clinical indexes. *Chest* 1984; 85:751–758.

39. Ripamonti C, Bruera E. Dyspnea: pathophysioloy and assessment. *J Pain Symp Manage* 1997; 13:220–232.

40. Piper B, Lindsey A, Dodd M, et al. The development of an instrument to measure the subjective dimensionof fatigue. In: Funk S, Tornquist E, Champange M, Gopp L, Wiese C, eds. *Key Aspects of Comfort. Management of Pain Fatigue and Nausea*. New York: Springer Publishing, 1989:199–208.

41. Lee K, Hicks G, Nino-Murcia G. Validity and reliability of a scale to assess fatigue. Psychiatric Research 1991; 36:291–298.

42. Kaasa T, Loomis J, Gillis K, Bruera E, Hanson J. The Edmonton Functional Assessment Tool: preliminary development and evaluation for use in palliative care. *J Pain Symp Manage* 1997; 13:10–19.

43. Reuben D, Mor V. Nausea and vomiting in terminal cancer patients. *Arch Intern Med* 1983; 146:2021–2023.

44. Morrow G. The assessment of nausea and vomiting. Past problems, current issues, and suggestions for future research. *Cancer* 1984; 53:2267–2278.

45. Melzack R. Measurement of nausea. *J Pain Symp Manage* 1989; 4:157–160.

46. Folstein M, Folstein S, McHugh P. Mini-mental state. *J Psychiatr Res* 1975; 12:189–198.

47. Katzman R, Brown T, Fuld P, Peck A, Schechter R, Schimmel H. Validation of a short orientation-memory-concentration test of cognitive impairment. *Am J Psychiatry* 1983; 140:734–739.

48. Inouye SK, van Dyck CH, Alessi CA, Balkin S, Siegal AP, Horwitz RI. Clarifying confusion: the confusion assessment method. A new method for detection of delirium. *Ann Intern Med* 1990; 113:941–948.
49. Trzepacz PT, Baker RW, Greenhouse J. A symptom rating scale for delirium. *J Psychiatry Res* 1988; 23:89–97.
50. Albert MS, Levkoff SE, Reilly CR, et al. The delirium symptom interview: an interview for the detection of delirium symtoms in hospitalized patients. *J Geriatr Psychiatry Neurol* 1992; 5:14–21.
51. Bruera E, Kuehn N, Miller MJ, Selmser P, Macmillan K. The Edmonton Symptom Assessment System (ESAS): a simple method for the assessment of palliative care patients. *J Palliat Care* 1991; 7:6–9.
52. McCorkle R, Young K. Development of a symptom distress scale. *Cancer Nurs* 1978; 1:373–378.
53. de Haes J, van Knippenberg F, Neijt J. Measuring psychological and physical distress in cancer patients: structure and application of the Rotterdam Symptom Checklist. *Br J Cancer* 1990; 62:1034–1038.
54. Aaronson NK, Ahmedzai S, Bergman B, et al. The European Organization for Research and Treatment of Cancer QLQ-C30: a quality-of-life instrument for use in international clinical trials in oncology. *J Natl Cancer Inst* 1993; 85:365–776.
55. Portenoy R, Thaler HT, Kornblith AB, et al. The Memorial Symptom Assessment Scale: an instrument for the evaluation of symptom prevalence, characteristics and distress. *Euro J Cancer* 1994; 30A(9):1:1326–1336.
56. Tamburini M, Rosso S, Gamba A, Mencaglia E, De Conno F, Ventafridda V. A therapy impact questionnaire for quality-of-life assessment in advanced cancer research. *Ann Oncol* 1992; 3:565–570.
57. Higginson IJ, McCarthy M. Validity of the support team assessment schedule: do staffs' ratings reflect those made by patients or their families? *Palliat Med* 1993; 7:219–228.
58. Peruselli C, Paci E, Franceschi P, Legori T, Mannucci F. Outcome evaluation in a home palliative care service. *J Pain Symp Manage* 1997; 13:158–165.
59. Higginson I, McCarthy M. Measuring symptoms in terminal cancer: are pain and dyspnoea controlled? *J R Soc Med* 1989; 82:264–267.
60. Mercadante S, Genovese G, Kargar J, et al. Home palliative care: results in 1991 versus 1988. *J Pain Symp Manage* 1992; 7:414–418.
61. Edmonds P, Stuttaford J, Penny J, Lynch A, Chamberlain J. Do hospital palliative care teams improve symptom control? Use of a modified STAS as an evaluation tool. *Palliat Med* 1998; 12:345–351.
62. Kane RL, Wales J, Bernstein L, Leibowitz A, Kaplan S. A randomised controlled trial of hospice care. *Lancet* 1984; 1:890–894.
63. Greer D, Mor V, Sherwood S, Morris J, Birnbaum H. National hospice study analysis plan. *J Chron Dis* 1983; 36:737–780.
64. Parkes CM. Terminal care: home, hospital, or hospice? *Lancet* 1985; 1:155–157.
65. Parkes CM. Terminal care: evaluation of an advisory domiciliary service at St Christopher's Hospice. *Postgrad Med J* 1980; 56:685–689.
66. Ventafridda V, De Conno F, Vigano A, Ripamonti C, Gallucci M, Gamba A. Comparison of home and hospital care of advanced cancer patients. *Tumori* 1989; 75:619–625.

67. Dunphy K, Amesbury B. A comparison of hospice and homecare patients: patterns of refferal, patient characteristics and predictors on place of death. *Palliat Med* 1990; 4:105–111.

68. Morris JN, Mor V, Goldberg RJ, Sherwood S, Greer DS, Hiris J. The effect of treatment setting and patient characteristics on pain in terminal cancer patients: a report from the national hospice setting. *J Chron Dis* 1986; 39:27–35.

69. Reuben DB, Mor V. Dyspnea in terminally ill cancer patients. Chest 1986; 89:234–236.

70. Ventafridda V, Ripamonti C, De Conno F, Tamburini M, Cassileth BR. Symptom prevalence and control during cancer patients' last days of life. *J Palliat Care* 1990; 6:7–11.

V

OPIOID TOLERANCE: REALITY OR MYTH?

13

Opioid Tolerance: A Clinical Perspective

LEIA PHIOANH NGHIEMPHU AND
RUSSELL K. PORTENOY

Although opioids play a central role in the treatment of chronic pain, under-treatment continues to be common. In part, undertreatment can be traced to persistent fears and misconceptions about opioid properties, such as tolerance. To optimize the use of these drugs, the mechanisms and clinical relevance of tolerance must be understood. The disparities between experimental research and clinical observations must be highlighted and can help inform future research.

Definition of Tolerance and Related Terminology

The term *tolerance* is a part of a nomenclature applied to opioids, which also includes terms such as physical dependence and addiction. These labels imply very diverse processes. This terminology must be appropriately defined for opioid-treated patients with pain (Table 13.1).

Tolerance

Tolerance refers to the diminishing effect of a drug after repeated exposure, or requirement of a higher dose to maintain the same effect.[1] The term is similarly defined by the World Health Organization[2] as a "decrease in response to a drug dose that occurs with continued use."

Both physical and psychological factors can contribute to tolerance.[2] Tolerance can be regarded as associative or nonassociative based on these factors. Associative tolerance refers to reduced drug effectiveness as a result of a learned behavior, such as operant conditioning. Nonassociative, or pharmacological, tolerance is independent of learning and relates to the physiological changes

Table 13.1. Definitions of nomenclature

Tolerance	Decreased drug effect after repeated exposure, requiring increased dose for same effect.
Associative	Tolerance as a result of a learned behavior, such as operant conditioning.
Nonassociative	Tolerance from pharmacological processes of the drug, also known as pharmacological tolerance.
Dispositional	Tolerance as a result of drug redistribution or metabolism, also known as pharmacokinetic tolerance.
Pharmacodynamic	Tolerance from adaptive changes in the neural system.
Physical dependence	Development of withdrawal symptoms upon cessation of drug use.
Addiction	A psychological and behavioral syndrome characterized by loss of control over drug use, compulsive use, and continual use despite harm; from the clinical perspective, therapy is characterized by aberrant drug-related behaviors.

induced by the drug. Nonassociative tolerance can be dispositional (i.e., pharmacokinetic) or pharmacodynamic. Dispositional tolerance would occur, for example, if repeated exposure to a drug caused an increase in metabolism or elimination, thereby lowering the drug concentration in the blood at the sites of action. In contrast, pharmacodynamic tolerance follows adaptive changes in the nervous system, such as changes at the receptor level, that change the sensitivity of the system to the drug.

For opioids, dispositional tolerance does not exist[3] and pharmacodynamic tolerance, which has been demonstrated in numerous animal models,[4-6] predominates. Associative tolerance also has been demonstrated in animal models.[7] It can be inferred that similar processes also occur in humans, and the need for increasing doses of opioids to maintain the same analgesic effect could be related to learning and to changes in the central nervous system.

Given the complexity of opioid dosing in the clinical situation, tolerance may be a problematic term when used to describe the need for a dose increase during the course of treatment with an opioid. Unfortunately, clinicians often label any patient tolerant whenever dose escalation is required to maintain analgesia. This usage ignores the fact that declining effects might not be attributable to either associative or nonassociative tolerance, but rather to other causes (Table 13.2).[8] Clinical observation, particularly in the population with cancer pain, suggests that a decreasing drug effect usually occurs because of increased pain associated with worsening pathology. For example, progression of a mass lesion, increasing inflammation, or the development of new pathophysiology that is relatively less opioid responsive could produce an increase in pain. Psychological processes can also influence the perception of pain, and changes in affect (e.g., anxiety or depression), or changes in cognitive states (causing altered pain reporting or shifts in the meaning attached to the pain or the responses of significant others) could be involved as well.

Table 13.2. Differential diagnosis for declining analgesic effects in the clinical setting

---

Increased activity in nociceptive pathways
   Increased activation of peripheral nociceptive pathways from
      Mechanical factors (e.g., tumor growth)
      Biochemical changes (e.g., inflammation)
      Peripheral neuropathic processes (e.g., neuroma formation)
   Increased activity in central nociceptive pathways from
      Central neuropathic processes (e.g., sensitization, shift in receptive fields, change in
modulatory processes)

Psychological processes
   Increasing psychological distress
   Change in cognitive state leading to altered pain perception or reporting (e.g., delirium)
   Conditioned pain behavior independent of the drug

Tolerance
   Pharmacodynamic processes
   Pharmacokinetic processes
   Psychological processes

Source: Adapted from Portenoy, 1994.[8]

Even though it is reasonable to speculate that pharmacodynamic tolerance to analgesic effects also could contribute to the need for dose escalation, the phenomenon should not be labeled tolerance without considering this differential diagnosis for worsening pain. If an alternative cause cannot be found, then it is possible that the decline in drug effect is caused solely by associative or pharmacodynamic tolerance. Stated in another way, pharmacodynamic tolerance cannot be assumed to be the driving force for dose escalation unless there is concurrent stability in the patient's baseline physical and psychological condition. Of course, there can be no direct proof of the neural changes that presumably cause tolerance in the patient, but the inference is reasonable under these conditions.

In the clinical setting, the term tolerance is often used in a manner that implies a negative outcome. Although tolerance to analgesic effects is indeed a concern, the phenomenon actually applies to all effects, including the undesirable, nonanalgesic effects of opioids such as respiratory depression, somnolence, and nausea.[9] Development of tolerance to these effects can open the therapeutic window and allow an increased range for dose titration. The rapid development of tolerance to some adverse effects, particularly respiratory depression and nausea, appears to be very common and greatly increases the proportion of patients who can benefit from opioids.

Physical dependence

Physical dependence and tolerance are physiologically related and misconceptions characterize both phenomena. In the addiction literature, for example, both

Table 13.3. Signs and symptoms of opioid abstinence in addicts

Signs	Symptoms
Hypertension	Pain (abdominal cramps, myalgia, allodynia)
Tachycardia	Dysphoria (fear, anger)
Tachypnea	Insomnia
Hyperthermia	Craving for opioids
Diarrhea	Nausea
Pupillary dilatation	Anxiety
Rhinorrhea	
Chills	
Vomiting	

Source: Adapted from Portenoy, 1994.[8]

tolerance and physical dependence are viewed as necessary for the development of addiction: tolerance would necessitate higher doses to maintain euphoric effects, while conditioned avoidance of withdrawal symptoms further sustains aberrant behavior.[10] Although this perspective has been included in the *Diagnostic and Statistical Manual, 4th Ed (DSM-IV) of the American Psychiatric Association*,[11] it is not appropriate for a definition of addiction relevant to patients with pain, as discussed in the next paragraphs.

Physical dependence is a physiological state characterized by withdrawal, or abstinence syndrome, after abrupt dose reduction, discontinuation of the opioid, or administration of an antagonist drug.[1] This condition has been studied extensively in both animals[12-14] and humans.[14-21] Abstinence symptoms are diverse (Table 13.3)[8,18,20] and the specific manifestations and the intensity of each symptom cannot be predicted in humans. Some patients experience a range of uncomfortable symptoms, whereas others experience just one or two. Some patients are so sensitive to withdrawal that they experience discomfort between opioid doses, whereas others remain entirely asymptomatic even if high dose therapy ceases altogether.

Both animal models and in vitro preparations suggest that the mechanisms for tolerance and physical dependence are interrelated.[22,23] In the clinical setting, however, these processes may or may not coexist to the same extent in individual patients. Although patients who are receiving relatively high doses are most likely to be both physically dependent and tolerant to at least some of the effects of opioids, this observation indicates only that the mechanisms for both of these phenomena are dose-related. In the absence of evidence in humans that links the physiology of physical dependence and tolerance, the two terms should be applied to distinct clinical phenomena.

Addiction

Clinicians tend to confuse physical dependence with addiction, mislabeling patients who have the potential for abstinence as addicts. This is a serious error, which stigmatizes patients and does not help clarify the defining characteristics of addiction. Tolerance and physical dependence do not imply addiction. The disease of addiction implies the loss of control over drug use, compulsive use, and persistent use despite harm.[1,9,24,25] Addiction is not an inherent property of opioids. Rather, it is a biopsychosocial phenomenon in which access to a potentially abusable drug leads a predisposed person to engage in a maladaptive pattern of use. To decrease the stigma associated with opioids and avoid patient distress, the distinction between physical dependence and addiction must be recognized[26] and the difficulty that may be involved in diagnosing addiction when the drug is a licit medicine given for an appropriate target symptom must be acknowledged.[24,27]

Basic Research Relevant to Opioid Tolerance

Experimental models have clarified the factors that may affect the development of both associative and nonassociative tolerance.[7] These factors include duration of drug exposure and dose, receptor selectivity of the drug, genetic make-up, and pain mechanism.[5,14,20,22,23,28–37]

Most studies have concentrated on pharmacodynamic opioid tolerance. A large number of investigations using in vivo and in vitro assays have established that tolerance can develop after acute dosing or accrue more gradually with repeated dosing, and that different opioid effects manifest tolerance at varying rates.[38,39] They have confirmed that pharmacodynamic processes make up most of nonassociative tolerance[18] and that the process is highly dose-dependent.[28,39,40] Further, these studies have observed that the rate of tolerance development can vary with different drugs, dosing schedules, routes of administration, and study paradigms.[5,37,41]

Studies of cross-tolerance among opioids have revealed that differences in intrinsic efficacy also play a role in the development of tolerance. In several animal models, intrinsic efficacy closely predicted both the pattern of tolerance to antinociceptive effects and the degree of cross-tolerance conferred by alternative opioid drugs.[6,40,42–45]

Drug-selective differences may relate to variations in drug-receptor interactions. A μ-receptor agonist induces minimal tolerance at κ and δ receptors.[46] In rats previously treated with levorphanol, a μ and κ receptor agonist, significant cross-tolerance developed to the μ agonist, morphine, whereas rats infused with morphine developed less cross-tolerance to levorphanol.[47] It is also possible that one receptor might influence the efficacy of a drug at another receptor site. For

example, a κ-opioid agonist has been shown to block the development of tolerance to morphine,[48,49] and the δ-receptor antagonist naltrindole inhibits tolerance and dependence to morphine in mice.[50] Receptor-selective interactions also
seem to affect abstinence phenomena.[51-53]

Variations in drug-receptor interaction are, in part, related to genetic differences in sensitivity.[54-55] In a recent study, different strains of rats had significantly
different sensitivity and rate of development of tolerance and dependence to
morphine.[56] Presumably, different species, or even strains within a single species,
can express different densities of receptor subtypes or have different affinities to
opioid receptors. This genetic variability may also explain the different responses
to opioids seen in humans.[57]

Nociception also might influence the development of analgesic tolerance. Rats with adjuvant-induced arthritis self-administered less morphine
overall than rats without a nociceptive lesion.[58] It is possible that this tolerance is receptor-selective. Different nociceptive stimuli (cutaneous thermal
versus visceral chemical)[59] and a model of neuropathic pain[60] respond in distinct
ways to drugs that bind the various opioid receptor subtypes. The degree to
which this receptor-selectivity affects the influence of nociception on tolerance
is unknown.

The mechanisms responsible for receptor-selective pharmacodynamic tolerance are presumably diverse. Among the possibilities are (1) a down-regulation
or decrease in number of opioid receptors, (2) uncoupling of the receptor from
its second messenger systems, especially the cyclic adenosine monophosphate
(cAMP) pathways, and (3) upregulation or activation of parallel systems.

In vitro studies have shown that the development of tolerance occurs in con-
junction with receptor desensitization after exposure to μ-opioid agonists,[61-63] but
not with change in the density of receptors.[29] Exposure to exogenous opioids also
can cause changes in endogenous opioid peptides, which might itself affect
receptors.[64] Changes in basal levels of endogenous peptides may also be a factor
in the development of abstinence syndrome following withdrawal of exogenous
opioids.[22] Although these observations suggest a direct role of the endogenous
peptides and receptor change in the development of tolerance, this has not been
consistently supported,[33] and more emphasis has been given to the other potential mechanisms.

Functional decoupling of opioid receptors from second messenger systems
appears to be an important mechanism. Binding of opioids to their receptors
activates a cascade of events via G-protein linkage to second messenger systems,
such as adenylate cyclase/cAMP, with subsequent activation of calcium-
dependent protein kinases such as protein kinase A (PKA) or protein kinase C
(PKC).[32] Uncoupling from G proteins could inhibit cell function,[29,65,66] possibly
through phosphorylation of the receptors or G protein subunits.[33] The system
directly involving PKC has been implicated in development of opioid tolerance.[67]
Changes in other steps along the second messenger pathways may also be
involved.[68]

The activation of parallel systems might also be involved. Binding of excitatory amino acids (EAA), such as glutamate, to the N-methyl-D-aspartate (NMDA) receptor, for example, causes a number of intracellular events, including increased PKC, that secondarily affect the sensitivity of the μ receptor.[69,70] Studies in animal models observed that noncompetitive and competitive NMDA antagonists, such as MK801, LY274614 and dextromethorphan, can reduce or prevent morphine tolerance.[69,71–75]

N-methyl-D-aspartate receptor activation also leads to release of nitric oxide, which might also play a role in the development of tolerance. Nitric oxide synthase (NOS) inhibitors such as NG-nitro-L-arginine can also block morphine tolerance in an animal model.[71,72,76] Similar results are not produced when the opioid agonist is κ-selective,[72,34] pointing to separate mechanisms of tolerance among different receptor subtypes.

Clinical Investigations and Observations

Unlike the extensive research on opioid tolerance in animals, few studies have specially addressed the development of tolerance in humans. One study suggested that acute tolerance, like that observed in animals, can also occur in humans.[77] This potential for rapid changes has also been suggested by studies of physical dependence in opioid addicts in recovery.[16,17] These observations were not supported, however, by a pharmacokinetic–pharmacodynamic study of methadone, in which brief infusions of methadone were given to patients with chronic cancer pain who had previously received chronic opioids.[78] Analysis of plasma concentration and analgesia during and after the infusion did not demonstrate a clockwise hysteresis, suggesting that acute tolerance, or any other process that would lessen analgesic efficacy during this brief period, did not occur. Given the limited data available, the likelihood and importance of acute opioid tolerance remains unproven.

A few other studies evaluated the development of tolerance after more prolonged administration of opioids. The most systematic of these studies have been performed in subjects without pain, specifically post-addicts who received opioids in a monitored inpatient setting for weeks or months.[18,20] In a group of studies, subjects were closely monitored for changes in vital signs, pupillary diameter, and psychological functions as they were given gradually increasing dosages of morphine for 5 weeks. They were maintained on 240 mg daily for 7 months, then tapered off morphine and monitored for several more months. These studies demonstrated that tolerance to the different opioid side effects develops at different rates and with great variability among individuals.

In a controlled study of patients with cancer pain, Houde and colleagues[79] evaluated the analgesic effects of graded single doses of morphine in 10 patients, before and after 2 weeks of regular morphine therapy. A shift to the right in the dose-response curve suggested that tolerance developed to the analgesic effects of morphine during this period. Another study by the same investigators compared morphine and metapon in 13 patients before and after 1 week of regular dosing with either drug.[80] Again, a rightward shift was demonstrated in the dose-response relationships for both drugs. The latter study also demonstrated the occurrence of cross-tolerance between these drugs, which occurred less rapidly and less completely than direct tolerance.

Although these limited clinical investigations suggest that some of the processes observed in experimental animal models also occur in humans, they are limited and do not adequately explain the range of reactions observed in clinical practice. Unlike the rapid development of tolerance to analgesic effects produced in animals,[4,5,45] most patients receiving chronic opioid treatment maintain a stable dose for long periods of time, with continued analgesia.[30,81-95]

The need for dose escalation may occur periodically during opioid treatment, however, and some patients even need continuously increasing doses to maintain analgesia. Usually, this need to increase the dose does not compromise the ability to have adequate analgesia.[28,96] Furthermore, the need for dose escalation usually relates to an identifiable process that could cause increasing pain, such as heightened nociceptive input from a worsening physical lesion.[91,97,98] The existence of a disease process in patients in pain thus complicates the effort to ascribe the need for dose escalation to tolerance. Although tolerance may contribute to declining efficacy, it cannot be said to be the predominating process if alternative reasons for escalating pain can be identified.

In clinical practice, opioid doses usually can be increased gradually with limited risk of most adverse effects, including respiratory depression and somnolence. Indeed, opioid doses have been known to reach extraordinary levels, many tens of thousands of morphine equivalent milligrams per day, without adverse results.[99] This observation confirms that pharmacodynamic tolerance to the adverse effects of opioids does occur. These effects are favorable and have mechanisms that are obscure. Ongoing pain also may be involved in the ability to tolerate dose escalation, but this process, like others involved in tolerance, is not understood.

Another observation in clinical practice is that opioid doses can be reduced dramatically with the effective use of a nonopioid analgesic method. For example, procedures such as nerve blocks or cordotomy reduce nociceptive afferent input and can allow prompt reduction in the opioid required to treat residual pain.[91,100] Similar findings occurred in delirious cancer patients who were given high doses for their crescendo pain; once the delirium improved from co-administration of a neuroleptic, the patients could be managed on much lower doses.[101] The ability to reduce the dose while maintaining effectiveness appears to indicate that analgesic tolerance had not occurred to the higher doses that were given before the nonanalgesic intervention was applied. It is also possible that analgesic tolerance did occur and quickly reversed once other factors contributing to pain were removed. Again, these observations support a possible relationship of pain or pain-related factors to changes in opioid response.

Abrupt reduction of nociceptive input via a procedure such as cordotomy can also result in development of adverse opioid effects that were not present prior to the procedure. This event would be unexpected if tolerance had occurred to the adverse effect. This observation again supports the importance of pain in the relationship between dose and response. Perhaps pain acts as an antagonist to the respiratory depressant effects of opioids via nociceptive input to the respiratory center in the medulla.[28] The ability to tolerate opioid dose escalation is, therefore, not an outcome of pharmacodynamic tolerance to adverse effects alone, but is rather likely to be some combination of nociceptive and tolerance mechanisms.

These clinical observations have not been investigated under controlled conditions. Presumably, analgesic tolerance does occur and contributes to the need for increasing dosages. Tolerance should not be viewed as an unimportant aspect of opioid treatment. Possibly, analgesic tolerance is more relevant in defining the dose-response relationship at the beginning of opioid treatment and it is also likely that patients differ vastly in their tendency to develop tolerance to analgesic and nonanalgesic effects. The few available observations must be generalized with caution.

Recent studies have begun to evaluate the combination of an opioid and an NMDA receptor antagonist in the hope that this formulation will provide synergy and, perhaps, reduce analgesic tolerance. The majority of these studies use either ketamine or dextromethorphan in combination with an opioid agonist.[70,102,103] Although these studies provide evidence that NMDA receptor blockade does potentiate analgesia, the extent to which the outcome relates to a change in tolerance remains to be investigated. Long-term studies that evaluate the need for dose escalation over time with these combinations are awaited.

Conclusion

From the clinical perspective, there is yet no unifying perspective on opioid tolerance. It is difficult to apply the findings in the laboratory and in pain-free patients to patients undergoing opioid treatment for pain, and the difficulty is compounded by the variability of response to opioids.

Clinical observations have become the main source of data for the development of guidelines for patient care. From these observations, several implications should be emphasized. First, tolerance to the analgesic effects of opioids rarely limits the course of pain treatment, and early administration of an opioid drug should be implemented as necessary. Second, tolerance presumably occurs to adverse effects and is a favorable phenomenon, widening the therapeutic window and creating a more favorable balance between analgesia and side effects. Third, tolerance should not be assumed to be the cause when a patient on a stable opioid dose begins to have increasing pain. The patient should always be evaluated for a change in pathology. Treatment with opioid drugs requires close follow-up, with repeated dose titration over time in an effort to maintain the optimal balance between analgesia and side effects. Fourth, tolerance is not a major element in a clinically relevant definition of addiction.

As more is learned about tolerance, basic and clinical research are needed to clarify the importance of tolerance in patient care and the strategies that might be used to prevent tolerance and improve the balance between analgesia and side effects. Additional studies are needed to evaluate the multiple opioid effects and the effect of chronic pain on opioid tolerance.

References

1. Jaffe JH. Drug addiction and drug abuse. In: Gilman AG, Goodman LS, Rall TW, Murad F, eds. *The Pharmacological Basis of Therapeutics, 7th ed.* New York: Macmillan, 1985:532–581.
2. World Health Organization. *Lexicon of Alcohol and Drug Terms.* Geneva: World Health Organization, 1994.
3. Jasinski DR. Tolerance and dependence to opiates. *Acta Anaethesiol Scand* 1997; 41:184–186.
4. Cochin J, Kometsky C. Development and loss of tolerance to morphine in the rat after single and multiple injections. *J Pharmacol Exp Ther* 1964; 1455:1–20.
5. Yaksh TL. Tolerance: factors involved in changes in the dose-effect relationship with chronic drug exposure. In: Basbaum AI, Besson JM, eds. *Towards a New Pharmacotherapy of Pain.* Chichester: John Wiley and Sons, 1991:157–180.
6. Sosnowski M, Yaksh TL. Differential cross-tolerance between intrathecal morphine and sufentil in the rat. *Anesthesiology* 1990; 73:1141–1147.
7. Tiffany ST, Maude-Griffen PM. Tolerance to morphine in the rat: associative and nonassociative effect. *Behav Neurosci* 1988; 102:534–543.
8. Portenoy RK. Opioid tolerance and responsiveness: research findings and clinical observations. In: Gebhart GF, Hammond DL, Jensen TS, eds. Proceedings of the 7th World Congress on Pain. *Progress in Pain Research and Management, vol. 2.* Seattle: IASP Press, 1994:595–619.
9. Zuckerman LA, Ferrante FM. Nonopioid and opioid analgesics. In: Ashburn MA, Rice LJ, eds. *The Management of Pain.* New York: Churchill Livingstone: New York, 1998:110–140.
10. Wikler A. *Opioid Dependence: Mechanisms and Treatment.* New York: Plenum Press, 1980.
11. American Psychiatric Association. *Diagnostic and Statistical Manual of Mental Disorders (DSM-IV).* American Psychiatric Association: Washington, DC, 1994.
12. Domino EF, Dahlstrom BE, Domino LE, et al. Relation of plasma morphine concentrations to severity of abrupt withdrawal in morphine-dependent monkeys. *J Pharmacol Exp Ther* 1987; 243:138–143.
13. Martin WR, Eades CG, Thompson WO, et al. Morphine physical dependence in the dog. *J Pharmacol Exp Ther* 1974; 189:759–771.
14. Redmond DE, Krystal JH. Multiple mechanisms of withdrawal from opioid drugs. *Ann Rev Neurosci* 1984; 7:443–478.

15. Creighton FJ, Ghodse AH. Naloxone applied to conjuctiva as a test for physical opiate dependence. *Lancet* 1989; 1:748–750.

16. Heishman SJ, Stitzer ML, Bigelow GE, et al. Acute opioid physical dependence in humans: effect of varying the morphine-naloxone interval. *J Pharmacol Exp Ther* 1989; 250:485–491.

17. Heishman, SJ, Stitzer, ML, Bigelow, GE, et al. Acute opioid physical dependence in humans: effect of varying the morphine-naloxone interval. *J Pharmacol Exp Ther* 1989; 250:127–134.

18. Jasinski DR. Assessment of the abuse of potentiality of the morphine like drugs (methods used in man). In: Martin WR, ed. *Drug Addiction I. Handbook of Experimental Pharmacology, Vol. 45.* New York: Springer-Verlag, 1977:197–258.

19. Judson BA, Himmelberger DU, Goldstein A. The naloxone test for opiate dependence. *Clin Pharmacol Ther* 1980; 27:492–501.

20. Martin WR. Neuropharmacology and neurochemistry of subjective effects, analgesia, tolerance and dependence produced by narcotic analgesics. In: Martin WR, ed. *Drug Addiction Handbook of Experimental Pharmacology, Vol 45.* New York: Springer-Verlag, 1977:43–158.

21. Martin WR, Jasinski DR. Physiological parameters of morphine dependence in man: tolerance, early abstinence, protracted abstinence. *J Psychiatr Res* 1989; 7:9–17.

22. Trujillo KA, Akil H. Opiate tolerance and dependence: recent findings and synthesis. *New Biologist* 1991; 3:915–923.

23. Way EL. Opioid tolerance and physical dependence and their relationship. In: Herz A, ed. *Opioids II. Handbook of Experimental Pharmacology, Vol 104.* New York: Springer-Verlag, 1993:573–595.

24. Portenoy RK, Payne R. Acute and chronic pain. In: Lowinson JH, Ruiz P, Millman RB, eds. *Comprehensive Textbook of Substance Abuse.* Baltimore: Williams and Wilkins, 1997:563–590.

25. Rinaldi RC, Steindler EM, Wilford BB, et al. Clarification and standardization of substance abuse terminology. *JAMA* 1988; 259:555–557.

26. Pappagallo M, Heinberg LJ. Ethical issues in the management of chronic nonmalignant pain. *Sem Neurol* 1997; 17:203–211.

27. Weissman DE and Haddox JD. Opioid pseudoaddiction: an iatrogenic syndrome. *Pain* 1989; 36:363–366.

28. Collett BJ. Opioid tolerance: the clinical perspective. *Br J Aaesth* 1998; 81:58–68.

29. Cox BM. Molecular and cellular mechanisms in opioid tolerance. In: Basbaum AI, Besson J-M, eds. *Towards a New Pharmacotherapy of Pain.* Chichester: John Wiley and Sons, 1991:137–156.

30. Foley, KM. Changing concepts of tolerance to opioids: what the cancer patient has taught us. In: Chapman CR, Foley, KM, eds. *Current and Emerging Issues in Cancer Pain: Research and Practice.* New York: Raven Press, 1993:331–350.

31. Johnson SM, Fleming WW. Mechanisms of cellular adaptive sensitivity changes: applications to opioid tolerance and dependence. *Pharmacol Rev* 1989; 41:435–488.

32. Kanjhan R. Opioids and pain. *Clin Exp Pharmacol Physiol* 1995; 22:397–403.

33. Nestler EJ. Under siege: the brain on opiates. *Neuron* 1996; 16:897–900.

34. Pasternak GW, Kolesnikov YA, Babey A. Perspectives on n-methyl-d-aspartate/nitric oxide cascade and opioid tolerance. *Neuropsychopharm* 1995; 13:309–313.

35. Puntillo K, Casella V, Reid M. Opioid and benzodiazepine tolerance and dependence: application of theory to critical care practice. *Heart & Lung* 1997; 26:317–324.

36. Smith AP, Law PY, Loh HH. Role of opioid receptors in narcotic tolerance/dependence. In: Pasternak GW, ed. *The Opiate Receptors.* Clifton, NJ, Humana, 1988: 441–485.

37. Vaught JL. What is the relative contribution of μ, δ, and κ opioid receptors to antinociception and is there cross-tolerance? In: Basbaum AI, Besson J-M, eds. *Towards a New Pharmacotherapy of Pain.* Chichester: John Wiley and Sons, New York, 1991:121–136.

38. Ling GSF, Paul D, Simantov R, et al. Differential development of acute tolerance to analgesia, respiratory depression, gastrointestinal transit and hormone release in a morphine infusion model. *Life Sci* 1989; 45:1627–1636.

39. Le Guen S, Catherine G, Besson J-M. Development of tolerance to the antinociceptive effect of systemic morphine at the lumbar spinal cord level: a c-Fos study in the rat. *Brain Res* 1998; 813:128–138.

40. Stevens CW. Perspectives on opioid tolerance from basic research: behavioural studies after spinal administration in rodents. In: *Cancer Surveys: Palliative Medicine: Problem Areas in Pain and Symptom Management,* 1994; 21:25–47.

41. Dafters R, Odber J. Effects of dose, interdose interval, and drug-signal parameters on morphine analgesic tolerance: implications for current theories of tolerance. *Behav Neurosci* 1989; 103:1082–1090.

42. Ivarsson M, Neil A. Differences in efficacies between morphine and methadone demonstrated in the guinea pig ileum: a possible explanation for previous observations of incomplete opioid cross-tolerance. *Pharm Toxicol* 1989; 65:368–371.

43. Paronis CA, Holtzman SG. Development of tolerance to the analgesic activity of μ agonists after continuous infusion of morphine, meperidine or fentanyl in rats. *J Pharmacol Exp Ther* 1992; 262:1–9.

44. Picker MJ, Yarbrough J. Cross-tolerance and enhanced sensitivity to the response rate-decreasing effects of opioids with varying degrees of efficacy at the μ receptor. *Psycho-pharmacology* 1991; 105:459–466.

45. Stevens CW, Yaksh TL. Potency of infused spinal antinociceptive agents is inversely related to magnitude of tolerance under continuous infusion. *J Pharmacol Exp Ther* 1989; 250:1–8.

46. Stevens CW and Yaksh TL. Studies of morphine and D-ala2-D-leu5-enkephalin cross-tolerance after continuous intrathecal infusion in the rat. *Anesthesiology* 1992; 76:596–603.

47. Moulin DE, Ling GSF, Pasternak GW. Unidrectional analgesia cross-tolerance between morphine and levorphanol in the rat. *Pain* 1988; 33:233–239.

48. Takahashi M, Senda T, Kaneto H. Role of spinal κ opioid receptors in the blockade of the development of antinociceptive tolerance to morphine. *Eur J Pharmacol* 1991; 200:293–297.

49. Su MT, Lin WB, Lue WM, et al. Blockade of the development of morphine tolerance by U-50,488, an AVP antagonist or MK-801 in the rat hippocampal slice. *Br J Pharmacol* 1998; 123: 625–630.

50. Abdelhamid EE, Sultana, M, Portoghese, PS, et al. Selective blockage of δ opioid receptors prevents the development of morphine tolerance and dependence in mice. *J Pharmacol Exp Ther* 1991; 258:299–303.

51. Adams JU and Holtzman SG. Pharmacologic characterization of the sensitization to the rate-decreasing effects of naltrexone induced by acute opioid pretreatment in rats. *J Pharmacol Exp Ther* 1990; 263:483–489.

52. Cowan A, Zhu XZ, Mosberg HI, et al. Direct dependence studies in rats with agents selective for different types of opioid receptor. *J Pharmacol Exp Ther* 1988; 246:950–955.

53. Fukagawa Y, Katz JL, and Suzuki T. Effects of a selective k-opioid agonist, U-50,488H, on morphine dependence in rats. *Eur J Pharmacol* 1989; 170:47–51.

54. Braun A, Shuster L, Elefterhiou BE, et al. Opiate receptors in mice: genetic differences. *Life Sci* 1975; 17:633–640.

55. Pick CG, Cheng J, Paul D, et al. Genetic influences in opioid analgesic senstivity in mice. *Brain Res* 1991; 566:295–298.

56. Hoffmann O, Plesan A, Wiesenfeld-Hallin Z. Genetic differences in morphine sensitivity, tolerance and withdrawal in rats. *Brain Res* 1998; 806:232–237.

57. Galer BS, Coyle N, Pasternak GW, et al. Individual variability in the response to different opioids: report of the five cases. *Pain* 1992; 49:87–91.

58. Lyness WH, Smith FL, Heavner JE, et al. Morphine self-administration in the rat during adjuvant-induced arthritis. *Life Sci* 1989; 45:2217–2224.

59. Schmauss C and Yaksh TL. In vivo studies on spinal opiate receptor systems mediating antinociception. II. Pharmacological profiles suggesting a differential association of μ, δ, and κ receptors with visceral, chemical and cutaneous stimuli in the rat. *J Pharmacol Exp Ther* 1983; 228:1–2.

60. Stevens CW, Kajander KC, Bennett GJ, and Seybold VS. Bilateral and differential changes in spinal μ, δ and κ opioid binding in rats with a painful, unilateral neuropahy. *Pain* 1991; 46:315–326.

61. Werling LL, McMahon PN, Cox BM. Selective changes in μ opioid receptor properties induced by chronic morphine exposure. *Proc Natl Acad Sci* 1989; 86:6393–6397.

62. Harris GC, Williams JT: Transient homologous μ-opioid receptor desensitization in rat locus coeruleus neurons. *J Neurosci* 1991; 11:2574–2581.

63. Tao PL, Han KF, Wang SD, et al. Immunohistochemical evidence of down-regulation of μ-opioid receptor after chronic PL-017 in rats. *Eur J Pharmacol* 1998; 344:137–142.

64. Harrison LM, Kastin AJ, Zadina JE. Opiate tolerance and dependence: receptors, G-proteins, and antiopiates. *Peptides* 1998; 19:1603–1630.

65. Christie MJ, Williams JT, North RA. Cellular mechanisms of opioid tolerance: studies in single brain neurons. *Mol Pharmacol* 1987; 32:633–638.

66. Puttfarcken PS, Werling LL, Cox BM. Effects of chronic morphine exposure on opioid inhibition of adnyl cyclase in 731c cell membranes: a useful model for the study of tolerance at μ opioid receptors. *Mol Pharmacol* 1988; 33:520–527.

67. Mayer DJ, Mao I, Price DD. The development of morphine tolerance and dependence in association with translocation of protein kinase C. *Pain* 1995; 61:365–374.

68. Nestler EJ, Hope BT, Widnell KL. Drug addiction: a model for the molecular basis of neural plasticity. *Neuron* 1993; 11:995–1006.

69. Koyuncuoglu H, Nurten A, Yamanturk P, et al. The importance of the number of NMDA receptors in the development of supersensitivity or tolerance to and dependence on morphine. *Pharmacol Res* 1999; 39:311–319.

70. Wiesenfeld-Hallin Z. Combined opioid-NMDA antagonist therapies: what advantages do they offer for the control of pain syndromes? *Drugs* 1998; 55:1–4.

71. Elliot K, Minami N, Kolesnikov Y, et al. The NMDA receptor antagonists, LY274614 and MK-801, and the nitric oxide synthase inhibitor, NG-nitro-L-arginine, attenuate analgesic tolerance to the μ-opioid morphine but not to κ opioids. *Pain* 1994; 56:69–75.

72. Elliott K, Kest B, Man A, et al. N-methyl-D-aspartate (NMDA) receptors, μ and κ opioid tolerance, and perspectives on new analgesic drug development. *Neuropsychopharmacol* 1995; 13:347–356.

73. McNally GP, Westbrook RF. Effects of systemic, intracerebral, or intrathecal administration of an N-methyl-D-aspartate receptor antagonist on associative morphine analgesic tolerance and hyperalgesia in rats. *Behav Neurosci* 1998; 112:966–978.

74. Tiseo PJ, Inturrisi CE. Attenuation and reversal of morphine tolerance by the N-methyl-Daspartate receptor antagonist, LY274614. *J Pharmacol Exp Ther* 1993; 264:1090–1096.

75. Trujillo KA, Akil H. Inhibition of morphine tolerance and dependence by the NMDA receptor antagonist MK-801. *Science* 1991; 251:85–87.

76. Highfield DA, Grant S. NG-nitro-L-arginine, an NOS inhibitor, reduces tolerance to morphine in the rat locus coeruleus. *Synapse* 1998; 29:233–239.

77. McQuay HJ, Bullingham RES, Moore RA. Acute opiate tolerance in man. *Life Sci* 1981; 28:2513–2517.

78. Inturrisi, CE, Portenoy, RK, Max, MB, et al. Pharmacokinetic-pharmacodynamic (PK-PD) relationships of methadone infusions in patients with cancer pain. *Clin Pharmacol Ther* 1990; 47:565–577.

79. Houde RW, Wallenstein SL, and Beaver WT. Evaluation of analgesics inpatients with cancer pain, In: Lasagna, L, ed. *International Encyclopedia of Pharmacology and Therapeutics*, sec. 6, vol. 1, Clinical Pharmacology. Oxford: Pergamon Press, 1966:59–98.

80. Houde RW and Nathan B. Eddy Memorial Lecture: The analgesic connection. In: Harris, LS, ed. Problems of drug dependence, NIDA Research Monograph, 55. Rockville, MD: National Institute of Drug Abuse, 1985:4–13.

81. Arner S, Rawal N, Gustafsson LL. Clinical experience of long-term treatment with epidural and intrathecal opiolds—a nationwide survey. *Acta Anaethesiol Scand* 1998; 32:253–259.

82. Bloomfield S, Hogg J, Ortiz O, et al. Analysis of breakthrough pain in 50 patients treated with intrathecal morphine infusion therapy. *Stereotact Funct Neurosurg* 1995; 65:142–146.

83. Brescia FJ, Portenoy RK, Ryan M, et al. Pain, opiold use and survival in hospitalized patients with advanced cancer. *J Clin Oncol* 1992; 10:149–155.

84. Dellemijn PL, van Duijn H, Vanneste JA. Prolonged treatment with transdermal fentanyl in neuropathic pain. *J Pain Symp Manage* 1998; 16:220–229.

85. France RD, Urban BJ, Keefe FJ. Long-term use of narcotic analgesics in chronic pain. *Soc Sci Med* 1984; 19:1379–1382.

86. Kanner RM, Foley KM. Patterns of narcotic drug use in a cancer pain clinic. *Ann NY Acad Sci* 1981; 362:161–172.

87. Onofrio BM, Yaksh TL. Long-term pain relief produced by intrathecal morphine infusion in 53 patients. *J Neurosurg* 1990; 72:200–209.

88. Pappagallo M, Campbell JN. Chronic opioid therapy as alternative treatment for post-herpetic neuralgia. *Ann Neurol* 1994; 35:S54–S56.

89. Plummer JL, Cherry DA, Cousins MF, et al. Long-term spinal administration of morphine in cancer and non-cancer pain: a retrospective study. *Pain* 1991; 44:215–220.

90. Portenoy RK, Foley KM. Chronic use of opioid analgesics in nonmalignant pain: report of 38 cases. *Pain* 1986; 25:171–186.

91. Schug SA, Zech D, Grond S, et al. A long-term survey of morphine in cancer pain patients. *J Pain Symp Manage* 1992; 7:259–266.

92. Taub A. Opioid analgesics in the treatment of chronic intractable pain of non-neoplastic origin. In: Kitahata LM, Collins D, eds. *Narcotic Analgesics in Anesthesiology.* Baltimore: Williams & Wilkins, 1982:199–208.

93. Twycross RG. Clinical experience with diamorphine in advanced malignant disease. *Int J Clin Pharmacol Ther Toxicol* 1974; 9:184–198.

94. Urban BJ, France RD, Steinberger DL, et al. Long-term use of narcotic/antidepressant medication in the management of phantom limb pain. *Pain* 1986; 24:191–197.

95. Winkelmuller M, Winkelmuller W. Long-term effects of continuous intrathecal opioid treatment in chronic pain of non-malignant etiology. *J Neurosurg* 1996; 85:4588–4667.

96. Sallerin-Caute B, Lazorthes Y, Deguine O, et al. Does intrathecal morphine in the treatment of cancer pain induce the development of tolerance? Neurosurgery 1998; 42:44–49.

97. Donner B, Zenz M, Strumpf M, et al. Long-term treatment of cancer pain with transdermal fentanyl. *J Pain Symp Manage* 1998; 15:168–175.

98. Gonzales GR, Elliot KJ, Portenoy RK, et al. The impact of a comprehensive evaluation in the management of cancer pain. *Pain* 1991; 47:141–144.

99. Coyle N, Adelhardt J, Foley KM, et al. Character of terminal illness in the advanced cancer patient: pain and other symptoms in the last 4 weeks of life. *J Pain Symp Manage* 1990; 5:83–93.

100. Macaluso C, Foley KM. Cordotomy for lumbosacral, pelvic and lower extremity pain of malignant origin: safety and efficacy. *Neurology* 1988; 38:110.

101. Coyle N, Weaver S, Breibart W, et al. Delirium as a contributing factor to "crescendo" pain: three case reports. *J Pain Symp Manage* 1994; 9:44–47.

102. Caruso FS, Mehlisch DR, Minn FL, et al. Synergistic analgesic interaction of morphine with dextromethorphan, an NMDA-receptor antagonist, in oral surgery pain [abstract]. *Clin Pharmacol Ther* 1998; 63:139.

103. Minn FL, Nelson SL, Brahim JS, et al. Superior analgesic activity of morphine with dextromethorphan, and NMDA receptor antagonist, in oral surgery pain [abstract]. Clin *Pharmacol Ther* 1998; 63:140.

14

Problems with Opioid Dose Escalation in Cancer Pain: Differential Diagnosis and Management Strategies

SEBASTIANO MERCADANTE

Chronic opioid therapy has been recognized as standard management for cancer pain. Analgesia can be achieved with different opioid dosages in individuals, as there is effectively no ceiling to their analgesic effect and the proportion of adverse effects that the patient can tolerate is usually the limiting factor of the dose used. Thus, analgesic dosage should be titrated to effect. However, opioid escalation may have different causes in the course of the illness, and several factors can interfere with an appropriate analgesic opioid response. The pain that requires increased opioid requirement poses assessment difficulties. The need for opioid escalation may indicate progression of the underlying disease, or reveal a previously unknown complication, indicating a change in the relation between dose and response. Other factors may play a role, including any process that reduces the efficacy of the current analgesic approach, the occurrence of tolerance, the appearance of intractable adverse effects and symptoms other than pain, type and temporal pattern of pain, morphine-metabolite ratio, individual factors, and primary psychological processes. Furthermore, the presence of far-advanced disease and associated multiorgan failure may confound the clinical picture.[1–4]

Disease Progression

Increasing activity in nociceptive pathways may occur with progression of a lesion or associated factors, like inflammatory change or evolution of peripheral or central process.[5] There appears to be general acceptance that the most common reason for escalating opioid doses is progression of the underlying malignant disease, which causes increasing pain.[6] Several studies have indicated that dose increases during chronic morphine treatment were related to particular events, such as surgery, invasive exploration, or progression of disease, generating an increase in pain,[7,8] supporting the view that development of tolerance to opioids is unlikely to be the driving force for loss of analgesia in patients who have alternative reasons for increasing pain. Notable examples of pain conditions with rapid onset over the course of days or weeks include prefracture pain from a weight-bearing bone, epidural compression, perforation of the gastrointestinal tract, and abscess formation.[9] Rapid increases in opioid requirements most often represent a harbinger of progressive cancer and not opioid tolerance, as described in preterminal rapid dose escalation.[10] However, progression of disease often occurs with little or no pain, as in the development of pulmonary or hepatic metastases, and opioid escalation can became unexpectedly rapid without evident progression of disease or modifications in the type of pain. Therefore, there is no clear relationship between the progression of disease and the associated pain syndrome, as a primary tumor mass or metastasis may not produce pain, whereas even small lesions can produce severe pain.[11] The differential diagnosis may be difficult in circumstances where there are no evident signs of tumor progression.

Five distinct patterns of opioid escalation have been reported. Whereas stable opioid use accounted for 30% of patients, 23% had a rapid escalation 24 hours prior to death or before a stabilization of dose. The other categories included 16% of patients reporting a varied pattern (zigzag) due to changing symptoms and medical status, 14% of patients with a slow increase in opioid requirements, and a minority of patients (9%) with a bell-shaped pattern—a gradual increase, then stabilization followed by a slow decrease in opioid requirement before death.[10] In another survey, most patients maintained or decreased the opioid dose in the last weeks of life, although maintaining acceptable pain relief, probably due to the worsening of the clinical condition.[12] A stable or decreasing dosage pattern has been reported in 50% of patients.[13]

Tolerance

Pharmacodynamic tolerance is pharmacologically defined as a reduced potency of the analgesic effects of an opioid following its repeated administration or the need for a higher dose to maintain the same effect, thus causing a shift to the right of the dose-response. It reflects some type of change in the neural systems activated by the drug, different from dispositional tolerance, which involves kinetic factors. A progressive diminution in antinociceptive responses is commonly observed with repeated opioid exposure.[14,15] This complex phenomenon is poorly understood. Pharmacodynamic tolerance seems not to be due to change in receptor number, which can be either up- or down-regulated following chronic exposure to opioids.[16] Rather, a functional decoupling of opioid receptors from second messenger-regulated cellular mechanisms occurs, possibly in addition to down-regulation of opioid receptors and adaptive behavioral changes.[17] Different observations suggest multiple involvement of opioid receptors in the development of tolerance. Other studies suggest that there may be important interactions among receptor subtypes. It has been postulated that non-mu compounds might be efficacious in limiting the development of opioid tolerance when given in an alternative regimen with mu-selective drugs.[18] Therefore, this function is to some extent a mixed-receptor function.[19] There is also evidence that parallel systems, including cholecystokinin and excitatory amino acids, are involved in tolerance. Finally, tolerance may be dependent on individual genetic differences in sensitivity to receptor-selective drugs.[5] For these reasons, a large intraindividual and interindividual variability in the development of tolerance exists that makes this phenomenon unpredictable. Tolerance remains obscure because data acquired in animals or pain-free subjects may not be applicable to patients who receive opioid drugs for pain.

In patients with cancer pain, a high baseline opioid requirement may be determined by prior opioid exposure.[4] Large increments are required to observe further analgesic effects during dose titration. Misinterpretation of poor analgesic response can be attributed to a low dose increment, as tolerance does not in itself reduce opioid responsiveness.[20] Dose escalation may be due to opioid analgesic tolerance rather than progressive disease.[21] This is also demonstrated by the reduction in the equianalgesic dose when switching opioids, because of possible incomplete cross-tolerance. An increasing trend in opioid requirement of 5% or greater of the initial dose, but not previous high doses, has been considered to be a risk factor for poor outcome.[4] With high dosages, there is a risk of metabolite accumulation and the occurrence of related adverse effects.[22] Thus, the possibility of rapid development of tolerance to the analgesic effects of opioids may be a problem in some circumstances.

There is no clear indication of what causes tolerance and what percentage of patients can be expected to develop tolerance in a presumed absence of disease progression. About 15% of 108 patients receiving parenteral opioids were reported to develop tolerance.[23] However, patients who are given opioids for cancer pain may remain on a stable dosage for a long period after achieving adequate analgesia.[24] In some circumstances, morphine doses can be decreased or stopped if pain is relieved by another treatment or the source of pain is abruptly eliminated. Studies of nonmalignant pain have shown that morphine doses may remain stable for a long time or occasionally may require escalation for pain exacerbation.[25] Another study showed that although mean morphine requirements increased 60% during the treatment period, the dose either remained stable throughout the course of therapy or could be reduced in more than 50% of patients.[6] Whereas the previous opioid dose did have univariate correlation with outcome, the results of a multivariate analysis showed that this correlation was probably due to the fact that patients with neuropathic pain were receiving significantly higher doses of opioids. Therefore, previous dose had no independent correlation with outcome.[26]

Tolerance develops to any opioid effect, including sedation, cognitive changes, respiratory depression, nausea and vomiting, and constipation. This is the favorable side of the coin, which may open the therapeutic window and facilitate successful individualization of therapy, allowing for an aggressive upward dose titration with a decline in dose-limiting toxicity.[27] Tolerance to adverse effects may not entirely be due to neural changes; rather, other mechanisms related to the pain may be involved. This observation is suggested by the occurrence of severe sedation after pain input had been removed by a neurolytic procedure in patients who were taking stable doses of opioids, with previously uncontrolled pain but who were alert.[27]

Tolerance to analgesic and nonanalgesic effects commonly occurs, although other factors may be operant that allow the patient to tolerate higher doses of opioids. Although the recognition of these unclear phenomena may have some clinical relevance, early and aggressive treatment of pain should be undertaken without concern that tolerance will inevitably compromise the efficacy of treatment. Tolerance may be predominant in some patients and minimal in others, or may be relevant in a patient for a short period. Escalating pain in a patient receiving a previously stable opioid dose should never be attributed, a priori, to the development of analgesic tolerance, unless a comprehensive evaluation has failed to disclose an alternative explanation.

Drug-Selective Effects

Opioid response may also be drug-selective, a possibility suggested by the remarkable individual variability of response to different drugs. Different receptorial attitudes may explain these differences. It has been suggested that the degree of tolerance is inversely related to the reserve of spare opioid receptors,[28] according to the law of mass action, which states that more potent drugs modify relatively fewer receptor–effector mechanisms to produce effects. It is possible to express the efficacy of a drug in terms of the fraction of the total receptor population (fractional receptor occupancy) that an agonist must occupy to yield a given effect. The number of receptors to be occupied is inversely proportional to the intrinsic activity. As the amount of the remaining unoccupied receptors depends on this property, the larger the receptor reserve, the greater the intrinsic efficacy. Characterization of various opioids into high efficacy and low efficacy agents has been proposed. Morphine has high occupancy characteristics and is considered a low intrinsic efficacy agonist. Thus, it may induce tolerance more readily than a high efficacy agonist, such as sufentanil, which has a higher receptor reserve.[28–30] The latter hypothesis also has been tested in relation to the dose-response changes with progressive increases in stimulus intensity.[31,32] The greater shift in morphine dose-response relative to sufentanil when stimulus intensity rises may support the receptor occupancy theory. Thus, whereas morphine acts as a full agonist at low stimulus intensity, it may become a partial agonist at high levels of pain stimulation, and the relative potency of sufentanil to morphine increases as tolerance develops.[29] Several opioids, including methadone, fentanyl, and sufentanil have been demonstrated to have much higher efficacy than morphine, due to their higher receptor reserve.[33] When acting through the same receptor, morphine, with its lower reserve, may lose its effectiveness as a result of tolerance, acting as a partial agonist when compared to methadone.[34] Although significant cross-tolerance for both sufentanil and morphine has been demonstrated, the magnitude of cross-tolerance from sufentanil to morphine was greater than from morphine to sufentanil, showing a unidirectional asymmetrical cross-tolerance.[29]

These observations may explain the loss of efficacy with increasing doses of morphine on the one hand, and the possibility of excitatory side effects produced by high doses of morphine itself or high concentrations of its metabolites, on the other hand (see Opioid Metabolites).

Pain Mechanisms

Nociception also may modulate or prevent the development of analgesic tolerance. The complexity of receptor heterogeneity, number, co-localizations, interactions, and plastic changes in response to pain stimulation and opioid exposure is extraordinary. The possible neurophysiological basis for the phenomenon of pain that is poorly responsive to opioids can be explored with specific reference to pain conditions consequent to a nerve injury. Both the mechanisms underlying tolerance and the plastic changes in the central nervous system after nerve injury are particularly relevant. When nerve injury occurs, there may also be loss of presynaptic opioid receptors. The importance of the latter outcome is not clear, however, as recent studies have globally shown a maintenance of opioid receptors after nerve injury.[35,36] Moreover, postsynaptic as well as supraspinal receptors will still be available and morphine can be effective with higher doses.[37,38] Experimental studies suggest similarities between a neuropathic pain state and opioid tolerance, and may explain why neuropathic pain states appear more resistant to opioid therapy.[39,40] The development of hyperalgesia and the rightward shift of the morphine antinociceptive dose-response curve can be prevented by the administration of NMDA receptor antagonists.[39]

Neuropathic pain has been shown to require higher doses of opioids to achieve acceptable analgesia, which is often accompanied by greater toxicity. Relatively high opioid doses and the need for a rapid increase in opioid dose predict a poor outcome for pain relief,[4] and rapid tolerance and opioid-related side effects are often associated in neuropathic cancer pain syndromes.[21] Although neuropathic mechanisms may reduce opioid responsiveness, pain can be still responsive to analgesic treatment and does not result in an inherent resistance to opioids.[26,41] The clinical characteristics of neuropathic pain do not predict response to opioids.[42] Indeed, patients with neuropathic pain did not show a particular disadvantage compared to those exhibiting nociceptive pain,[43] unless associated with neurological impairment.[44] As mentioned above, opioids with high efficacy should also be potentially more effective in neuropathic pain conditions. In a recent randomized, double-blind, crossover study of intravenous fentanyl in neuropathic pain, fentanyl was reported to relieve neuropathic pain. The beneficial effect of fentanyl may be independent of the type of neuropathic pain and the degree of sedation, and was attributed to its efficacy.[42]

Pharmacokinetic Processes

Dispositional tolerance is defined by changes in opioid plasma concentrations caused by different pharmacokinetic factors. Absorption of morphine may be poor due to different conditions. A low blood concentration of morphine has been found in patients with stomatitis or with cancer of the oral cavity and poor appetite.[45] Patients with mucosal damage in the gastrointestinal tract may have a reduction in absorption of drugs, requiring an increase in opioid dosage. Pain flare also may be caused by regurgitation of medication causing an unwanted decrease in analgesic plasma concentration. Large surgical resections of the gastrointestinal tract may reduce the intestinal surface for absorption. The administration of opioids through a digestive stoma may be less effective. An elimination effect with an abrupt decrease in plasma concentration of morphine can be anticipated in some circumstances, such as in the case of bleeding, a pathological condition in which morphine may be rapidly eliminated from the body. A decreased consciousness level due to hypotension may render it difficult to determine plasma concentrations, as these patients seldom complain of pain. Pathological conditions may also influence the distribution of morphine. Whereas in patients without fluid retention there is a correlation between the plasma concentration of morphine and dosage, in patients with pleural fluid, ascites or edema, the plasma concentration of morphine shows a different correlation with dosage. This is because in patients with fluid retention the distribution volume is about twice as large as that in patients without fluid retention. Edema at the site of infusion may produce poor absorption of opioids given by the subcutaneous route because of a local dilution effect and poor blood circulation.

The metabolite : morphine ratio is markedly altered in renal failure as a result of a decrease in the clearance of metabolites and an increase in their elimination half-life. In this condition, an increase in the dose of morphine is associated with a small rise in plasma morphine concentration but a sharp increase in M6G concentration. Renal failure also affects morphine pharmacokinetics in other ways, including impairment of intestinal absorption, reduction of the volume of distribution, increase in hepatic blood flow with an increased clearance of morphine, and increased deconjugation. Hepatic disease, which potentially reduces the efficiency of glucuronidation, may explain cases in which a higher concentration of morphine than M6G has been found, although no significant association between hepatic dysfunction and plasma concentrations of morphine or metabolites has been found.[46] Glucuronidation may be inhibited by the concomitant administration of ranitidine.[47]

Effect of Tumor

A possible relationship between opioid drugs and tumor growth has been hypothesized, suggesting that the tumor itself may play a role in reducing the effects of opioids, mimicking opioid tolerance. μ-receptors have been found in cancer cells of neural origin as well as in different cancer lines of human non-neural origin, with effects on cell growth.[48] Moreover tumor cells may also develop resistance and may mediate intracellular events by binding with opioid drugs, through mechanisms similar to those reported with chemotherapeutic agents.[49] The trapping of the drug in tumor cells may result in the drug being diverted from specific sites of the nervous system.[50] This hypothesis should be tested in appropriate study designs for the interesting implications it may have in explaining the unpredictability of opioid therapy in cancer patients.

Primary tumors may have a different evolution in terms of distant metastases and then pain mechanisms.[51] High doses of opioids and adjuvants are necessary to achieve an acceptable pain relief in patients with mesothelioma. Patients with head and neck tumor presented a high opioid escalation index.[44] Prevalence of moderate or severe pain was highest in gynecological cancer.[52] Similarly, significant differences in the prevalence of most symptoms depending on the primary site have been found. Nausea has been found most prevalent in gynecological cancer, or typical gender-related cancer.[51–54] This may limit or influence an appropriate opioid escalation.

A metastatic involvement of midbrain periaquaductal gray, which plays a key role in analgesia via caudal projecting pathways to pain-related regions of the spinal cord, has been also hypothized to explain massive opioid resistance, requiring increasing doses.[55] Structural lesions in the brain may be associated with allodynia.

Age and Sex

Gender and age can influence opioid requirements. Women report severe levels of pain, more frequent pain, and pain of longer duration than do men,[56] and have been reported to more likely have inadequate pain management.[57] Gender differences in morphine analgesia might be due to interactions between opioid and steroid receptors, different production of metabolites, or a different involvement of the NMDA system. Women also have been reported to present with a high prevalence of nausea and vomiting.[53,54] The presence of these side effects may limit dose escalation and the achievement of adequate analgesia. The opioid escalation index was lower and intervals without changing therapy were longer in the presence of higher VAS and frequency of intestinal symptoms in women than in men.[44]

Elderly patients are more likely to be affected by the acute and chronic toxicities of opioids. Opioid requirements for acute pain decrease with age, and plasma concentrations tend to be higher after morphine dosing in the elderly.[58,59] With advanced age, elimination of metabolites tends to be prolonged, probably as a result of a reduced renal function.[46] Concomitant organ dysfunction is commonly present in older patients, thus facilitating the occurrence of undesirable effects.[60] Although this group of patients could be considered at risk for developing more adverse effects during opioid therapy, an appropriate dosage of opioids has been associated with a lower intensity of opioid-related symptoms, but similar pain relief and fewer opioid doses.[53] In a recent survey, elderly patients have been reported to have lower opioid doses than younger adults, although experiencing a similar level of pain intensity.[61]

Temporal Factors and Breakthrough Pain

Breakthrough pain has been defined as a transitory increase in pain intensity on a baseline pain of moderate intensity in patients on regularly administered analgesic treatment. Intermittent pain may be induced by movement, defined as incident pain, or may not be related to activity and, therefore, less predictable.[62] These transient pains have been reported to reduce opioid responsiveness. Most terminally ill patients with incident pain found that it was a major limiting factor to activity. Freedom from pain was particularly difficult to achieve in patients with bone metastasis and incident pain.[2]

The difficulty with incident pain is not a lack of response to systemic opioids, but rather that the doses required to control the incident pain produce unacceptable side effects when the patient is at rest. Pain control is usually excellent if the patient remains immobile or refrains from performing the pain-causing maneuver. Some breakthrough pains may be related to a low baseline opioid dose or long intervals between doses.[63]

Opioid Metabolites

Morphine metabolites are involved in various ways in determining the complex effects of morphine, both favorable and adverse, and may complicate the clinical use of morphine in the treatment of cancer pain. While morphine-6-glucuronide (M6G) binds the opioid receptors exerting a relevant analgesic activity, morphine-3-glucuronide (M3G), the principal morphine metabolite, has been shown to functionally antagonize the analgesic effects of morphine, possibly contributing to the development of tolerance.[64–66] Moreover, M3G has been reported to have excitatory effects and may induce hyperalgesia, myoclonus, agitated delirium respiratory stimulation, and behavioral excitation by non-opioid mechanisms via an antiglycinergic effect at the spinal cord level.[67]

Studies suggest that analgesic response is dependent on the M3G:M6G ratio on an individual basis.[68] Chronic morphine therapy may induce high levels of M3G placing a self-limitation on morphine therapy, with a paradoxical requirement of higher doses. This antianalgesic effect of M3G, however, remains controversial. In subsequent clinical studies, this hypothesis was not confirmed. In patients with morphine resistant-pain who elected to have invasive procedures, M3G:M6G ratios, either in blood and cerebrospinal fluid, were similar to those of patients with well-controlled pain.[69] No relationship between M3G concentration in CSF and pain relief was detected in patients treated by epidural morphine.[70]

Although the hypothesis that M3G plays a major role in morphine resistance is weak, it does not exclude the possibility of the occurrence of important toxic effects limiting opioid responsiveness.[71–74] Changes in production, distribution, and metabolism of morphine and its metabolites, due to varying degrees of renal insufficiency, may account for the variability of the morphine:metabolite ratio observed.[1,75] A progressive increase in the concentration of M3G and of M6G in the CSF of patients with renal failure has been reported.[1,76] Patients who predominantly accumulate **morphine-6-glucuronide** would be expected to develop progressive sedation, whereas patients significantly accumulating **morphine-3-glucuronide** would be expected to exhibit excitatory symptoms with decreased analgesia. More likely, mixed syndromes may be expected when both types of metabolites accumulate.[77] Taking into account these clinical observations, it has been suggested that the accumulation of toxic metabolites during chronic opioid therapy can reduce the opioid response, leading to severe and intolerable adverse effects, even in patients with apparently normal renal function.[46]

Opioids with Extra-Opioid Effects

According to several experimental observations, neuropathic pain and hyperalgesia as well as tolerance development in cancer pain patients may potentially be prevented or decreased by repeated treatment with NMDA antagonists, so that any manipulation targeted to prevent NMDA receptor activation, its intracellular consequences, or calcium influx would inhibit the induction of tolerance and hyperalgesia.[39,78] Morphine has no affinity for NMDA or monoamine receptors. Its analgesic effects, and many of its adverse effects (an exception is its central excitatory effects, which probably involve a non-opioid receptor), seem mainly to be mediated via the mu receptor. In contrast, it is now clear that some opioids have appreciable affinity for the NMDA receptor. Methadone, ketobe-midone, meperidine, and dextropropoxyphene have been reported to have an independent effect on NMDA receptors, inducing antagonist effects,[79–82] These drugs may potentially be more effective in circumstances in which a NMDA receptor activation develops, such as in patients with neuropathic pain who seem to develop tolerance. Thus, differences in the selectivity of opioids toward these other receptors may produce varied opioid responses, especially in the presence of some mechanisms.[83]

Predisposition to Side Effects

Upward dose titration is often difficult due to the development of adverse effects. Pharmacokinetic factors or pharmacodynamic factors may favor the occurrence of adverse effects because of higher than anticipated plasma concentration or exaggerated responses at low plasma opioid concentrations.

Sedation is commonly observed when patients initially receive opioid anal-gesics or after a significant increase in dose. This effect tends to disappear with stable opioid doses. In some patients, severe sedation persists and poses a limi-tation to further opioid escalation, although the data may be confounded by the disease and concomitant drugs as well as the beliefs, personality, and motivation of the patient.

Nausea and vomiting are frequent complications at the beginning of opioid therapy, but usually disappear within a few days of treatment. These symptoms may persist, however, beyond the first few days of treatment or develop during long-term opioid therapy.[84,85] The presence of these gastrointestinal symptoms may render the treatment less effective because of pharmacokinetic holes pro-duced by the low absorption of oral opioids.

Delirium, which is a process of global brain dysfunction, should be included in the differential diagnosis of possible causes of opioid escalation for uncon-trolled pain. Delirium, including perceptual distortions and hallucinations, which can occur in the absence of significant confusion, attention deficits, or psy-chomotor changes, tends to disappear after some days of stable dosing, but may occur again after a rapid opioid escalation. A differential diagnosis include post-anoxic lesions, uremia, cerebral metastases, chronic use of steroids, and many others.[86] Although the occurrence of confusion is attributed to multiple factors in advanced cancer patients, especially in the last week of life, it often appears specifically related to opioids when it occurs acutely.

Delirium may be an important and frequently unrecognized factor associated with crescendo pain, and opioids can contribute to exacerbate delirium. It may also be speculated that delirium can increase pain through associated emotional lability and affective disinhibition, increased anxiety, and altered ability to report pain accurately.[87] There is a poor response to opioids during cognitive failure episodes. Cancer patients with pain who are at risk for developing delirium should be identified using simple screening methods such as the Mini-Mental Status Examination.[88] Specific treatment for agitation should be appropriate in these circumstances. Confusional states were associated with an increased opioid escalation index and neuropathic pain. The response of these patients may be less than that observed in patients with nociceptive pain, because the neurological impairment is more likely when a quick escalation is required.[44]

Neuroexcitatory symptoms, such as myoclonus and hyperalgesia, are occasionally reported to limit opioid escalation, and are attributed to both opioid and extra-opioid effects.[46,89] Many authors speculate that the neuroexcitatory metabolites of morphine may be responsible for the simultaneous development of myoclonus and a hyperalgesic state in cancer pain patients treated with high doses of opioids.[65,68,72,90] However, myoclonus may also occur after the administration of other opioids[67,91] or the use of concomitant drugs.[92]

As mentioned above, with hepatic or renal insufficiency, opioid effects are less predictable. Metabolic derangement produced by major organ dysfunction may predispose patients to additive central toxicity because of changes in drug or drug metabolite concentration. Most adverse effects occurring during chronic opioid therapy have been explained by metabolite production and accumulation, possibly dependent on individual factors, regardless of the renal condition. Metabolic and cerebral derangement, commonly present in older patients, may facilitate the occurrence of undesirable effects. Significant associations between increasing age, elevated bilirubin or LDH levels, and the occurrence of cognitive impairment have been found.[60] However, results of a multivariate analysis suggest that cognitive function did not have any univariate or multivariate correlation with outcome.[93]

Concurrent administration of other neurotropic drugs may predispose patients to opioid adverse effects. Sedation from opioids may be additive or synergistic with sedation from many other central nervous system depressants, including antidepressants, anxiolytic, and neuroleptic agents.[94]

Psychological Factors

Worsening pain may also occur as a consequence of psychological processes, such as anxiety or depression, changes in cognitive state leading to altered pain perception or reporting, or conditioned pain behavior independent of the drug.[5] Affective and cognitive factors can modify a patient's pain compliant. Although difficult to assess, psychological status plays an important role in the experience of cancer pain.[44] The degree of psychological distress has been reported as the major negative prognostic factor and addictive personalities were considered at risk of a poor prognosis for pain control. A history of drug addiction or severe alcoholism may result in misuse of opioids and in the rapid development of tolerance.[4] However, patient misinformation may be a source of inadequate dosage.

Pain severity correlated with the patient's belief that his or her pain was due to cancer.[95] The clinical implications are obvious for cancer patients who often not only ignore the pain cause but also their diagnoses and prognoses. A false opioid resistance with inadequate pain relief may be due to patients' or physicians' fears of the risks of using opioids. Inadequate self-care or family care may substantially contribute to an ineffective outcome for opioid therapy. Misconceptions and lack of knowledge deficit, motivation, and performance capabilities should be detected in clinical practice to avoid cases of pseudo-opioid resistant pain.[96] Moreover, inadequate treatment of the patient's pain may lead to behavioral changes similar to those seen with addiction. Inadequate prescription of analgesics and the consequent escalation demands by the patient may induce a crisis of mistrust between the patient and the health care team, with disastrous consequences.[97] The suspicion of addiction in patients who are receiving opioids for the treatment of pain may arise from some predictive aberrant drug-related behaviors, including selling prescription drugs, forging prescriptions, stealing drugs from others, injecting oral formulations, obtaining prescription drugs from nonmedical sources, concurrent abuse of illicit drugs, multiple dose escalations despite warning, and multiple episodes of loss of prescription.[5]

Infection

Occult local infection may prove to be the cause of worsening pain and escalating opioid requirement.[98–100] Infection may be an underrecognized cause of progressive pain in the cancer population, because of associated immunologic deficits with absence of febrile response, variable value of white count due to tumor stimulation or use of steroids, concurrent anticancer therapy, or bone marrow infiltration. Moreover local signs of infection may be absent because of a depressed inflammatory response.

Management Strategies

The analysis of the factors influencing opioid escalation may be useful in explaining the loss of efficacy with increasing doses, although multiple causes are commonly involved. The interpretation of these data may be difficult. A comprehensive evaluation of the causes that can contribute to worsening pain or altered pain perception, including recurrent disease, psychological distress, pain characteristics, and the history of previous opioid use, should be performed before making any therapeutic decisions. Patients with organ dysfunction and aged populations should be treated cautiously, with low initial doses, relatively small increments, and frequent reevaluation. Attempts should be made to check and normalize the metabolic and hydration status.[101]

Treatment strategies also include establishing trust with the patient and educating the family. Although difficult to assess, psychological status plays an important role in the experience of cancer pain. It is possible to attain better analgesia following the introduction of psychological interventions or psychotropic medication.[20] Appropriate explanation and reassurance should be offered distressed patients. For example, a patient with a pain syndrome resistant to 12 g of oral morphine responded to listening, explanation, 60 mg of morphine daily, and low doses of diazepam.[102] Moreover cancer-related organic factors can present as depression. Antidepressant medications are the mainstay of management in patients who meet criteria for major depressive episodes and the judicious use of benzodiazepines is the mainstay of the pharmacologic treatment of severe anxiety.[103]

From a clinical point of view, different strategies have been proposed to shift the dose-response curve when dose escalation fails, because of inefficacy or production of adverse effects. These strategies may involve aggressive treatment of adverse effects or symptoms associated with pain or methods to enhance analgesia when opioids alone are ineffective at maximally tolerated doses. These approaches may produce either a leftward shift of the analgesia curve or a rightward shift of the toxicity curve.

Drugs That Reduce Opioid Side Effects

As adverse effects may limit further opioid escalation, aggressive management may allow higher and more effective opioid doses. Opioid-induced nausea and vomiting occur in an unpredictable way in many patients, especially ambulatory patients. Tolerance to nausea and vomiting usually develops after a few days. However, these symptoms can persist in some patients and reduce the patient's compliance with opioid escalation. Moreover, nausea and vomiting should be aggressively treated because they may also reduce opioid absorption when the opioid is given by oral route. Persistent nausea should be managed according to its putative triggering mechanism.[104,105] Aggressive therapy with antiemetics is indicated while changing the route of administration until tolerance to these side effects occurs.[106] A combination of drugs with different mechanisms can be more effective.

In patients in which a confusional state may mimic pain, an appropriate assessment may abort the pattern of crescendo pain with the use of a therapeutic trial of neuroleptic drugs, switching to an alternative drug, or using a different route of opioid administration.[87] Symptoms can be relieved in some cases by hydration or psychotropic drugs, including benzodiazepines or neuroleptics.[86,107,108] Benzodiazepines must be used cautiously because they may exacerbate sedation and the confusional state in some patients.[94] Midazolam seems to be the drug of choice, allowing easy titration and reversal of sedation by decreasing the dose. Haloperidol is a well-recognized neuroleptic that can reduce some cognitive disturbances.[106] The drug dose is titrated to the level required to control symptoms.[88]

Myoclonus is generally managed with opioid dosage reduction, but in some cases this is not possible because of existing pain. A specific treatment to control myoclonus may allow continued opioid escalation when pain is uncontrolled. For example, myoclonic activity can be reduced by drugs with peripheral muscle relaxant effects, such as dantrolene.[91] A change to a different opioid, and the addition of a benzodiazepine, such as diazepam, clonazepam, or midazolam, may be useful. In one report, clonazepam dramatically reduced myoclonus after lorazepam failed to control the contractions in a patient treated with high doses of opioids.[109] In another report, severe multifocal myoclonus and seizures associated with high dose opioid therapy responded to parenteral midazolam, and rotation to alternative opioids.[22] A continuous infusion of midazolam may be useful because of the rapid effect after midazolam administration, the maintenance of the analgesia achieved with a specific dose of morphine, the physical compatibilty of morphine with midazolam, and the short half-life of midazolam during short-term administration that allows for rapid titration to an effective dose.[110] However, benzodiazepines may act by masking the effects of metabolites rather than clearing them, and lead to a down-regulation of endogenous GABA.[74]

The sedative effects of opioid therapy may be manageable using psychostimulants. Methylphenidate has been shown to increase the analgesic effectiveness and to decrease sedation in cancer patients taking opioids.[107] The use of methylphenidate has been demonstrated to allow patients to tolerate higher doses of opioids during the period between incident pain episodes.[108] Other studies, however, did not definitively demonstrate a significant benefit for methylphenidate in opioid-induced drowsiness.[111] Although psychostimulants may be useful, they should be administered cautiously. Sedation caused by other factors could potentially respond poorly to psychostimulants and worsen neurological status.[112]

Drugs to Enhance Analgesia

One approach to the patient with pain that is poorly responsive to escalating doses of opioids may be the administration of a nonopioid analgesic. Most of these drugs, however, may add further problems because of additive or synergistic effects on opioid-related adverse effects or produce further problems in the cancer population. Because the nature of dose-related analgesic effects is poorly characterized for these drugs, a stepwise titration to effect is recommended.

Antidepressants may improve depression, enhance sleep, and provide decreases in perception of pain. While the analgesic effect of the tricyclic antidepressants is not directly related to antidepressant activity, efficacy has been established in many painful disorders with a neuropathic mechanism. Neuro-pathic pain characterized by continuous dysesthesias is believed to be the most favorable indication for antidepressant therapy.[106] However, in meta-analyses conducted to clarify the effectiveness of amitriptyline in chronic pain, partial or insignificant relief and a number of disagreeable side effects were evidenced.[113–115] Adverse effects, including antimuscarinic effects, such as dry mouth, impaired visual accommodation, urinary retention, constipation, antihis-taminic effects (sedation), and anti-alpha-adrenergic effects (orthostatic hypotension), may limit clinical application in cancer pain.

The evidence supporting analgesic efficacy is particularly strong for amitriptyline. Amitriptyline has been shown to induce analgesia and potentiate morphine analgesia; it also increases the plasma concentration of morphine.[116] Nevertheless, alternative drugs with lower incidences of side effects should be considered in patients predisposed to its sedative, anticholinergic, or hypoten-sive effects.[106]

Local anesthetics (lidocaine and mexiletine), carbamazepine, phenytoin, and open sodium channel blockers have been reported to relieve neuropathic pain states. Although the exact mechanism of these drugs is not known, they all inhibit sodium channels of hyperactive and depolarized nerves while not interfering with normal sensory function. Mechanisms other than sodium-channel blockade have been advocated for the systemic analgesic effect, including the modification of presynaptic calcium channels and postsynaptic receptors, involvement of the opioid system, an central action mediated by glycine.[117]

Evidence suggests that sodium channel-blocking agents act both centrally and peripherally within the nervous system. The analgesic response to lidocaine was characterized by a precipitous break in pain over a narrow dosage and con-centration range.[118] Oral mexiletine is more convenient because of its oral prepa-ration and has been used empirically. The response to intravenous lidocaine infusion has been reported to predict the response to oral mexiletine.[119] Although cancer patients with neuropathic pain have been reported to benefit from lido-caine,[120] one double-blind, crossover, placebo-controlled study failed to demon-strate any benefit from 5 mg/kg of lidocaine administered as an intravenous infusion over 30 minutes for neuropathic pain syndromes related to cancer.[121] Although sodium channel-blocking agents are useful for the management of chronic neuropathic pain, no conclusive clinical study has statistically verified these observations in cancer pain. Flecainide may be useful in the management of neuropathic pain of advanced cancer patients, although concern about pos-sible cardiac complications has limited its use.[122]

Other anticonvulsant agents, such as carbamazepine, phenytoin, valproate, and clonazepam, have been reported to relieve pain in numerous peripheral and central neuropathic pain conditions, although contradictory results have been found.[85,106,123] The efficacy of these drugs could be explained by the inhibitory effects exerted on NMDA-receptors,[124] and other mechanisms, including sodium channel blockade for some. However, no measurable differences in the analgesic benefit of anticonvulsants and antidepressants were evidenced in a systematic review of available trials in neuropathic pain.[115]

Topical approaches may also be useful in neuropathic pain. Capsaicin depletes substance P in small primary afferent neurons. Patients with neuropathic pain presumed to have a strong peripheral input, including postmastectomy syndrome and postherpetic neuralgia, may benefit from topical capsaicin cream. A cream of eutectic mixture of local anesthetics (EMLA) applied under an occlusive dressing to increase skin penetration, also has been reported to produce skin anesthesia and to reduce neuropathic pain with a strong peripheral component.[125]

Nonsteroidal anti-inflammatory drugs (NSAIDs) may be effective in some breakthrough pains, such as headache and incident pain due to bone metastases.[11] Thus, NSAIDs may be useful to increase basal analgesia or provide short-lived analgesia for breakthrough pain (rescue drugs). The opioid-sparing effect of NSAIDs may be helpful in conditions in which it is necessary to reduce the opioid dose on account of the occurrence of adverse effects.[126] However, prolonged use is associated with complications at the gastrointestinal and renal levels, and often requires drugs to prevent gastric damage.[12] In a recent survey, however, severe gastrointestinal bleeding was attributed to the advanced disease rather than to NSAID use.[127]

The bisphosphonates potentiate the effects of analgesics in metastatic bone pain by inhibiting the cascade of cellular, biochemical, and physiochemical events that lead to osteoclastic bone resorption. Incident pain due to bone metastases may potentially benefit directly or through prevention of pathological fractures. Pamidronate, a potent bisphosphonate, significantly reduced morbidity caused by bone metastases, including a 30% to 50% reduction in pain, impending pathological fractures, and the need for radiotherapy. Best results are obtained with doses of 60 mg or 90 mg of pamidronate every 4 weeks. This treatment is generally well tolerated; side effects include transient low grade fever, nausea, myalgia, and mild infusion site reactions.[11,128]

Nitrous oxide has properties that might enable prompt control of breakthrough pain. It is an analgesic, anxiolytic, and sedative agent with a rapid onset of action. Nitrous oxide delivered in 50%–50% with oxygen by a patient-controlled mechanism was safely and effectively used by advanced cancer patients with breakthrough pain because of bone metastases.[129] Environmental exposure to caregivers was minimal. It should not be used in the presence of bowel distension.[63]

Drugs That Enhance Analgesia Produced by Opioids

Another strategy to address poor responsiveness is to target analgesic tolerance and attempt to reduce or prevent it. Agents that block the activity of NMDA-receptors may provide new tools for the treatment of poorly responsive pain syndromes, particularly in the presence of opioid tolerance or neuropathic mechanisms.[130] These drugs may have both direct analgesic effects or reverse tolerance.

Most clinical experience is with ketamine, a noncompetitive NMDA receptor blocker. Ketamine significantly influences central hyperexcitability and inhibits the wind-up phenomenon in spinal cord neurons. In this way, ketamine may inhibit central temporal summation and have a marked hypoalgesic effect on high intensity stimuli.[131] A synergistic effect between ketamine and opioids has been observed in cancer pain patients who no longer responded to high doses of morphine.[132–139] Ketamine should be given at an initial starting dose of 100–150 mg daily, whereas the dose of opioids should be reduced by 50%, with the dose being titrated against the effect. Psychotomimetic effects should be monitored and prevented using haloperidol in doses of 2–4 mg daily, or minimal doses of diazepam.[140] In a recent double-blind study, ketamine was highly effective in enhancing morphine analgesia in neuropathic cancer pain.[141] Moreover, intrathecal ketamine 1 mg daily has been shown to enhance intrathecal morphine analgesia in advanced cancer patients with pain.[142]

Dextromethorphan, a potent NMDA-antagonist, has been considered a promising drug because it does not appear to produce psychotomimetic side effects.[143] However, studies of cancer patients with pain with doses of 90 mg daily, did not show significant analgesic activity.[144]

Some broad spectrum opioids, such as methadone, kerobemidone, meperidine, and dextropropoxyphene, possess NMDA-antagonist activity, and, as a consequence, may be potentially more effective in circumstances in which an NMDA-receptor activation develops, such as in cases of neuropathic mechanism associated with tolerance.[83]

Magnesium ions are natural blockers for ion channels that are permeated by calcium and opened by NMDA-receptor activation. However, exogenously administered magnesium failed to reduce pain and allodynia significantly in patients with different neuropathic syndromes.[145]

In a double-blind, randomized, controlled study, the NMDA-receptor antagonist amantadine was safe and partially effective for surgical neuropathic pain in cancer patients. Further trials with a long-term design, higher dose, and different neuropathic mechanisms should be conducted to confirm this observation.[146]

Proglumide, a cholecystokinin antagonist, has been shown to have significant effects at low doses on opioid analgesia. In a short, double-blind, crossover study in cancer patients with pain, no differences between full opioid dosage with placebo and one-half opioid dose with proglumide were found. Different designs are necessary to establish the real additive analgesic effect of proglumide.[147]

Many investigators have shown that calcium channel blockers may potentiate opioid nociception, as pharmacological interference with calcium-related events may modify chronic opioid effects, including the expression of tolerance. Controversial results have been reported in patients with cancer pain. In a clinical series, nimodipine succeeded in reducing the daily dose of morphine in 16 of 23 patients, although it failed in 2 patients and was withdrawn in 5 patients.[148] However, nimodipine given orally at a dose of 30 mg every 8 hours failed to enhance the analgesic effect of slow-release morphine in cancer patients with pain.[149] Subsequently, in a double-blind, placebo-controlled study, nimodipine enhanced opioid analgesia in cancer patients requiring morphine dose escalation.[150] However, the design of study and a high rate of patient withdrawal before the end of study may limit the value of these findings.

Emergencies Due to Abrupt Disease Progression

In cases of rapid progression of disease, a protocol for management of cancer pain emergencies has been suggested. A loading dose of 10–20 mg of intravenous morphine administered over 15 minutes, a rapid upward dose titration doubling the dose every one-half hour, with careful monitoring over time for dose-related toxicity, allowed for a safe management of acute cancer pain presentation.[9] Such rapid escalation of dose would be difficult to manage orally, although a protocol has been reported previously.[105] However, a continuous infusion is characterized by slow increases in plasma concentrations, which is inadequate to manage emergencies. The risk of respiratory depression is low, because the presence of severe pain despite a bolus of morphine predicts that the dose can be safely doubled, although careful observation and frequent assessment are required to ensure that dose escalation may be stopped when adequate pain control is achieved.[9] Nevertheless, a delay occurs between the peak blood level and the time of peak analgesia with morphine. This hysteresis, because of the relatively poor lipid solubility, may be overcome by choosing more lipophilic opioids with an immediate effect, such as fentanyl or, better, alfentanil. This is even more useful when very high doses of morphine are ineffective and may induce severe hyperexcitation of the central nervous system.[22] Remifentanil may provide an immediate effect, within seconds, but it poses some problems in titration, because of lack of experience in the setting of cancer pain management.[63]

Route of Administration

The route of administration has an important role in determining the morphine:metabolite ratio both in plasma and CSF. The prevalence of myoclonus among patients receiving oral morphine was threefold higher than those receiving parenteral morphine.[60] Concentrations of M3G and M6G in relation to morphine were found to be greater following oral administration than after intravenous administration.[151] Therefore, switching from oral administration to parenteral administration may change the morphine:metabolite relationship and reduce toxicity caused by accumulation of the metabolites. The use of nonoral routes of opioid administration as the patient's pain problems progress is often necessary for other reasons as well.[152]

Adverse effects also may be reduced in intensity with the use of the spinal route. In a prospective randomized comparative study in patients with an involvement of the brachial or lumbar plexus, the epidural route for opioid administration was superior to oral opioids because of a lower incidence of adverse effects. However, complete pain relief was not achieved in all patients and technical problems arose in the group treated by epidural route.[153] Patients chronically treated with oral morphine showed all reaction time percentiles significantly longer than controls, whereas the epidural opioid group showed only the involvement of the longest reaction times.[154] However, epidural and subcutaneous administration of morphine were comparable in terms of both effectiveness and acceptability. Both treatments provided better pain relief with less adverse effects compared with the previous oral morphine treatment.[155] Moreover, continuous pain originating from deep somatic tissues is equally well controlled by both oral and spinal opioids, whereas somatic pain from mucocutaneous ulcers and from fractures, from intestinal distension as well as neuropathic pain, respond poorly to spinal opioids, suggesting a lack of improved analgesic activity by spinal morphine.[156] Even when opioids are administered intrathecally, pain relief can still be insufficient, especially when neuropathic or incident pain components are present. The use of local anesthetics and other adjuvants, such as clonidine and neostigmine, by the intrathecal route is decisive in recapturing patients unresponsive to opioid escalation given either systemically or spinally, who did not benefit from previous opioid substitution or change of route of administration.[157]

Modality of Administration

Some pain with a typical temporal pattern needs to be treated with rescue doses rather than with increases in the basal regimens, to avoid increased opioid plasma concentrations when the pain crisis disappears. However, intervals between the pain flares still are at risk for adverse effects. A rescue dose of opioid can provide a means to treat breakthrough pain in patients already stabilized on a baseline opioid regimen.[63] Although orally administered patient-controlled analgesia (PCA) is currently a standard practice in cancer pain management, with a dose equivalent to 5%–10% of the total opioid dose administered every 2 to 3 hours,[62] the onset of action of an oral dose may be too slow and better results may be obtained with a parenteral rescue dose. A subcutaneous administration is associated with a slower onset of effect compared to an intravenous one, but should be considered equivalent in terms of efficacy.[152]

Oral transmucosal dosing is a noninvasive approach to the rapid onset of analgesia. Highly lipophilic agents may pass rapidly through the oral mucosa avoiding the first-pass metabolism, therefore achieving active plasma concentrations within minutes.[158–160] In a randomized, double-blinded, placebo-controlled trial, oral transmucosal fentanyl appeared effective in the treatment of cancer-related breakthrough pain.[161]

Opioid Switching

As opioids have differential effects on selective subsets of opioid receptors in the central nervous system, and cross-tolerance between opioids is incomplete, a shift from one opioid to another is a useful option when the side effect–analgesic relationship is inconvenient; also, it allows for elimination of possible toxic metabolites. Patients who experience dose-limiting adverse effects during opioid escalation may benefit from a trial of an alternative opioid.[77,162,163] In a switch from one opioid to another, the latter drug is often observed to be relatively more potent than would be anticipated, given published estimates. Hydromorphone is often used. However, the presence of a renal disease suggests a choice of opioid with no active metabolites.[83] Moreover, alternative opioids with high intrinsic efficacy, such as fentanyl and methadone, may be more effective in conditions characterized by a rapid development of tolerance or sustained by a neuropathic pain mechanism, or both.[101] This is much more relevant when switching to methadone, because it has a high efficacy when compared with morphine, extra opioid anti-NMDA effects, and interesting pharmacokinetic properties, that make its use unique. Methadone can be particularly beneficial in patients on doses of opioids requiring rapid dose escalation, in which NMDA-receptor activation is likely to develop, such as in the case of neuropathic mechanisms associated with tolerance.[83,101,164,165]

Methadone has been reported to be useful in restoring opioid responsiveness in patients whose pain ceases to be controlled by morphine, hydromorphone or diamorphine[163,166–172] at doses much lower than those suggested by the opioid conversion charts. The clinical benefit will depend on the degree to which cross-tolerance exists to analgesia as well as to side effects. As the degree of cross-tolerance may change as opioid doses are escalated, it is advisable to proceed with caution when switching from one opioid to another in patients receiving very high opioid doses. Data suggest that switching to methadone using current proposed ratios may lead to severe toxicity. A strongly positive correlation between dose ratio and previous morphine dose suggests the need for a highly individualized and cautious approach when rotating from morphine to methadone in patients with cancer pain on high doses of morphine.[173–175] To circumvent this problem, different methods have been proposed. A gradual switch over has been suggested, using 1/3 of the previous opioid dose for oral methadone, and using an oral methadone/parenteral hydromorphone ratio of 1:1.[171] If extra doses are not required, the previous opioid may be reduced without a concomitant increase of methadone. Other authors suggest an initial dose of methadone of one tenth of the total daily morphine dose, but not greater than 30 mg at intervals determined by the patient, but no more frequently than 3 hours, and then to divide the steady-state total daily dose (after 6 days) into a twice daily regimen.[176] If long-acting opioid metabolites are considered responsible for adverse effects;[71,164] a rapid switch using a morphine-methadone ratio of 5 : 1, and monitoring of the dosage in the following days, may be useful and is currently used at our institution. The subsequent titration process should take into account the characteristics of the pain syndromes and the individual clinical situation.[101]

Fentanyl series also have been used successfully for opioid switching. Fentanyl has been shown to relieve neuropathic pain by its intrinsic analgesic effect.[42] Patients with cancer pain requiring a cessation of morphine therapy due to unacceptable opioid side effects, and switched to subcutaneous fentanyl, obtained an improvement in adverse effects, and adequate pain relief was observed in almost all patients.[177,178] An approximate equivalence of 68 : 1 of morphine to fentanyl has been reported clinically. Sufentanil, a more potent opioid than fentanyl, was effective when the dose necessitated too large a volume for a syringe-driver, with a relative potency of sufentanil to fentanyl of about 10 : 1.[178,179] Subcutaneous fentanyl was convenient in patients with terminal bowel obstruction associated with renal failure.[180] Uremic patients, suspected to have an accumulation of active morphine metabolites, who developed increasing agitation on a continuous subcutaneous infusion of diamorphine within the last few days of life, were switched to subcutaneous alfentanil using an alfentanil-diamorphine conversion ratio of 10 : 1, and doses very much towards the lower end of the range of alfentanil were commonly used.[181]

Other Measures

An occult infection should be pursued aggressively as a potentially reversible cause of intractable pain and increasing opioid requirements. Appropriate investigations include blood cultures, diagnostic imaging, and needle aspiration and culture. If a specific focus of infection is not clearly demonstrated, but the suspicion is high, a trial of broad spectrum antibiotics may be appropriate. Antibiotic therapy and drainage of the abscess resulted in markedly improved pain control, decreased analgesic requirements, and improved quality of life in a patient with metastatic breast cancer.[99]

Radiotherapy provides an effective symptomatic treatment for local bone pain and can be another method for treating a breakthrough pain that may be result from poor opioid responsiveness. Treatments with single fractions may be more convenient and equally effective in terms of pain relief in advanced cancer patients.[182] Hemibody radiation has been suggested in the presence of multiple areas of pain, although toxicity is of concern.[183] Although radioisotopes are more imprecise in delivering specific dose irradiation, their advantages include less toxicity, easy administration, and effectiveness in subclinical sites of metastases.[11]

Breakthrough pain may be reduced with effective bracing. Unfortunately, the lower extremities are rarely amenable because of the high degree of load. In some circumstances, mobility aids, bracing of the painful part, instruction in ergonomic principles, and adaptation of the patient's home may be more productive than a pharmacologic approach. Orthopedic intervention may restore mobility in bed-bound patients. Impending fractures require surgical stabilization using fixation devices or prosthetic reconstruction. Surgical stabilization of the spine and extremities may dramatically improve quality of life, decrease incident pain and prevent complications associated with immobility. However, risks should be balanced against the benefits of such interventions.[11,63]

Selected well-localized pain syndromes with breakthrough somatic and neuropathic mechanisms may benefit from an intermittent or continuous administration of local anesthetics by a catheter.[184–189] Location and type of pain are of primary importance in considering patient seletion.

Some neurolytic blocks, such as celiac plexus block, have fewer complications. Although it has been recommended in the early stage of the illness,[190,191] the use of a nociceptive pathway block has not gained general acceptance. Rather, this procedure should be considered an opioid sparing technique, which may convert a patient with poorly responsive pain into a patient who achieves good comfort with lower and more tolerated doses.[192]

A percutaneous cervical cordotomy by radiofrequency has been utilized in patients with unilateral bone pain. This technique usually produces good relief in most patients for unilaterally well-localized pain of any origin except for some neuropathic pains. However, some pain may persist or develop below or above the level of analgesia, with worsening pain at the opposite side of the body. Moreover, the risk of serious complications, including mirror pain, general fatigue or hemiparesis, and respiratory failure, with a deterioration in performance status, is high.[11,193]

References

1. Portenoy RK, Foley KM, Stulman J, et al. Plasma morphine and morphine-6-glucuronide during chronic morphine therapy for cancer pain: plasma profiles, steady-state concentrations and the consequences of renal failure. *Pain* 1991; 47:13–19.
2. Banning A, Sjogren P, Henriksen H. Treatment outcome in a multidisciplinary cancer pain clinic. *Pain* 1991; 47:129–134.
3. Mercadante S. Predictive factors and opioid responsiveness in cancer pain. *Eur J Cancer* 1998; 34:627–631.
4. Bruera E, MacMillan D, Hanson J, MacDonald RN. The Edmonton staging system for cancer pain : preliminary report. *Pain* 1989; 37:203–210.
5. Portenoy RK. Opioid tolerance and responsiveness: research findings and clinical observations. In: Gebhart GF, Hammond DL, Jensen TS, eds. *Proceedings of the 7th World Congress on Pain*. Seattle: IASP Press, 1994:595–619.

6. Schug SA, Zech D, Grond S, Jung H, Meuser T, Stobbe B. A long term survey of morphine in cancer pain patients. *J Pain Symptom Manage* 1992; 7:259–266.

7. Foley KM. Controversies in cancer pain. *Cancer* 1989; 63:2257–2265.

8. Collin E, Poulain P, Gauvain-Piquard A, Petit G, Pichard-Leandri E. Is disease progression the major factor in morphine "tolerance" in cancer pain treatment? *Pain* 1993; 55:319–326.

9. Hagen NA, Elwood T, Ernst S. Cancer pain emergencies: a protocol for management. *J Pain Symptom Manage* 1997; 14:45–50.

10. Coyle N, Adelhardt J, Foley KM, Portenoy RK. Character of terminal illness in the advanced cancer patient: pain and other symptoms during the last four weeks of life. *J Pain Symptom Manage* 1990; 5:83–93.

11. Mercadante S. Malignant bone pain: physiopathology, assessment and treatment. *Pain* 1997; 69:1–18.

12. Mercadante S. Treatment and outcome of cancer pain in advanced cancer patients followed at home. *Cancer*, 1999; 85:1849–1858.

13. Zech DFJ, Grond S, Lynch J, Hertel D, Lehmann KA. Validation of World Health Organization guidelines for cancer pain relief: a 10-year prospective study. *Pain* 1995; 63:65–76.

14. Stevens CW, Yaksh TL. Potency of infused spinal antinociception agents is inversely related to magnitude of tolerance after continuous infusion. *J Pharmacol Exper Res* 1989; 250:1–8.

15. Yaksh TL. Tolerance: factors involved in changes in the dose-effect relationship with chronic drug exposure. In: Basbaum AI, Besson JM, eds. *Towards a New Pharmacotherapy of Pain*. Chichester: John Wiley & Sons, 1991:157–179.

16. Collin E, Cesselin F. Neurobiological mechanisms of opioid tolerance and dependence. *Clin Pharmacol* 1991; 14:465–488.

17. Trujillo KA, Akil H. Opiate tolerance and dependence: recent findings and synthesis. *New Biologist* 1991; 3:915–923.

18. Russell RD, Chang KJ. Alternated delta and mu receptor activation: a stratagem for limiting opioid tolerance. *Pain* 1989; 36:381–389.

19. Desmeules JA, Kayser V, Guilbaud G. Selective opioid receptor agonists modulate mechanical allodynia in an animal model of neuropathic pain. *Pain* 1993; 53:277–285.

20. Portenoy RK, Foley KM, Inturrisi CE. The nature of opioid responsiveness and its implications for neuropathic pain : new hypothesies derived from studies of opioid infusions. *Pain* 1990; 43 :273–286.

21. Fainsinger RL, Bruera E. Is this opioid analgesic tolerance? *J Pain Symptom Manage* 1995; 10:573–577.

22. Hagen NA, Swanson R. Strychnine-like multifocal myoclonus and seizures in extremely high dose opioid administration: treatment strategies. *J Pain Symptom Manage* 1997; 14:51–58.

23. Bruera E, Brenneis C, Michaud M. Use of the subcutaneous route for the administration of narcotics in patients with cancer pain. *Cancer* 1998; 62:407–411.

24. Portenoy RK. Chronic opioid therapy in non-malignant pain. *J Pain Symptom Manage* 1990; 6:S56-S62.

25. Portenoy RK, Foley KM. Chronic use of opioid analgesics in non-malignant pain: report of 38 cases. *Pain* 1986; 25:171–186.

26. Bruera E, Schoeller T, Wenk R, et al. A prospective multicenter assessment of the Edmonton staging system for cancer pain. *J Pain Symptom Manage* 1995; 10:348–355.

27. Portenoy RK. Tolerance to opioid analgesics: clinical aspects. *Cancer Surveys* 1995; 21:49–65.

28. Duttaroy A, Yoburn BC. The effect of intrinsic efficacy on opioid tolerance. *Anesthesiology* 1995; 82:1226–1236.

29. Sosnowski M, Yaksh TL. Differential cross-tolerance between intrathecal morphine and sufentanil in the rat. *Anesthesiology* 1990; 73:1141–1147.

30. Saeki S, Yaksh TL. Suppression of nociceptive responses by spinal mu opioid agonists: effects of stimulus intensity and agonist efficacy. *Anesth Analg* 1993; 77:265–274.

31. Dirig DM, Yaksh TL. Differential right shifts in the dose-response curve for intrathecal morphine and sufentanil as a function of stimulus intensity. *Pain* 1995; 62:321–328.

32. Kissin I, Brown P, Bradley E. Magnitude of acute tolerance to opioids is not related to their potency. *Anesthesiology* 1991; 75:813–816.

33. Frenk H, Watkins LR, Mayer DJ. Differential behavioral effects induced by intrathecal microinjection of opiates: comparison of convulsive and cataleptic effects produced by morphine, methadone, and D-ala-methionine-enkephalinamide. *Brain Res* 1984; 299:31–42.

34. Ivarsson M, Neil A. Differences in efficacies between morphine and methadone demonstrated in guinea pig ileum. *Pharmacol Toxicol* 1989; 65:368–371.

35. Besse D, Lombard MC, Perrot S, Besson JM. Regulation of opioid binding sites in the superficial dorsal horn of the rat spinal cord following loose ligation of the sciatic nerve: comparison with sciatic nerve section and lumbar dorsal rhizotomy. *J Neurosci* 1992; 50:921–933.

36. Devor M. (1989) The pathophysiology of damaged peripheral nerves. In: Wall PD, Melzack R, eds. *Textbook of Pain*. New York: Churchill Livingstone, 1989:68–81.

37. Dickenson A. Neurophysiology of opioid poorly responsive pain.(1995) In: Hanks GW, ed. *Palliative Medicine. Problem Areas in Pain and Symptom Management*, Vol. 21. New York: Cold Spring Harbor Laboratory Press, 1995:5–16.

38. Miaskowski C, Taiwo YO, Levine JD. Contribution of supraspinal mu and delta opioid receptors to antinociception in the rat. *Eur J Pharmacol* 1991; 205:247–252.

39. Mao J, Price D, Mayer DJ. Experimental mononeuropathy reduces the antinociceptive effects of morphine: implications for common intracellular mechanisms involved in morphine tolerance and neuropathic pain. *Pain* 1995; 61:353–364.

40. Mayer DJ, Mao J, Price DD. The development of morphine tolerance and dependence is associated with translocation of protein kinase C. *Pain* 195; 61:365–374.

41. Jadad AR, Carroll D, Glynn CJ, Moore RA, McQuay HJ. Morphine responsiveness of chronic pain : double blind randomized crossover study with patient-controlled analgesia. *Lancet* 1992; 339:1367–1371.

42. Dellemjin PL, Vanneste JA. Randomized double-blind active-placebo-controlled crossover trial of intravenous fentanyl in neuropathic pain. *Lancet* 1997; 349:753–758.

43. Mercadante S, Maddaloni S, Roccella S, Salvaggio L. Predictive factors in advanced cancer pain treated only by analgesics. *Pain* 1992; 50 :151–155.

44. Mercadante S, Dardanoni G, Salvaggio L, Armata MG, Agnello A. Monitoring of opioid therapy in advanced cancer pain patients. *J Pain Symptom Manage* 1997; 13:204–212.

45. Yokokawa N, Hiraga K, Oguma T, Konishi M. Relationship between plasma concentration of morphine and analgesic effectiveness. *Postgrad Med* 1991; 67(suppl.2):S50-S54.

46. Mercadante S. The role of morphine metabolites in cancer pain. *Palliat Med* 1999; 13:95–104.

47. Aasmundstad TA, Storset P. Influence of ranitidine on the morphine-3-glucuronide to morphine-6-glucuronide ratio aftre oral administration of morphine in humans. *Hum Exp Toxicol* 1990; 17:347–352.

48. Zagon IS, Hytrek SD, McLaughlin P. Opioid growth factor tonically inhibits human colon cancer prolifaration in tissue culture. *Am J Physiol* 1996; 271:R511–518.

49. Callaghan R, Riordan JR. Synthetic and natural opiates interact with P-glycoprotein in multi-drug-resistant celss. *J Biol Chem* 1993; 268:16059–16064.

50. Arcuri E. Can tumors act as opioid traps, mimicking opioid tolerance? *J Pain Symptom Manage* 1998; 16:78–79.

51. Mercadante S, Casuccio A, Pumo S, Fulfaro F. Opioid response-primary diagnosis relationship in advanced cancer patients followed at home. *J Pain Symptom Manage* 2000; 20:21–34.

52. Vainio A, Auvinen A. Prevalence of symptoms among patients with advanced cancer. An international collaborative study. *J Pain Symptom Manage* 1996; 12:3–10.

53. Mercadante S, Casuccio A, Pumo S. Factors influencing the opioid response in advanced cancer patients with pain followed at home: the effects of age and gender. *Support Care Cancer* 2000; 8:123–130.

54. Grond S, Zech D, Diefenbach C, Bischoff A. Prevalence and pattern of symptoms in patients with cancer pain: a prospective evaluation of 1635 cancer patients referred to a pain clinic. *J Pain Symptom Manage* 1994; 9:372–382.

55. Collins JJ, Berde CB, Grier H, Nachmanoff DB, Kinney HC. Massive opioid resistance in an infant with a localized metastasis to the midbrain periaqueductal gray. *Pain* 1995; 63:271–275.

56. Unruh AM. Gender variations in clinical pain experience. *Pain* 1996; 65:123–167.

57. Cleeland CS, Gonin R, Hatfield AK, et al. Pain and its treatment in outpatients with metastatic cancer. *N Engl J Med* 1994; 330:592–596.

58. MacIntyre PE, Jarvis DA. Age is the best predictor of postoperative morphine requirements. *Pain* 1995; 64:357–368.

59. McQuay HJ, Carroll D, Faura CC, Gavaghan DJ, Hand CH, Moore RA. Oral morphine in cancer ain: influences on morphine and metabolite concentration. *Clin Pharmacol Ther* 1990; 48:236–244.

60. Tiseo PJ, Thaler HT, Lapin J, Inturrisi CE, Portenoy RK, Foley KM. Morphine-6-glucuronide concentrations and opioid-related side effects: a survey in cancer patients. *Pain* 1995; 61:47–54.

61. Viganò A, Bruera E, Suarez-Almazor M. Age, pain intensity, and opioid dose in patients with advanced cancer. *Cancer* 1998; 8:83–1244–1250.

62. Portenoy RK, Hagen NA. Breakthrough pain: definition, prevalence and characteristics. *Pain* 1990; 41:273–281.

63. Mercadante S, Arcuri E. Breakthrough pain in cancer patients: pathophysiology and treatment. *Cancer Treat Rev*, 1998; 24:425–432.

64. Smith GD, Smith MT. Morphine-3-glucuronide: evidence to support its putative role in the development of tolerance to the antinociceptive effects of morphine in the rat. *Pain* 1995; 62:51–60.

65. Gong QL, Hedner J, Bjorkman R, Hedner T. Morphine-3-glucuronide may functionally antagonize morphine-6-glucuronide induced antinociception and ventilatory depression. *Pain* 1992; 48:249–255.

66. Faura CC, Olaso MJ, Cabanes CG, et al. Lack of morphine-6-glucuronide antinociception after morphine treatment. Is morphine-3-glucuronide involved? *Pain* 1996; 65:25–30.

67. Werz MA, MacDonald RL. Opiate alkaloids antagonize postsynaptic glycine and GABA responses: correlation with convulsant action. *Brain Res* 1982; 236:107–119.

68. Morley JS, Miles JB, Bowsher D. Paradoxical pain. *Lancet* 1992; 340:1045.

69. Gourcke CR, Hackett LP, Ilett KF. Concentrations of morphine, morphine-6-glucuronide and morphine-3-glucuronide in serum and cerebrospinal fluid following morphine administration to patients with morphine-resistant pain. *Pain* 1994; 56:145–149.

70. Samuelsson H, Hedner T, Venn R, Michalkiewicz A. CSF and plasma concentrations of morphine and morphine glucuronides in cancer patients receiving epidural morphine. *Pain* 1993; 51:179–185.

71. Sjogren P, Jensen NH, Jensen TS. Disappearance of morphine-induced hyperalgesia after discontinuing or substituting with other opioid agonists. *Pain* 1994; 59:313–316.

72. Sjogren P, Jonsson T, Neils-Henrik J, Neils-Erick D, Jensen TS. Hyperalgesia and myoclonus in terminal cancer patients treated with continuous intravenous morphine. *Pain* 1993; 55:93–97.

73. Zaw-Tun N, Bruera E. Active metabolites of morphine. *J Palliat Care* 1992; 8:48–50.

74. Jenkins C, MacMillan K, Bruera E. Increasing pain and ascalating opioid dose in a patients with cancer. *J Palliat Care* 1997; 13:43–47.

75. Portenoy RK, Khan E, Layman M, et al. Chronic morphine therapy for cancer pain: plasma and cerebrospinal fluid morphine and morphine-6-glucuronide concentrations. *Neurology* 1991; 41:1457–1461.

76. D'Honneur G, Gilton A, Sandouk P, Scherrman JM, Duvaldestin P. Plasma and cerebrospinal fluid concentrations of morphine and morphine glucuronides after oral morphine. The influence of renal failure. *Anesthesiology* 1994; 81:87–93.

77. Bruera E, Pereira J. Neuropsychiatric toxicity of opioids. In: Jensen TS, Turner JA, Wiesenfeld-Hallin Z, eds. *Proceedings of the 8th World Congress on Pain*. Seattle: IASP Press, 1996; 717–738.

78. Wegert S, Ossipov MH, Nichols ML, et al. Differential activities of intrathecal MK-801 or morphine to alter responses to thermal and mechanical stimuli in normal or nerve-injury rats. *Pain* 1997; 71:57–64.

79. Andersen S, Dickenson AH, Kohn M, Reever A, Rahman W, Ebert B. The opioid ketobemidone has a NMDA blocking effect. *Pain* 1996; 67:369–374.

80. Ebert B, Andersen S, Krogsgaard-Larsen P. Ketobemidone, methadone and pethidine are non-competitive N-methyl-D-aspartate (NMDA) antagonists in the rat cortex and spinal cord. *Neurosci Lett* 1995; 187:165–168.

81. Ebert B, Thorkildsen C, Andersen S, Christrup LL, Hjeds H. Opioid analgesics as noncompetitive N-methyl-D-aspartate (NMDA) antagonists. *Biochem Pharmacol* 1998; 56:553–559.

82. Ebert B, Andersen S, Hjeds H, Dickenson AH. Dextropropoxyphene acts as a noncompetitive N-methyl-D-aspartate antagonist. *J Pain Symptom Manage* 1998; 15:269–274.
83. Mercadante S. Methadone in cancer pain. *Eur J Pain* 1997; 1:77–85.
84. Portenoy RK, Coyle N. Controversies in the long-term management of analgesic therapy in patients with advanced cancer. *J Pain Symptom Manage* 1990; 5:307–319.
85. Mercadante S, Portenoy RK. Opioid poorly responsive cancer pain. Part 3. Clinical strategies to improve opioid responsiveness. *J Pain Symptom Manage*, in press.
86. Fainsinger R, Bruera E. The management of dehydration in terminally ill patients. *J Palliat Care* 1994; 10:55–59.
87. Coyle N, Breitbart W, Weaver S, Portenoy RK. Delirium as a contributing factor to "crescendo" pain: three case reports. *J Pain Symptom Manage* 1994; 9:44–47.
88. Bruera E, Fainsinger R, Miller MJ, Kuehn N. The assessment of pain intensity in patients with cognitive failure: a prelimanry report. *J Pain Symptom Manage* 1992; 7:267–270.
89. Mercadante S. Pathophysiology and treatment of myoclonus in cancer. *Pain* 1998; 74:5–9.
90. Sjogren P, Dragsted L, Christensen CB. Myoclonic spasm during treatment with high doses of intravenous morphine in renal failure. *Acta Anaesthesiol Scand* 1993; 37:780–782.
91. Mercadante S. Dantrolene sodium in treating myoclonus associated with morphine therapy. *Anesth Analg* 1995; 81:1307–1308.
92. Potter JM, Reid DB, Shaw RJ, Hackett P, Hickmann PE. Myoclonus associated with treatment with high doses of morphine. the role of supplemental drugs. *Br Med J* 1989; 299:150–153.
93. Bruera E, Schoeller T, Montejo G. Organic hallucinosis in patients receiving high doses of opioids for cancer pain. *Pain* 1992; 48:397–399.
94. Ripamonti C, Bruera E. CNS adverse effects of opioids in cancer patients. Guidelines for treatment. *CNS Drugs* 1997; 8:21–37.
95. Daut RL, Cleeland CS. The prevalence and severity of pain in cancer. *Pain* 1982; 50:1913–1918.
96. Evers GCM. Pseudo-opioid-resistant pain. *Support Care Cancer* 1997; 5:457–460.
97. Weissman DE, Haddox JD. Opioid pseudoaddiction—an iatrogenic syndrome. *Pain* 1989; 36:363–366.
98. Coyle N, Portenoy RK. Infection as a cause of rapidly increasing pain in cancer patients. *J Pain Symptom Manage* 1991; 6:266–269.
99. Mackey JR, Birchall I, MacDonald N. Occult infection as a cause of hip pain in a patient with metastatic breast cancer. *J Pain Symptom Manage* 1995; 10:569–572.
100. Bruera E, MacDonald RN. Intractable pain in patients with advanced head and neck tumors: a possible role of local infection. *Cancer Treat Rep* 1986; 70:691–692.
101. Mercadante S. Opioid rotation in cancer pain. *Curr Rev Pain* 1998; 3:131–142.
102. Twycross RG. Attention to detail in palliative care. *Prog Palliat Care* 1994; 2:222–227.
103. Breitbart W. Psycho-oncology: depression, anxiety, delirium. *Sem Oncol* 1994; 21:754–769.

104. Peroutka SJ, Snyder SH. Antiemetics: neurotransmitter receptor binding predicts therapeutic actions. *Lancet* 1982; i:658–659.
105. Lichter I. Accelerated titration of morphine for rapid relief of cancer pain. *N Zeal Med J* 1994; 107:488–490.
106. Portenoy RK. Adjuvant analgesic agents. *Hematol/Oncol Clin North Am* 1996; 10:103–119.
107. Bruera E, Miller Ml, MacMillan D, Kuhen N. Neuropsychological effects of methylphenidate in patients receiving a continuous infusion of narcotics for cancer pain. *Pain* 1992; 48:163–166.
108. Bruera E, Fainsinger R, MacEachern T, Hanson J. The use of methylphenidate in patients with incident cancer pain receiving regular opiates: a preliminary report. *Pain* 1992; 50:75–77.
109. Eisele JH, Grisby EJ, Dea G. Clonazepam treatment of myoclonic contractions associated with high-dose opioids: case report. *Pain* 1992; 49:213–232.
110. Holdsworth M, Adamsa VR, Chvez CM, Vaughan LJ, Duncan MG. Continuous midazolam infusion for the management of morphine-induced myoclonus. *Ann Pharmacother* 1995; 29:25–29.
111. Wilweiding MB, Loprinzi CL, Mailliard JA, et al. A randomized, crossover evaluation of methylphenidate in cancer patients receiving strong narcotics. *Support Care Cancer* 1995; 3:135–138.
112. O'Neill WM. The cognitive and psychomotor effects of opioid drugs in cancer pain management. *Cancer Surv* 1995; 21:67–84.
113. Onghena P, Van Houdenhove B. Antidepressant-induced analgesia in chronic non-malignant pain: a meta-analysis of 39 placebo-controlled studies. *Pain* 1992; 49:205–219.
114. McQuay HJ, Carroll D, Glynn CJ. Low dose amitryptiline in the treatment of chronic pain. *Anesthesia* 1992; 47:646–652.
115. McQuay HJ, Tramèr M, Nye BA, Carroll D, Wiffen PJ, Moore RA. A systematic review of antidepressants in neuropathic pain. *Pain* 1996; 68:217–227.
116. Ventafridda V, Ripamonti C, De Conno F, Bianchi M, Pazzucconi F, Panerai AE. Antidepressants increase bioavailability of morphine in cancer patients. *Lancet* 1987; 1:1204.
117. Backonja M. Local anesthetics as adjuvant analgesics. *J Pain Symptom Manage* 1994; 9:491–499.
118. Ferrante FM, Paggioli J, Cherukuri S, Arthur GR. The analgesic response to intravenous lidocaine in the treatment of neuropathic pain. *Anesth Analg* 1996; 82:91–97.
119. Galer BS, Harle J, Rowbotham MC. Response to intravenous lidocaine infusion predicts subsequent response to oral mexiletine: a prospective study. *J Pain Symptom Manage* 1996; 12:161–167.
120. Brose WG, Cousins MJ. Subcutaneous lidocaine for treatment of neuropathic cancer pain. *Pain* 1991; 45:145–148.
121. Bruera E, Ripamonti C, Brenneis C, Macmillan K, Hanson J. A randomized double-blind crossover trial of intravenous lidocaine in the treatment of neuropathic cancer pain. *J Pain Symptom Manage* 1992; 7:138–140.
122. Dunlop RJ, Hockley JM, Tate T, Turner P. Flecainide in cancer nerve pain. *Lancet* 1994; 337:1347.

123. Tanelian DL, Victory RA. Sodium channel-blocking agents. *Pain Forum* 1995; 4:75–80.

124. Catterall WA, Common modes of drug action on sodium chennels: local anesthetics, antiarrhytmics and anticomvulsamts. *Trends Pharmacol Sci* 1987; 7:167–169.

125. Rowbotham MC. Topical analgesic agents. In: Fields HJL, Liebeskind JC, eds. *Pharmacological Approachs to the Treatment of Chronic Pain: New Concepts and Critical Issues.* Seattle: IASP Press, 1994:211–220.

126. Mercadante S, Sapio, Caligara M, Serretta R, Dardanoni G, Barresi L. Opioid-sparing effect of diclofenac in cancer pain. *J Pain Symptom Manage* 1997; 14:15–20.

127. Mercadante S, Barresi L, Casuccio A. Gastrointestinal bleeding in advanced cancer patients. *J Pain Symptom Manage* 2000; 19:160–162.

128. Fulfaro F, Casuccio A, Ticozzi C, Ripamonti C. The role of bisphosphonates in the treatment of painful metastatic bone disease. A review of phase III trial. *Pain* 1998; 78:157–169.

129. Keating HJ, Kundrat M. Patient-controlled analgesia with nitrous oxide in cancer pain. *J Pain Symptom Manage* 1996; 11:126–130.

130. Mercadante S, Portenoy RK. Opioid poorly responsive cancer pain. Part 2. Basic mechanisms that could shift dose-response for analgesia. *J Pain Symptom Manage*, in press.

131. Aredt-Nielsen L, Peterson-Felix S, Fischer M, Bak P, Bjerring P, Zbinden AM. The effect of N-Methyl-D-aspartate antagonists (ketamine) on single and repeated nociceptive stimuli: a placebo-controlled experimental human study. *Anesth Analg* 1995; 81:63–68.

132. Oshima F, Tei K, Kayazawa H, Urabe N. Continuous subcutaneous injection of ketamine for cancer pain. *Can J Anaesth* 1990; 37:385–392.

133. Sosnowski M, Lossignol D, Fodderie L. Reversibility of opioid insensitive pain. Proceedings of the 7th World Congress on Pain, Paris, August 22–27, 1993:16.

134. Ogawa S, Kanamaru T, Noda K, et al. Intravenous microdrip infusion of ketamine in subanaesthetic doses for intractable terminal cancer pain. *Pain Clin* 1994; 7:125–129.

135. Mercadante S, Caligara M, Sapio M, Serretta R, Lodi F. Long-term ketamine subcutaneous continuous infusion in neuropathic cancer pain. *J Pain Symptom Manage* 1995; 10:564–568.

136. Persson J, Axelsson G, Hallin RG, Gustafsson LL. Beneficial effects of ketamine in a chronic pain state with allodynia, possibly due to central sensitization. *Pain* 1995; 60:217–222.

137. Edmonds P, Davis C. Experience of the use of subcutaneous ketamine in patients with cancer-related neuropathic pain. *Eur J Palliat Care.* Abstracts of the 4th Congress of the European Association for Palliative Care, Barcelona, 1995; 68.

138. Clark JL, Kalan GE. Effective treatment of severe cancer pain of the head using low-dose ketamine in an opioid-tolerant patients. *J Pain Symptom Manage* 1995; 10:310–314.

139. Luczak J, Dickenson AH, Kotlinska-Lemieszek A. The role of ketamine, an NMDA receptor antagonist, in the management of pain. *Progress Palliat Care* 1995; 3:127–134.

140. Mercadante S. Ketamine in cancer pain: an update. *Palliat Med* 1996; 10:225–230.

141. Mercadante S, Arcuri E, Tirelli W. The analgesic effect of ketamine in cancer patients on opioid therapy: a randomized, controlled, double-blind, cross-over, double dose study. *J Pain Symptom Manage* 2000; 20:246–252.

142. Yang CY, Wong CS, Chang JY, Ho ST. Intrathecal ketamine reduces morphine requirements in patients with terminal cancer pain. *Can J Anaesth* 1996; 43:379–383.

143. Mao J, Price DD, Caruso FS, Mayer D. Oral administration of dextromethorphan prevents the development of morphine tolerance and dependence in rats. *Pain* 1996; 67:361–368.

144. Mercadante S, Casuccio A, Genovese G. Ineffectiveness of dextromethorphan in cancer pain. *J Pain Symptom Manage* 1998; 16:317–322.

145. Felsby S, Nielsen J, Arendt-Nielsen L, Jensen TS. NMDA receptor blockade in chronic neuropathic pain: a comparison of ketamine and magnesium chloride. *Pain* 1995; 64:283–291.

146. Pud D, Eisenberg E, Spitzer A, Adler R, Fried G, Yarnitsky D. The NMDA receptor antagonist amantadine reduces surgical neuropathic pain in cancer patients: a double blind, randomized, placebo controlled trial. *Pain* 1998; 75:349–354.

147. Bernstein ZP, Yucht S, Battista E, Lema M, Spaulding MB. Proglumide as a morphine adjunct in cancer pain management. *J Pain Symptom Manage* 1998; 15:314–320.

148. Santillan R, Maestre JM, Hurlé MA, Florez J. Enhancement of opiate analgesia by nimodipine in cancer patients chronically treated with morphine: a preliminary report. *Pain* 1994; 58:129–132.

149. Roca G, Aguilar JL, Gomar C, Mazo V, Costa J, Vidal F. Nimodipine fails to enhance the analgesic effect of slow release morphine in the early phases of cancer pain treatment. *Pain* 1996; 68:239–243.

150. Santillàn R, Hurlè MA, Armijo JA, de los Mozos R, Flòrez J. Nimodipine-enhanced opiate analgesia in cancer patients requiring morphine dose escalation: a double-blind, placebo-controlled study. *Pain* 1998; 76:17–26.

151. Peterson GM, Randall CTC, Peterson J. Plasma levels of morphine and morphine glucuronides in the treatment of cancer pain: relationship to renal function and route of administration. *Eur J Clin Pharmacol* 1990; 38:121–124.

152. Mercadante S, Fulfaro F. Alternative routes to oral morphine in cancer pain. *Oncology*, 1999; 13:215–225.

153. Vainio A, Tigerstedt I. Opioid treatment for radiation cancer pain: oral vs. epidural techniques. *Acta Anesthesiol Scand* 1988; 32:179–185.

154. Sjogren P, Banning A. Pain, sedation and reaction time during long-term treatment of cancer patients with oral and epidural opioids. *Pain* 1989; 39:5–11.

155. Kalso E, Heiskanen T, Rantio M, Rosenberg PH, Vainio A. Epidural and subcutaneous morphine in the management of cancer pain: a double-blind cross-over study. *Pain* 1996; 67:443–449.

156. Samuelsson H, Hedner T. Pain characterization in cancer patients and the analgesic response to epidural morphine. *Pain* 1991; 46:3–8.

157. Mercadante S. Problems of long-term spinal opioid treatment in advanced cancer patients. *Pain* 1999; 79:1–13.

158. Coluzzi PH. Oral patient-controlled analgesia. *Semin Oncol* 1997; 24 (suppl.16):35–42.

159. Cleary JF. Pharmacokinetic and pharmacodynamic issues in the treatment of break-through pain. *Semin Oncol* 1997;24 (suppl.16):13–19.

160. Fine PG. Fentanyl in the treatment of cancer pain. *Semin Oncol* 1997; 24 (suppl.16):20–27.

161. Farrar JT, Cleary J, Rauck R, Busch M, Nordbrock E. Oral transmucosal fentanyl citrate: randomized, double-blinded, placebo-controlled trial for treatment of break-through pain in cancer patient. *J Natl Cancer Inst* 1998; 90:611–616.

162. Cherny NJ, Chang V, Frager G, et al. Opioid pharmacotherapy in the management of cancer pain. *Cancer* 1995; 76:1288–1293.

163. de Stouz ND, Bruera E, Suarez-Alazor M. Opioid rotation for toxicity reduction in terminal cancer patients. *J Pain Symptom Manage* 1995; 10:378–384.

164. Galer BS, Coyle N, Pasternak GW, Portenoy RK. Individual variability in the response to different opioids: report of five cases. *Pain* 1992; 49:87–91.

165. Crews JC, Sweeney N, Denson DD. Clinical efficacy of methadone in patients refractory to other mu-opioid receptor agonist analgesics for the management of ter-minal cancer pain. *Cancer* 1993; 72:2266–2272.

166. Portnow JM, Corbett RJ. Oral methadone for relief of chronic pain from cancer. *N Engl J Med* 1982; 306:889–990.

167. Leng G, Finnegan MJ. Successful use of methadone in nociceptive cancer pain unre-sponsive to morphine. *Palliat Med* 1994; 8:153–155.

168. MacDonald N, Der L, Allen S, Champion F. Opioid hyperexcitability: the applica-tion of an alternate opioid therapy. *Pain* 1993; 53:353–355.

169. Rimmer T, Trotman I. Methadone restores opioid sensitivity in cancer pain. *Palliat Med* 1996; 10:58.

170. Manfredi PL, Borsook D, Chandler SW, et al. Intravenous methadone for cancer pain unrelieved by morphine and hydromorphone: clinical observation. *Pain* 1997; 70:99–101.

171. Viganò A, Fan D, Bruera E. Individualized use of methadone and opioid rotation in the comprehensive management of cancer pain associated with poor prognostic indicators. *Pain* 1996; 67:115–119.

172. Morley JS, Watt JWG, Wells JC, Miles JB, Finnegan MJ, Leng G. Methadone in pain uncontrolled by morphine. *Lancet* 1993; 342:1243.

173. Lawlor P, Turner K, Hanson J, Bruera E. Dose ratio between morphine and methadone in patients with cancer pain: a retrospective study. *Cancer* 1998; 82:1167–1173.

174. Bruera E, Pereira J, Watanabe S, Belzile M, Kuehn N, Hanson J. Opioid rotation in patients with cancer pain. A retrospective comparison of dose ratios between methadone, hydromorphone, and morphine. *Cancer* 1996; 78:852–857.

175. Ripamonti C, Groff L, Brunelli C, Polastri D, Stavrakis A, De Conno F. (1998) Switching from morphine to oral methadone in treating cancer pain: what is the equianalgesic dose ratio? *J Clin Oncol* 1998; 16:3216–3221.

176. Morley JS. Makin MK. Comments on Ripamonti et al. *Pain* 1997; 73:14.

177. Watanabe S, Pereira J, Hanson J, Bruera E. Fentanyl by continuous subcutaneous infusion for the management of cancer pain: a retrospective study. *J Pain Symptom Manage* 1998; 16:323–326.

178. Paix A, Coleman A, Lees J, et al. Subcutaneous fentanyl and sufentanil infusion substitution for morphine intolerance in cancer pain management. *Pain* 1995; 61:263–269.

179. Singer M, Noonan KR. Continuous intravenous infusion of fentanyl: case reports of use in patients with advanced cancer and intractable pain. *J Pain Symptom Manage* 1993; 8:215–220.

180. Mercadante S, Caligara M, Sapio M, Serretta R, Lodi F. Subcutaneous fentanyl infusion in obstructed patient with renal failure. *J Pain Symptom Manage* 1997; 13:241–244.

181. Kirkham SR, Pugh R. Opioid analgesia in uraemic patients. *Lancet* 1995; 345:1185.

182. Hoskin PJ. Radiotherapy for bone pain. *Pain* 1995; 63:137–139.

183. Needham PR, Hoskin PJ. Radiotherapy for painful bone metastases. *Palliat Med* 1994; 8:95–104.

184. Mercadante S, Sapio M, Villari P. Suprascapular nerve block by catheter for breakthrough shoulder cancer pain. *Reg Anaesth* 1995; 20:343–346.

185. Aguilar JL, Montes A, Samper D, Roca G, Vidal F. Interpleural analgesia through a Du Pen catheter in lung cancer pain. *Cancer* 1992; 70:2621–2623.

186. Fischer HBJ, Peters TM, Fleming IM, Else MB. Peripheral nerve catheterization in the management of terminal cancer pain. *Reg Anesth* 1996; 21:482–485.

187. Myers DP, Lema MJ, de Leon-Casasola OA, Bacon DR. Interpleural analgesia for the treatment of severe cancer pain in terminally ill patients. *J Pain Symptom Manage* 1993; 8:505–510.

188. Sato S, Yamashita S, Iwai M, Mizuyama K, Satsumae T. Continuous interscalene block for cancer pain. *Reg Anesth* 1994; 19:73–75.

189. Boys L, Peat SJ, Hanna MH, Burn K. Audit of neural blockade for palliative care patients. *Palliat Med* 1993; 7:205–212.

190. Polati E, Finco G, Gottin L, Bassi C, Pederzoli P, Ischia S. Prospective randomized double-blind trial of neurolytic coeliac plexus block in patients with pancreatic cancer. *Br J Surg* 1998; 85:199–201.

191. Lillemoe KD, Cameron JL, Kaufman HS, Yeo CJ, Pitt HA, Sauter PK. Chemical splanchnicectomy in patients with unresectable pancreatic cancer. A prospective randomized trial. *Ann Surg* 1993; 217:447–457.

192. Mercadante S, Nicosia F. Celiac plexus block: a reappraisal. *Reg Anesth Pain Med* 1998; 23:37–48.

193. Mercadante S. Analgesic blocks in palliative care. *Eur J Palliat Care* 1995; 2:103–106.

VI

PAIN AND OTHER SYMPTOMS: TREATMENT CHALLENGES

15

Dose Ratios Among Different Opioids: Underlying Issues and an Update on the Use of the Equianalgesic Table

PETER LAWLOR, JOSE PEREIRA, AND
EDUARDO BRUERA

In patients with cancer pain, a change of opioid is recognized as a useful strategy in the management of either opioid toxicity alone or the combination of opioid toxicity and failure to achieve adequate analgesia with an existing opioid.[1–3] Terms such as opioid rotation,[2] sequential opioid trials,[4] or opioid substitution[5,6] are used to describe this strategy. The frequency of opioid rotation varies in different centers with rates as high as 40%.[7] To assist physicians with dose calculation for an opioid switch, guidelines in the form of equianalgesic tables are available in health agency publications,[8,9] major textbooks,[10,11] and major reviews.[12]

This chapter initially clarifies relevant terminology and briefly summarizes the putative underlying mechanisms and factors associated with opioid cross-tolerance. The basis of the current equianalgesic tables is discussed, followed by an outline of their limitations, particularly in the light of recently published studies. Finally, suggestions are made regarding potential revision of specific areas of these tables, and also regarding methodological aspects of future clinical research on equianalgesic dose ratios.

Clarification of Terminology

Tolerance is defined as the decrease in a drug affect, such as analgesia or an adverse effect, as a result of prior exposure to the drug. Cross-tolerance between two opioids refers to the phenomenon whereby tolerance to a particular opioid effect from an existing opioid is conferred to a newly substituted opioid. The extent to which this occurs is commonly referred to as complete or incomplete. The order or direction in which they are administered can influence the level of cross-tolerance between two opioids. Cross-tolerance is not necessarily the same in both directions, hence the term asymmetrical cross-tolerance,[13] or it may only exist in one direction, hence the term unidirectional cross-tolerance.[14] True pharmacological tolerance implies a pharmacodynamic or a neuroadaptive process. This is in contrast to pharmacokinetic or dispositional tolerance, which refer more to drug bioavailability rather than neuroadaptive processes.

Potency of an opioid refers to the dose required to produce a given opioid effect. This is not synonymous with intrinsic efficacy, which refers to the degree of receptor occupancy in order to achieve a certain level of effect. The relative potency of two opioids is determined by the respective doses required to achieve the same level of effect, and in the case of analgesia, this ratio is commonly referred to as either the dose ratio or equianalgesic dose ratio.

Relevance of Tolerance and Cross-Tolerance

While the phenomenon of tolerance is well recognized in animal models of opioid exposure,[15-17] its existence with regard to analgesia in cancer pain patients is debated.[18,19] However, the development of tolerance in cancer patients to opioid side effects is well recognized.[11,19] This allows for dose increases to occur without intolerable sedation, nausea, or respiratory depression. Although clinical use of the term cross-tolerance commonly tends to refer exclusively to analgesic effects, the term also encompasses the level of tolerance to adverse effects. Differences between opioids in the balance between analgesic cross-tolerance level and the level of cross-tolerance to adverse effects can be exploited to clinical advantage. Switching opioids can possibly achieve a more favorable balance between analgesia and adverse effects, hence the rationale for trial of a different opioid in the event of toxicity or inadequate analgesia.[2,19,20]

Pharmacodynamic Basis of Opioid Cross-Tolerance

Putative pharmacodynamic mechanisms and factors implicated in opioid tolerance and cross-tolerance are outlined in Table 15.1. Although the combination of these mechanistic variables, their interrelationships and in turn, their relationships with associated factors in parallel systems are highly complex, the 1990s has revealed greater insight into these phenomena. This insight has occurred primarily because of the development of techniques such as receptor cloning[21] and antisense oligonucleotide sequences that "knockdown" specific opioid receptors.[22] Clinical experience suggests that tolerance is generally not a major problem in the treatment of chronic pain.[19,23] Therefore, cross-tolerance in this

Table 15.1. Potential pharmacodynamic mechanisms and factors implicated in opioid tolerance and cross-tolerance

Levels of operation	Potential mechanism or factor
Opioid receptors	Differential receptor selectivity of opioid agonist
	Receptor occupancy and intrinsic efficacy of opioid
	Downregulation of receptor numbers—internalization
	Altered receptor affinity and uncoupling of G protein link
	Modulatory role of δ-receptoractivation
NMDA receptor	Increased intracellular calcium levels
	Nitric oxide production
Intracellular	Protein kinases: receptor phosphorylation adenylyl cyclase phosphorylation
	Protein kinase C activation—NMDA activation
Other parallel systems	? Cholecystokinin (CCK)
	? α 2-adrenoreceptor
	? Adenosine (A_1) receptor
	? 5-HT receptors
	? Dopamine (D) receptors
Genetic	c-fos proto-oncogene activation

NMDA, *N*-methyl-D-aspartate.

setting is possibly of greater importance, particularly in relation to switches among currently available opioids but also in relation to the potential development of new drugs, whose receptor targeting will possibly entail greater selectivity than those currently available. Although, the preponderance of research has focussed on opioid tolerance rather than cross-tolerance, there is a considerable degree of conceptual duality in the mechanisms underlying both tolerance and cross-tolerance. Reviewing these pharmacodynamic mechanisms provides potential explanations for incomplete cross-tolerance and asymmetrical or unidirectional cross-tolerance.

The differential level of opioid receptor selectivity ascribed to individual opioid agonists is recognized as a potential explanation for the level of cross-tolerance among opioids.[19,23,24,25] Both animal and in vitro studies of opioid cross-tolerance between μ- and κ-receptor selective agonists have largely demonstrated a lack of cross-tolerance.[26–29] However, some studies have demonstrated a degree of cross-tolerance between selective μ- and κ-receptor agonists.[30,31] The occurrence of either cross-tolerance or lack of cross-tolerance in one direction between two opioids does not imply a similar occurrence in the opposite direction.[14,30,32] Hence in rats treated with levorphanol, a mixed μ and κ agonist, cross-tolerance was conferred to both levorphanol and morphine, a μ agonist, but the reverse failed to occur when morphine was administered first.[14]

The δ opioid receptor has been suggested as having a modulatory role in the development of morphine tolerance.[33] Studies involving selective blockage of the δ receptor in mice, using either a selective opioid antagonist[34] or an antisense oligonucleotide to "knockdown" the receptor,[35] suggest a consequent attenuation of morphine tolerance. Interaction or "cross-talk" between μ and δ receptors has also been proposed, in addition to a possible μ–δ receptor complex.[36] The heterogeneity of the δ opioid receptor is demonstrated by the opposing actions of its subtypes.[37] Collectively, studies examining the differential receptor selectivity associated with different opioids suggest a potential role for this mechanism in relation to incomplete cross-tolerance.

Opioid receptors are coupled to effector proteins such as adenylyl cyclase through G-proteins (guanine nucleotide regulatory protein).[38,39] Opioid agonists promote receptor signaling via G-proteins, including inhibition of adenylyl cyclase and regulation of calcium and potassium channels.[39,40] Regulation of opioid receptor activity following agonist binding can be achieved by endocytotic internalization, resulting in a downregulation or decrement of receptor number,[41–43] or by desensitization, a process involving an uncoupling of the link between receptor and effector protein.[44,45] An in vivo study of tolerance development in mice exposed to an opioid with high intrinsic efficacy showed initially a receptor downregulation but following the opioid infusion there was a 55%–65% increase in μ receptor mRNA associated with a decrease in tolerance level.[46] Differences in the level of rapid internalization or downregulation of opioid receptors relates to both type specific receptor mechanisms[43,47] and variations in the ability of different opioids to bind to these receptors.[48–50] Morphine is exceptional in its inability to promote rapid internalization of μ receptors.[48,51,52]

A study involving chronic administration of morphine to rats showed that desensitization of μ and δ opioid receptors in different brain structures is not identical.[37] Desensitization of both μ and δ receptors has been linked to the phosphorylation activity of G-protein–coupled receptor kinases.[53,54] Other kinases, including protein kinase C have also been implicated in μ receptor desensitization.[45] While the relative contribution of desensitization and internalization to the development of opioid tolerance is not entirely clear, some authors have suggested an interrelationship between these two mechanisms.[55] A recent animal study revealed that chronic morphine exposure is associated with phosphorylation of adenylyl cyclase, which is likely to be protein kinase C–mediated.[56] As an earlier study of chronic morphine exposure showed an increased G-protein stimulatory effect on adenylyl cyclase,[57] the authors propose that phosphorylation of certain adenylyl cyclase isoforms increases their responsiveness to the stimulatory effects of these G-proteins. Hence tolerance would involve a shift from inhibition to stimulation of adenylyl cyclase.

The influence of the intrinsic efficacy of different opioids on the development of tolerance and cross-tolerance has been examined in animal and in vitro studies. The level of intrinsic efficacy of an opioid is reflected in the number of "spare receptors" available for opioid binding. In the case of methadone, its high intrinsic efficacy has been associated with the development of relatively less tolerance,[58,59] and in addition it has been suggested to play a role in the asymmetric cross-tolerance between morphine and methadone.[58,60,61] In a comparison study of intrathecally administered fentanyl and morphine in rats, the lower level of tolerance development with fentanyl and in turn, the greater level of cross-tolerance as a result of pretreatment with morphine, was attributed to the greater intrinsic efficacy of fentanyl.[13] A study examining tolerance to morphine, etorphine, and fentanyl in mice showed that tolerance development was inversely related to intrinsic efficacy when administered by continuous but not intermittent infusion.[62] In the case of acute opioid tolerance, a study of the analgesic effects of morphine, alfentanil, and sufentanil in rats concluded that the magnitude of acute tolerance to these opioids was not inversely related to their relative potency.[63]

Many studies using N-methyl-D-aspartate (NMDA) receptor antagonists have demonstrated a role for activation of the NMDA receptor in the development of tolerance to morphine.[64–67] The role of NMDA activation in opioid tolerance has been linked with activation of protein kinase C,[65,68,69] elevation of intracellular calcium levels,[69,70] and nitric oxide production.[71,72] Promotion of immediate early gene (IEG) expression such as c-fos has been associated with NMDA receptor activation, and is likely mediated by an increase in intracellular calcium.[73] An association between c-fos proto-oncogene expression and the neuronal ability to convert short-term stimulation to longer-term plasticity changes, similar to those involved in memory formation has been suggested.[74] N-methyl-D-aspartate antagonism has been suggested to play a role in opioid potency, in addition to differentially modulating μ and κ receptor tolerance.[75]

Methadone has been shown to act as a noncompetitive NMDA antagonist.[76,77] This property of methadone has been queried by many authors as contributing to its greater relative analgesic potency when substituted in the case of chronic as opposed to acute administration of morphine and hydromorphone.[78–80] A recent prospective randomized study comparing morphine and methadone in 40 advanced patients suggested escalation of opioid dose over time was less likely to occur with methadone than with morphine.[81] The mechanism of pain warrants consideration, as neuropathic pain has generally been reported to be less responsive to opioids,[82–84] or in the case of some studies, nonresponsive to opioids.[85] Methadone is possibly more effective in the treatment of neuropathic pain, an observation that has been attributed to its recognized NMDA receptor antagonist properties.[6] Moreover, an explanatory model of shared mechanisms (predominantly NMDA receptor activation) subserving both the neuronal plasticity of hyperalgesia and opioid tolerance has been suggested.[70]

Apart from the NMDA system, many studies have investigated the complex interplay of other parallel systems in relation to their potential role in opioid tolerance and cross-tolerance. A study of cross-tolerance between α_2-adrenoceptor agonists and selective opioid receptor agonists in mice demonstrated differential cross-tolerance between α_2 receptors and opioid receptor types or subtypes.[86] Symmetrical cross-tolerance has been shown to exist between adenosine (A_1) and μ peripheral antinociceptive mechanisms.[87] A further study of peripheral antinociception showed cross-tolerance between μ and α_2 receptors, and between α_2 and A_1, suggesting that their underlying mechanisms are related.[88] The authors of the latter study proposed the existence of an A_1, α_2, and μ receptor complex. Cross-tolerance has also been demonstrated between intrathecal fentanyl, a potent μ agonist and 5-HT.[89] The phenomenon of cross-tolerance between opioidergic and at least some of the parallel systems is likely to relate to convergence and sharing of second messenger systems. Interaction between the opioid and cholecystokinin systems has been proposed.[90] Animal studies suggest that cholecystokinin antagonists attenuate morphine tolerance.[91–93] A randomized double-blind, cross-over study in patients with cancer pain suggested beneficial analgesic effects with the addition of proglumide, as an adjunct to opioid therapy.[94]

In the mouse, chronic morphine administration has been shown to lead to increased dopamine receptor sensitivity,[95] whereas bromocriptine has been shown to attenuate the development of tolerance to morphine analgesia.[96] The complexity of interaction between opioidergic and dopaminergic systems was highlighted in a recent study in rats.[97] Chronic morphine administration resulted in desensitization of both dopamine D_2 and δ opioid receptors in striato-pallidal neurons, but failed to induce μ receptor tolerance in the striato-nigral pathway.

Opioids differ in their intrinsic efficacy, potency, relative receptor selectivity, and in turn receptors differ in their regulatory processes such as phosphorylation, uncoupling, and internalization. These factors combined with the potential interactions of other parallel systems could contribute in varying degrees to the pharmacodynamic phenomenon of tolerance, whereas their contribution to opioid cross-tolerance has been less well-studied and consequently is less well-known.

Nonpharmacodynamic Issues in Opioid Cross-Tolerance

The predominantly nonpharmacodynamic factors worthy of consideration in the context of opioid cross-tolerance are summarized in Table 15.2. The role of ongoing nociception on the development of opioid tolerance is controversial.[98] Although there has been a profusion of both in vitro and animal experimental model studies of opioid tolerance, the translation of their findings to the clinical context of humans with advanced cancer is extremely challenging. Tolerance development with opioid treatment in animal studies can occur within hours to days,[99,100] or even after a single dose.[101] In humans, the duration of opioid treatment required for tolerance development and the influence of route of administration on this duration are less clear. Clinical experience in humans suggests that using different routes of administration, plateaus of stable dosing are maintained for long periods of time, usually days to weeks.[23,102,103] Animal studies suggest that the presence of chronic nociceptive stimulation does not prevent the development of tolerance[17] but might significantly facilitate the development of morphine

Table 15.2. Nonpharmacodynamic factors to consider in relation to opioid tolerance and cross-tolerance

Pain related	Disease progression or infection at tumor site
	Incidental versus non-incidental
	Impact of other therapies and adjuvant drugs
Dispositional or pharmacokinetic factors	Absorption of opioid—change of route of administration
	Drug interactions
	Drug biotransformation and metabolism
	Antinociceptive metabolites (e.g., morphine-6-glucuronide)
	? Antagonist metabolites (e.g., morphine-3-glucuronide)
	Renal function
	Genetic enzymatic deficiencies
Patient behavior and psychological state	Somatization and psychological distress
	Chemical coping
	Cognitive status and delirium

tolerance.[104] While there is some control over the level of pain stimulus in animal studies, this rarely occurs in clinical practice. In patients who appear tolerant to opioid side effects, a neurolytic procedure can result in the emergence of side effects such as sedation if the opioid dose is not reduced.[19] The presence of tolerance therefore often warrants the use of adjuvant therapies,[23] and in turn, the continued use or discontinuation of these therapies in the context of opioid rotation could influence the apparent level of opioid cross-tolerance. Disease progression is considered the most likely reason for dose escalation in patients with advanced cancer.[102,105] Clinical experience suggests that escalation in opioid analgesic requirements is likely to relate to disease factors such as the mechanical effects of tumor growth and the biochemical effects of inflammation,[19] or local infection.[106,107] The presence of predominantly incidental pain has a recognized association with greater difficulty in achieving analgesia,[108] and the use of opioid doses high enough to control episodes of incident pain but in excess of analgesic requirements between these episodes, thereby resulting in the manifestation of adverse effects.[109] Incidental pain can therefore play a role in the manifestation of tolerance levels to both analgesic and adverse effects. Neuropathic pain, discussed previously in relation to methadone and NMDA activation, similarly warrants clinical consideration in relation to opioid cross-tolerance, albeit that the complex relationship between neuronal modulatory processes and tolerance development is not completely understood.

Problems with delivery of an opioid or its active metabolite to its site of action can result in escalation of opioid dose to maintain the same level of analgesia, hence the development of dispositional or pharmacokinetic tolerance. Many factors in the absorption, metabolism, and elimination sequence can influence this type of tolerance. Specifically these factors include pharmacokinetic properties such as route of administration, partition coefficient, pKa, degree of ionization, unbound fraction of dose, apparent volume of distribution, and clearance.[110] A change in route of opioid administration is required in approximately 60% of advanced cancer patients in their last 4 weeks of life,[111] often because of impediments in relation to the mode of administration and absorption.

Current equianalgesic dose tables quote the oral to parenteral potency ratios for most opioids. In the case of morphine, single-dose studies showed a 6:1 oral to parenteral dose ratio.[112] However, clinical practice in cancer patients (reflected also in most equianalgesic tables) exposed to repeated dosing suggests this ratio is 2:1 or 3:1.[113,114] The different oral to parenteral dose ratios of morphine in single dosing and chronic dosing has been attributed to the accumulation of the active analgesic metabolite, morphine-6-glucuronide (M-6-G),[113] possibly facilitated by an enterohepatic circulation.[115]

The potential role of morphine metabolites in the generation of morphine tolerance is controversial. Morphine is largely metabolized to morphine-3-glucuronide (M-3-G) and to a lesser extent to M-6-G and normorphine.[115] Morphine-6-glucuronide has an analgesic potency in the range of 2 to 800 times that of morphine, depending on route of administration, species studied, and study design.[116] A study of morphine infusions in humans showed a significant correlation between M-6-G/morphine ratio and pain relief.[117] In contrast, animal studies suggest that M-3-G administered intracerebroventricularly can antagonize morphine analgesia.[118] Studies have also suggested that M-3-G can functionally antagonize both the antinociceptive and respiratory depressive effects of M-6-G via intrathecal and intracerebroventricular routes,[119] but does not do so via intravenous administration.[120,121] Morphine-3-glucuronide has been associated with a number of neuroexcitatory phenomena such as allodynia, hyperalgesia, "wet-dog shakes" and myoclonus in animals.[118] Similar neuroexcitatory effects, including seizures have been reported in humans on high dose morphine or hydromorphone.[112–126] The hydromorphone metabolite, hydromorphone-3-glucuronide (H-3-G)[127] and the morphine metabolite, normorphine-3-glucuronide[128] also have neuroexcitatory and antinociceptive effects in rats, and therefore these metabolites could potentially influence tolerance development. In the case of morphine, some authors have suggested an imbalance in the ratio of M-3-G to M-6-G, with a disproportionate amount of M-3-G giving rise to paradoxical pain.[129] A study of M-6-G antinociception in mice showed a rightward shift of the dose response curve with prior administration of M-3-G.[130] However, a study of cancer patients with morphine-resistant pain revealed ratios of M-6-G/morphine in plasma and cerebrospinal fluid (CSF) that were similar to those previously reported for patients in good pain control.[131] Furthermore, a systematic review of the M-6-G/M-3-G ratio in a variety of study populations suggested that this ratio remains virtually constant.[132] A study of morphine metabolite levels in hospice patients showed significantly higher levels of both M-3-G and M-6-G in patients with renal impairment, and all of these patients had associated nausea and delirium.[133] Given the recognized role of the NMDA receptor in opioid tolerance and the recognized low affinity binding of M-3-G to this receptor,[134] a study in rats failed to show that this metabolite's neuroexcitatory effects were elicited through the NMDA receptor.[135] In the setting of high opioid dose administration there is growing evidence suggesting that accumulation of these metabolites is associated with the development of adverse neuroexcitatory effects.[122,123,136] In the context of renal impairment, there is clear evidence of accumulation of morphine metabolites,[116,137,138,132,133] and in humans this accumulation has been documented in association with adverse effects such as nausea,[133,139] respiratory depression,[140] multifocal myoclonus,[122,136] and delirium.[133] An opioid switch could therefore allow for the clearance of these metabolites and restoration of a more favorable balance between analgesia and adverse effects, often at a much lower dose of opioid than standard dose ratios would suggest,[4,125,141] especially where hyperalgesia has occurred in relation to the previous opioid.[122,126,142]

A study of cancer pain management in humans examined the relationship between analgesia and CSF levels of morphine and its metabolites following a switch from oral or subcutaneous to intracerebroventricular (ICV) administration of morphine.[143] The CSF level of morphine increased 50-fold in the first 24 hours following ICV administration of morphine. This was the main reason proposed for the improved analgesia, on the grounds that morphine was delivered closer to one of its main sites of action and was in higher concentration in this region. Despite detection of M-6-G in plasma, CSF levels of M-6-G were undetectable in 9 out of 20 patients with poor pain control on systemic morphine, suggesting that M-6-G contributes to the analgesic effects of systemically administered morphine. Because the ICV dosage requirements did not increase over time, and because reduction in side effects coincided with a 90% decrease in CSF levels of M-3-G, the authors suggest that both morphine tolerance and its neuroexcitatory side effects are unlikely to be caused by morphine itself but rather involve the active glucuronide metabolites. A study of the disposition of morphine in cancer patients receiving long-term subcutaneous infusions of morphine showed large intra- and interindividual variability.[144] In a pharmacokinetic study of 151 cancer patients undergoing chronic treatment with oral morphine, morphine dose, age, sex, renal and hepatic dysfunction, and concomitant medications as explanatory variables accounted for 70% of the variance in plasma concentrations of morphine, M-6-G and M-3-G.[145] In the case of concomitant medications, raised creatinine and coadministration of tricyclic antidepressants increased plasma M-3-G concentrations, ranitidine increased morphine plasma concentrations, and raised creatinine plus coadministration of ranitidine increased M-6-G plasma concentrations. The pharmacodynamic relevance of the coadministration of tricyclic antidepressants or ranitidine with morphine or other opioids in clinical practice is less clear. Overall, on the basis of current evidence, it is likely that morphine metabolites are involved in both adverse effects and analgesic tolerance, although their precise contribution remains unclear.

Genetic polymorphism in relation to the enzymatic ability to metabolize opioids can possibly influence both the level of analgesia and the emergence of adverse effects. In the case of codeine, an estimated 7%–10% of caucasians lack the cytochrome P-450 enzyme, CPY 2D6 to allow O-demethylation to its active analgesic metabolite, morphine.[146,147] Poor metabolizers of codeine that lack the CPY 2D6 enzyme therefore achieve a poorer level of analgesia but surprisingly have the same level of adverse effects.[148] This enzymatic deficiency could have a significant impact on cross-tolerance between codeine and other opioids. Oxycodone undergoes demethylation to oxymorphone using the same cytochrome enzyme but the amount produced[149,150] and the role of this metabolite in the analgesic effects of oxycodone are not entirely clear,[151] albeit that oxymorphone has a relative analgesic potency 10 times that of morphine.[152] Poor pain control has been documented in a known poor metabolizer of oxycodone lacking the CPY 2D6 enzyme.[153] Severe respiratory depression and sedation reported in a cancer patient following an opioid switch from oxycodone to hydromorphone was postulated to be because of an inadvertently high dose of hydromorphone in the case of a poor metabolizer of oxycodone.[154] Apart from these examples, the interindividual variability in opioid responsiveness has been postulated to be due in part to genetic differences,[155] Hence it is possible that genetic differences could potentially influence cross-tolerance between opioids.

The impact of psychological state and behavioral patterns on pain expression and consequently on opioid dosing and possible tolerance development is well recognized but difficult to quantify. Somatization or psychological distress, and a history of drugs or alcohol abuse have been identified as risk factors for poor pain control in cancer patients.[156] Delirium in cancer patients is often manifested as disinhibition with the consequent risk of misinterpreting pain level and administering opioids inappropriately.[157]

Earlier Clinical Studies of Opioid Cross-Tolerance and Basis of Current Equianalgesic Tables

Some of the earlier clinical studies of cross-tolerance in humans were conducted in cancer pain patients on relatively low doses of opioid.[158] One of these studies involved an initial double-blind relative potency comparison using placebo and graded doses of morphine and metopon on two groups of patients. One group were administered morphine for a week, whereas the other received metopon. At the end of this period, a relative potency estimate was again conducted with graded doses similar to the initial relative potency assay. Although their sample sizes were too small to allow definitive conclusions, their findings demonstrated a trend that direct tolerance developed to both opioids and cross-tolerance also occurred, albeit to a lesser degree.

The current equianalgesic tables are based largely on the pioneering work of Houde et al.[112] Originally the tables were developed to provide the pharmaceutical industry with dose guidelines when introducing new analgesics. These early studies involved single dosing with an elegant study design, incorporating

Table 15.3. Characteristics of earlier studies on relative analgesic potency of opioids

---

Single-dose studies
Low doses used
Wide confidence intervals for dose ratios
Limited follow-up in relation to tolerance or toxicity

---

double-blind and cross-over features. The studies involved cancer patients with postoperative and chronic pain. The patients were largely either opioid naïve or else had limited opioid exposure to low-dose opioids. Broad confidence intervals accompanied most of the relative potency estimates derived from these studies, indicating a wide interindividual variability. In summary, the early studies did not involve long-term treatment, high doses, and systematic monitoring of toxicity, and therefore did not capture potential ratio changes over time. Current equianalgesic tables, incorporating much of the data derived from these early studies, express the relative potency of different opioids in relation to route of administration and also in relation to a standard dose of morphine. However, current tables usually do not include the standard deviation or range of dose ratios. The characteristics of the current tables are summarized in Table 15.3. In daily clinical practice, the equianalgesic tables require the user to make three basic assumptions: (1) that the ratio is fixed over a variety of opioid doses; (2) that the ratio is unchanged whether the switch takes place in one or other direction; (3) that the variation is not extensive enough to justify not starting at the recommended ratio.

More Recent Studies of Cross-Tolerance and Relative Analgesic Potency of Opioids

In the last decade there have been numerous studies reported on the relative analgesic potency of different opioids. These studies are summarized in Tables 15.4–15.7. The studies in relation to morphine, hydromorphone, methadone, oxycodone, and fentanyl are discussed. A comprehensive discussion of conversion ratios for the various routes of administration of an opioid is beyond the scope of this chapter.

Studies of Morphine and Hydromorphone

Three studies of the relative potency between these two opioids are summarized in Table 15.4. The consumption of morphine and hydromorphone by patient controlled analgesia for the treatment of oral mucositis in two different groups of

Table 15.4. Studies of morphine and hydromorphone

Study authors	Study design [Stable dosing]	N	Direction of switch and routes studied°	Dose ratio[†]
Bruera et al.[78]	Retrospective [48 hours]	36	M : HM (po—sc and sc—po)	5.3 (4.9–6.4)
		12	HM : M (po—sc and sc—po)	3.6 (5.0–3.3)
Dunbar et al.[180]	Prospective [4-day minimum]	36	M iv—PCA	3.5[‡]
		21	HM iv—PCA	
Lawlor et al.[32]	Retrospective [48 hours]	44	M : HM sc—sc and po—po	5.0 (4.2–5.9)
		47	HM : M sc—sc and po—po	3.7 (2.9–4.5)

° M, morphine; HM, hydromorphone; po, oral; sc, subcutaneous; iv, intravenous.

[†] Expressed as median (first–third quartiles) in the direction M : HM.

[‡] Mean value.

patients was studied over a 7-day period.[180] This was not a cross-over study but rather a comparison between two separate groups. Although there was a similar level of satisfaction between the two groups in relation to the opioid that was administered, resting pain scores for mouth pain and throat pain, and scores for throat pain on swallowing were different between the morphine and hydromorphone groups. The mean dose ratio of 3.55 (M : HM) derived from this study contrasts markedly with the ratios given in the current equianalgesic tables, which quote either 7 : 1[9–11,159] or 5 : 1 ratios.[8] This study also suggested that the dose ratio changes over time reflecting a lesser potency of hydromorphone with repeated use. The other two studies in Table 15.4 come from the same center but relate to patients from different time periods. Both of these studies involved switches from morphine to hydromorphone or vice versa, the previous opioid being administered for at least 48 hours before the opioid switch, a time to reach stabilization of 24[78] or 48[32] hours, and then a 48-hour period where stable dosing was maintained. The earlier study involved opioid switches that also involved a change of administrative route, whereas the most recent study involved opioid switches without a change in route of administration. Our most recent study showed no statistically significant difference in dose ratios between the same opioid switches that involved either oral to oral or subcutaneous to subcutaneous administrations. Both of these studies showed marked interindividual variability and no correlation between the previous opioid dose and the dose ratio. The M : HM dose ratios derived from these two studies were 5 and 5.3. However, the dose ratio (expressed as M : HM) for the HM to M switches were 3.5 and 3.7, differing significantly from the ratio for M to HM switches ($p = 0.0001$).[32] This suggests a differential level of cross-tolerance between these two opioids. Alternatively, the authors suggest that a unified median dose ratio of 4.29,

Table 15.5. Studies of switches to methadone from other opioids

Study authors (design)	Prior opioid (route)[a]	Dose range [mg/day]	N	Median dose ratio (1st–3rd quartiles)
Bruera et al.[78] (Retrospective)	HM (sc)	[13–300]	49	0.95 (0.2–12.3)
		[≥300]	16	1.6 (0.3–14.4)[b]
		[13–2,076]	65	1.14 (0.5–2.04)[b]
Lawlor et al.[79] (Retrospective)	M (iv, po, sc)	[42–12,012][c]	14	11.36 (5.9–16.3)
	ME (po, pr)	[3–240]	6	8.25 (4.37–11.3)
	Combined		20	11.20 (5.06–13.24)
Ripamonti et al.[160] (Retrospective)	HM (sc)	[36–1,080]	(37)	1.47 (0.81–2.47)
	Others[d]		(51)[e]	0.25 (0.17–0.44)
			88	0.51 (0.20–1.38)
Ripamonti et al.[80] (Cross-sectional, prospective)	M (po)	[30–90]	10	3.7 (2.5–8.8)[b]
		[90–300]	20	7.75 (4–10)[b]
		[≥300]	8	12.25 (10–14.3)[b]
		[30–800]	38	7.75 (5–10)[b]

[a] po = oral, iv = intravenous, sc = subcutaneous, pr = rectal.
[b] Median (range).
[c] Expressed as morphine equivalent subcutaneously (sc).
[d] Morphine (15), Oxycodone (15), Codeine (8) orally and Buprenorphine sublingual (8).
[e] Doses of initial opioid were converted to a hydromorphone equivalent.

based on a total of 91 switches between morphine and hydromorphone, would accommodate the possibility that cross-tolerance is the same in both directions, M to HM and HM to M. The concept of a unified dose ratio is a contrived mathematical explanation and is less in keeping with the real life study findings, which suggest an inequality of bidirectional cross-tolerance between these two opioids.

Studies of Methadone and Other Opioids

Four studies examining the relative potency of methadone, and reported in the last 3 years are summarized in Table 15.5. The dose ratio of oral morphine to oral methadone quoted in the current equianalgesic tables is as low as 3:1.[9,11] In each of the four studies summarized in Table 15.5, the relative potency of methadone to the other opioids was higher than anticipated on the basis of ratios quoted in the current equianalgesic tables. One of these studies involved a comparison of retrospectively collected data from centers in Edmonton and Milan.[160] In 37 switches from hydromorphone to methadone conducted by the Edmonton group the median (range) hydromorphone dose in mg was 236 (36–1080), and in 51 switches from other opioids to methadone conducted by the Milan group the median hydromorphone equivalent dose prior to switching was 3 (1–60) ($p < 0.001$). In this study as well as the three other studies summarized in Table 15.5, the dose ratio was correlated positively with the opioid dose prior to switching to methadone. Many other case series and case reports also suggest that the relative potency of methadone is much greater than the current equianalgesic tables would suggest.[125,126,161–165]

The most recent study demonstrates differing dose ratios in relation to the different dose ranges of morphine prior to rotation.[80] The correlation of previous opioid dose and dose ratio was highly positive, reflected in a Pearson correlation coefficient, $r = 0.91$. The authors of this and other studies propose a phased switch over protocol over a 3-day period when switching from another opioid to methadone.[78–80,160] During each of these 3 days approximately 33% of the estimated final methadone dose is added whereas the original opioid dose is reduced by approximately 33%. Morley and Makin[166] propose a protocol that involves stopping the prior opioid on the day of switching to methadone and then in the case of patients on a prior oral morphine equivalent dose of more than 300 mg daily, the dose of methadone is given as 30 mg on a prn basis (not more than 3-hourly) for 6 days. For those patients on a prior morphine equivalent dose of less than 300 mg daily, the corresponding dose of methadone given on a prn basis (not more than 3-hourly) for 6 days is 10% of the oral morphine equivalent of the opioid prior to switching. At the end of this 6-day period they recommend continuing with a mean 12-hourly dose based on the last 2 days use of methadone. Further prospective studies are required to determine the most appropriate protocol to use in switching from other opioids to methadone.

Studies of Oxycodone and Other Opioids

Recent studies examining the relative potency of oxycodone (Oxy) are summarized in Table 15.6. Earlier single-dose studies in cancer patients by Beaver et al. suggested that the parenteral:oral dose ratio for oxycodone was $1:2$[167] and the dose ratio between parenteral morphine and oxycodone was in the range of $2:3$ and $3:4$.[168] Current equianalgesic tables quote a dose ratio for oxycodone: morphine of $1.5:1$ for parenteral administration[10,11,159] and $1:1$ to $3:2$[10] or $1:1$[9,11,159] for oral administration. Kalso and Vainio's randomized double-blind study of morphine and oxycodone in cancer patients suggested that the consumption of intravenous oxycodone was a median of 30% higher than that of morphine to achieve equianalgesia, and the order in which the drugs were administered had no effect on the consumption.[169] In contrast, the inferred ratio of oral M:oral Oxy based on consumption levels was $1.48:1$, suggesting that oral oxycodone was more potent than oral morphine. A further study by Kalso et al.[170] in postoperative patients suggested a $2:3$ ratio for intravenous Oxy:intravenous M. Two further studies suggested equipotency between morphine and oxycodone, in the case of oral to oral switch,[171] and in the case of intravenously administered morphine and oxycodone to two similar patient groups without a cross-over feature.[172] The remaining three studies in Table 15.6 case conducted in cancer

Table 15.6. Studies of morphine or hydromorphone and oxycodone

Study authors	Study design (dosing period)[a]	N	Direction of switch and routes studied[b]	Dose ratio[c]
Kalso and Vainio[169]	RDBXO (48 hours)	20	Oxy iv—Oxy po M iv—M po M po—Oxy po M iv—Oxy iv	0.7 (0.49–0.78) 0.31 (0.17–0.35) 1.48[d] 0.7 (0.6–0.88)
Kalso et al.[170]	RDB (2 hours)		Oxy iv or M iv	Oxy:M, 2:3
Glare and Walsh[171]	Prospective, open	10/24	Oxy po—M po Oxy po—M iv	1:1 3:1
Heiskanen and Kalso[174]	RDBXO (3–6 days)	27/45	Oxy po—M po M po—Oxy po	2:3 4:3
Bruera et al.[173]	RDBXO (7 days)	23/31	M po—Oxy po Oxy po—M po	M:Oxy, 1.5:1 (1–2.3:1)
Silvasti et al.[172]	RDB (24 hours)	24 25	Oxy iv (PCA) M iv (PCA)	M:Oxy, 1:1
Gagnon et al.[175]	Retrospective (24 hours minimum)	8 11 19	M sc—Oxy sc HM sc—Oxy sc M sc—Oxy sc[e]	1.0 0.4 1.4

[a] RDB, randomized, double-blind; XO, cross-over study.

[b] M, morphine; HM, hydromorphone; Oxy, oxycodone; po, oral; iv, intravenous; sc, subcutaneous; PCA, patient-controlled analgesia.

[c] Ratios expressed in the direction of the switch unless otherwise stated. Ratios are quoted as per original papers and their values as median and (range) where available.

[d] Ratio was inferred from median doses given in the original paper.

[e] Expressed as morphine equivalent.

patients and included two randomized double-blind cross-over studies,[173,174] and a retrospective study. They all suggested a 2:3 dose ratio for Oxy:M, when given orally[173,174] or subcutaneously.[175] The study by Heiskanen and Kalso[174] found that the direction of the opioid switch with oral administration resulted in a different dose ratio, 2:3 for an oxycodone to morphine switch and 4:3 for a morphine to oxycodone switch. The authors of this cross-over study suggest the possibility of a period effect relating to the previous opioid, particularly as the study design did not involve a wash-out phase. This bidirectional difference was not found in the study by Bruera et al.[173]

Fentanyl and Other Opioids

The use of fentanyl in advanced cancer patients has increased, particularly with the advent of a transdermal mode of administration. Studies that examined the relative potency of fentanyl in relation to other opioids are summarized in Table

Table 15.7. Morphine or hydromorphone and fentanyl studies

Study authors	Study design	N	Direction of switch and routes studied[°]	Dose ratio
Paix et al.[182]	Retrospective	8	M sc—F sc	68[†] (Range, 15–100)
Donner et al.[176]	Prospective Open	38	M po—F td	70[†]
Watanabe et al.[183]	Retrospective	4	M sc—F sc	85.4 (65–112.5)[‡]
		6	HM sc—F sc	23 (10–29)[‡]

[°] HM, hydromorphone; F, fentanyl; sc, subcutaneous; po, oral; td, transdermal.
[†] Mean value.
[‡] Median value (range).

15.7. The mean ratios quoted in these studies show relatively close agreement. The largest study to date that examined fentanyl's relative potency with chronic use, involved a prospective study of the transdermal route.[176] Although this study found a mean ratio of 70:1 for M:F, the authors concluded that a ratio of 100: 1 provides for a relatively safe conversion in the direction from oral morphine to fentanyl. Although the manufacturers of the fentanyl transdermal patch have provided a slide table with dose ranges of other opioids and the recommended dose of fentanyl relative to these ranges, there is a paucity of data in the literature concerning the use of fentanyl in chronic therapy. Furthermore, there is some controversy over the most appropriate protocol for switching either from or to the fentanyl transdermal delivery system in relation to other opioids.[177,178]

Limitations of the Current Equianalgesic Tables in the Light of Recent Clinical Studies

There are several limitations to the current equianalgesic tables.[3,179] These tables represent essentially an effort to provide a cookbook-styled guide for physicians when switching from one opioid to another. Given the potential interplay and complexity of pharmacodynamic and nonpharmacodynamic factors described earlier in this chapter, it is hardly surprising that such a cookbook-styled table would inherently entail certain limitations when used in the context of chronic opioid administration. Switching opioids in advanced cancer patients is often done against a background involving one or more of the following factors: cognitive impairment or delirium, hepatic or renal dysfunction, other concomitant metabolic disturbances, and finally the influence of often many concomitant treatments. The context in which an opioid switch takes place in palliative care is therefore often in contrast to the relatively controlled environment in the early relative potency studies.

With the current equianalgesic tables there are at least five major areas with limitations that warrant recognition:

1. These tables do not reflect the tremendous interindividual variability in relative potency estimates.[32,78]

2. Although Houde et al. recognized that tolerance development with repetitive dosing could influence the relative potency estimate between two opioids, this message is often inadequately portrayed or absent from many of the current equianalgesic tables. However, in the text accompanying these tables many authors have recommended equianalgesic dose reductions in the range of 25%–75% to allow for incomplete cross-tolerance.[10,159]

3. The current equianalgesic tables assume that the same relative potency ratio operates irrespective of the level of opioid dose reached prior to an opioid switch. The relative potency ratio in switching to methadone has been shown to vary in relation to the previous opioid dose.[78–80,160] The earlier studies of Houde et al.[158] involved single doses and the doses used were relatively low and hence the rather unique finding in relation to methadone, where the dose ratio is correlated positively with the previous opioid dose, might not have been manifested.

4. The current equianalgesic tables do not account for the possibility of unidirectional cross-tolerance, for example, the relative potency ratio for a switch from morphine to hydromorphone is considered to be the same as the reverse switch. Recent studies however suggest that this might not be the case and that the level of cross-tolerance is not equal when switching in both directions.[32,78]

5. The current equianalgesic tables do not take into account the possibility of the accumulation of active metabolites, particularly in the case of renal impairment.[133]

Proposals for Updating the Current Equianalgesic Tables

While the cookbook concept has obvious flaws in relation to equianalgesic tables, there is nonetheless a need to present information for the busy physician in a readily accessible format. We suggest that the following areas warrant consideration for revision in relation to the opioid pharmacotherapy of chronic pain:

1. There is compelling evidence to suggest that methadone is more potent than previously appreciated. The correlation of dose ratio with the previous opioid dose is paramount. We therefore suggest different dose ratios depending on the dose of previous opioid similar to that used by Ripamonti et al.[80] in their most recent study outlined in Table 15.5. Although there is no universally agreed protocol for switching to methadone, all equianalgesic tables should in the meantime carry a warning concerning methadone's long half-life and the need for experience on the part of a physician making opioid switches involving methadone.

2. Both earlier and more recent studies, as outlined in this chapter, have demonstrated tremendous interindividual variability in dose ratios. We suggest that this warning should be stated directly in the equianalgesic tables and the need for careful individual titration be stated emphatically.

3. Regarding oxycodone, the bulk of available evidence from randomized controlled trials[169,173,174] suggests that oral oxycodone has a dose ratio of 2:3 when compared to oral morphine. Different bidirectional cross-tolerance possibly also exists[174] but warrants further study. In the meantime we suggest that a ratio of 1:2 for oral oxycodone to oral morphine would serve for safe initial titration.[173]

4. The best available evidence relating to the inequality of bidirectional cross-tolerance between morphine and hydromorphone[32,78] (see Table 15.3) and the dose ratio of 3.5 between these two opioids with chronic use[180] could be of particular significance with higher opioid doses. We therefore suggest that there should be at least a footnote warning placed in relation to the dose ratio between these two opioids, most commonly quoted as 7:1 for M:HM.[9–11,159]

5. The reports of severe opioid toxicity (including hyperalgesia) in renal impairment, associated with the accumulation of pharmacologically active metabolites[122,133,136,181] merit a footnote warning concerning the use of those opioids with active metabolites such as morphine and hydromorphone in renal impairment.

Methodological Issues and Future Research

The dangers of misinterpreting data from single-dose studies in relation to the chronic use of opioids in cancer patients is highlighted in this chapter. In a somewhat similar way, the interpretation of randomized controlled trials examining dose ratios in the context of advanced cancer warrant caution. In clinical practice, the reason for switching opioids in a palliative care setting is often adverse side effects such as delirium.[141,153] This contrasts markedly with many of the randomized controlled trials where the titration of opioid doses do not reach the point of toxicity, which is the particular juncture where opioid switching is likely to occur in clinical practice. Although randomized controlled trials are considered the "gold standard" of evidence, it is possible therefore that they might not capture the real clinical context of switching opioids in advanced cancer. Randomized controlled trials in the context of repeated opioid dosing, and incorporating a cross-over feature will still provide more useful information than single-dose studies. To incorporate a cross-over feature in the clinical context of opioid toxicity, anticipatory consent would have to be obtained from the patient in a cognitively intact state, or alternatively proxy consent from a relative or other designated proxy could be obtained at the time of occurrence of opioid toxicity. Clearly the design of such studies are challenging in both a pragmatic and ethical sense. In the interim some of the best possible evidence might emanate from systematic and sequential observations of dose patterns in cohorts of patients, who are on chronic opioid treatment and require a switch in the event of toxicity.

The advent of patient-controlled analgesia provides a useful mechanism for studying relative potency of opioids but again might not represent the clinical context of opioid switching in an effort to manage opioid toxicity. Furthermore, studies that calculate the consumption of two opioids over an extended number of days, do not necessarily reflect the actual dose of opioid needed directly at the time of switching, where there is likely to be a carry-over or period effect, which can relate to a plethora of pharmacodynamic and pharmacokinetic factors, as discussed previously. In the context of clinical practice it would seem wise to adopt a study methodology that has an arm incorporating a cross-over feature and hence captures the early carry-over effect associated with the previous opioid, which could have a significant impact in clinical practice.

The issue of equianalgesia also poses some difficulties in interpreting the findings of some studies.[169,174] In clinical practice in the setting of palliative care, the patient is often cognitively impaired and unable to give a reliable account of pain perception through visual analog or other descriptor scales.

The role of morphine as a reference opioid for all other opioids is probably related to its frequency of use and many years of clinical experience with its use. The issue of the correct oral to parenteral dose ratio for morphine with repeated dosing warrants further research as relatively few studies have examined this in a systematic way.

Conclusions

The issue of cross-tolerance among opioids is highly complex and reflects the interplay of many pharmacodynamic and pharmacokinetic factors. Hence there are appreciable difficulties in reaching a simple ratio or value regarding the relative potency of two opioids, particularly in the context of chronic opioid treatment. The current equianalgesic tables were based largely on single-dose studies and therefore have definite limitations in their applicability to chronic opioid pharmacotherapy. We suggest that revisions be considered regarding opioid switches involving methadone, particularly in relation to the underappreciated potency of methadone, and the correlation of methadone dose with the dose of prior opioid, which is best reflected by presenting different dose ratios for different dose ranges. Current evidence suggests that oxycodone is more potent than previously appreciated, this in turn warrants recognition in the equianalgesic tables. The inequality of bidirectional cross-tolerance between morphine and hydromorphone in chronic therapy also merits recognition. The findings of randomized controlled clinical trials have limited applicability to the context of opioid toxicity in clinical practice.

Ultimately, the equianalgesic tables can be no more than guidelines for physicians. The emphasis should be placed on initial safe-dose conversions and the need to follow up with careful titration of opioid dose in each individual case, as evidenced by the extensive interindividual variability in relative potency ratios obtained to date.

References

1. Lawlor PG, Bruera E. Side-effects of opioids in chronic pain treatment. *Curr Opin Anaesthesiol* 1998; 11:539–545.
2. De Stoutz ND, Bruera E, Suarez-Almazor M. Opioid rotation for toxicity reduction in terminal cancer patients. *J Pain Symp Manage* 1995; 10:378–384.
3. Derby S, Chin J, Portenoy RK. Systemic opioid therapy for chronic cancer pain. Practical guidelines for converting drugs and routes of administration. *CNS Drugs* 1998; 9:99–109.
4. Watanabe S. Intraindividual variability in opioid response: a role for sequential opioid trials in patient care. In: Portenoy RK, Bruera E, eds. *Topics in Palliative Care*. New York, Oxford University Press, 1997:195–203.
5. Makin MK, Ellershaw JE. Substitution of another opioid for morphine. Methadone can be used to manage neuropathic pain related to cancer. *BMJ* 1998; 317:81.
6. Morley JS, Makin MK. The use of methadone in cancer pain poorly responsive to other opioids. *Pain Rev* 1998; 5:51–58.
7. Bruera E, Franco JJ, Maltoni M, Watanabe S, Suarez-Almazor M. Changing pattern of agitated impaired mental status in patients with advanced cancer: association with cognitive monitoring, hydration, and opioid rotation. *J Pain Symp Manage* 1995; 10:287–291.
8. *Cancer Pain: a Monograph on the Management of Cancer Pain.* (H42-2/5). 1984. Ottawa: Health & Welfare Canada: Minister of Supply and Services, Canada.
9. Jacox A, Carr DB, Payne R. *Pharmacologic Management, Clinical Practice Guidline: Management of Cancer Pain.* Rockville, U.S. Department of Health and Human Services, 1994:39–74.
10. Hanks GWC, Cherny NI. Opioid analgesic therapy. In: Doyle D, Hanks GWC, Macdonald N, eds. *The Oxford Textbook of Palliative Medicine*. Oxford, Oxford University Press, 1998:331–355.
11. Foley KM. Supportive care and quality of life. In: DeVita VT Jr., Hellman S, Rosenberg SA, eds. *Cancer: Principles & Practice of Oncology*. Philadelphia, Lippincott-Raven, 1997:2807–2841.
12. Levy MH. Pharmacologic treatment of cancer pain. *N Engl J Med* 1996; 335: 1124–1132.
13. Sosnowski M, Yaksh TL. Differential cross-tolerance between intrathecal morphine and sufentanil in the rat. *Anesthesiology* 1990; 73:1141–1147.
14. Moulin DE, Ling GS, Pasternak GW. Unidirectional analgesic cross-tolerance between morphine and levorphanol in the rat. *Pain* 1988; 33:233–239.
15. Albrecht E, Heinrich N, Lorenz D, et al. Influence of continuous levels of fentanyl in rats on the mu-opioid receptor in the central nervous system. *Pharmacol Biochem Behav* 1997; 58:189–194.

16. Ouellet DM, Pollack GM. A pharmacokinetic-pharmacodynamic model of tolerance to morphine analgesia during infusion in rats. *J Pharmacokinet Biopharm* 1995; 23:531–549.

17. Yu W, Hao JX, Xu XJ, Wiesenfeld-Hallin Z. The development of morphine tolerance and dependence in rats with chronic pain. *Brain Res* 1997; 756:141–146.

18. Jasinski DR. Tolerance and dependence to opiates. *Acta Anaesthesiol Scand* 1997; 41:184–186.

19. Portenoy RK. Tolerance to opioid analgesics: clinical aspects. *Cancer Surv* 1994; 21:49–65.

20. Fallon M. Opioid rotation: does it have a role? *Palliat Med* 1997; 11:177–178.

21. Kieffer BL. Recent advances in molecular recognition and signal transduction of active peptides: receptors for opioid peptides. *Cell Mol Neurobiol* 1995; 15:615–635.

22. Pasternak GW, Standifer KM. Mapping of opioid receptors using antisense oligodeoxynucleotides: correlating their molecular biology and pharmacology. *Trends Pharmacol Sci* 1995; 16:344–350.

23. Foley KM. Changing concepts of tolerance to opioids: what the cancer patient has taught us. In: Chapman CR, Foley KM, eds. *Current and Emerging Issues in Cancer Pain: Research and Practice*. New York, Raven Press, 1993:331–350.

24. Pasternak GW. Progress in opiate pharmacology. In: Chapman CR, Foley KM, eds. *Current and Emerging Issues in Cancer Pain: Research and Practice*. New York, Raven Press, Ltd, 1993:113–127.

25. Vaught JL. What is the relative contribution of mu, delta, and kappa opioid receptors to antinociception and is there cross-tolerance? In: Basbaum AI, Besson JM, eds. *Towards a New Pharmacotherapy of Pain*. New York, Wiley, 1991:121–136.

26. Jin W, Terman GW, Chavkin C. Kappa opioid receptor tolerance in the guinea pig hippocampus. *J Pharmacol Experimental Therapeutics* 1997; 281:123–128.

27. Craft RM, Dykstra LA. Differential cross-tolerance to opioids in squirrel monkeys responding under a shock titration schedule. *J Pharmacol Exp Ther* 1990; 252: 945–952.

28. Bhargava HN, Ramarao P, Gulati A. Effects of morphine in rats treated chronically with U-50, 488H, a kappa opioid receptor agonist. *Eur J Pharmacol* 1989; 162:257–264.

29. Bhargava HN, Matwyshyn G, Ramarao P. The effect of U-50, 488H, a kappa-opiate receptor agonist on tolerance to the analgesic and hyperthermic effects of morphine in the rat. *Gen Pharmacol* 1991; 22:429–434.

30. Laurido C, Hernandez A, Perez H. Cross-tolerance to acute administration of mu and kappa opioid agonists at the spinal cord level in the rat. *Int J Neurosci* 1996; 87:191–199.

31. Garaulet JV, Milanes MV, Laorden ML. Cross-tolerance between kappa and mu opioid agonists in the guinea pig ileum myenteric plexus. *J Pharmacol Exp Ther* 1995; 272:658–662.

32. Lawlor P, Turner K, Hanson J, Bruera E. Dose ratio between morphine and hydromorphone in patients with cancer pain: a retrospective study. *Pain* 1997; 72:79–85.

33. Inturrisi CE. Opioid pharmacology: tolerance, receptor modulation, and new analgesics. In: Payne R, Patt RB, Hill CS, eds. *Assessment and Treatment of Cancer Pain*. Seattle, IASP Press, 1998:275–288.

34. Abdelhamid EE, Sultana M, Portoghese PS, Takemori AE. Selective blockage of delta opioid receptors prevents the development of morphine tolerance and dependence in mice. *J Pharmacol Exp Ther* 1991; 258:299–303.

35. Kest B, Lee CE, McLemore GL, Inturrisi CE. An antisense oligodeoxynucleotide to the delta opioid receptor (DOR-1) inhibits morphine tolerance and acute dependence in mice. *Brain Res Bull* 1996; 39:185–188.

36. Traynor JR, Elliott J. Delta-opioid receptor subtypes and cross-talk with mu-receptors. *Trends Pharmacol Sci* 1993; 14:84–86.

37. Noble F, Cox BM. Differential desensitization of mu- and delta-opioid receptors in selected neural pathways following chronic morphine treatment. *Br J Pharmacol* 1996; 117:161–169.

38. Raynor K, Kong H, Mestek A, et al. Characterization of the cloned human mu opioid receptor. *J Pharmacol Exp Ther* 1995; 272:423–428.

39. Yaksh TL. Pharmacology and mechanisms of opioid analgesic activity. *Acta Anaesthesiol Scand* 1997; 41:94–111.

40. Grudt TJ, Williams JT. Opioid receptors and the regulation of ion conductances. *Rev Neurosci* 1995; 6:279–286.

41. Rogers NF, el-Fakahany E. Morphine-induced opioid receptor down-regulation detected in intact adult rat brain cells. *Eur J Pharmacol* 1986; 124:221–230.

42. Cvejic S, Devi LA. Dimerization of the delta opioid receptor: implication for a role in receptor internalization. *J Biol Chem* 1997; 272:26959–26964.

43. Chu P, Murray S, Lissin D, von Zastrow M. Delta and kappa opioid receptors are differentially regulated by dynamin-dependent endocytosis when activated by the same alkaloid agonist. *J Biol Chem* 1997; 272:27124–27130.

44. Tao PL, Chang LR, Chou YP, Law PY, Loh HH. Chronic opioid treatment may uncouple opioid receptors and G-proteins: evidence from radiation inactivation analysis. *Eur J Pharmacol* 1993; 246:233–238.

45. Mestek A, Hurley JH, Bye LS, et al. The human mu opioid receptor: modulation of functional desensitization by calcium/calmodulin-dependent protein kinase and protein kinase C. *J Neurosci* 1995; 15:2396–2406.

46. Sehba F, Duttaroy A, Shah S, Chen B, Carroll J, Yoburn BC. In vivo homologous regulation of mu-opioid receptor gene expression in the mouse. *Eur J Pharmacol* 1997; 339:33–41.

47. Chakrabarti S, Yang W, Law PY, Loh HH. The mu-opioid receptor down-regulates differently from the delta-opioid receptor: requirement of a high affinity receptor/G protein complex formation. *Mol Pharmacol* 1997; 52:105–113.

48. Sternini C, Spann M, Anton B, et al. Agonist-selective endocytosis of mu opioid receptor by neurons in vivo. *Proc Natl Acad Sci U S A* 1996; 93:9241–9246.

49. Blake AD, Bot G, Li S, Freeman JC, Reisine T. Differential agonist regulation of the human kappa-opioid receptor. *J Neurochem* 1997; 68:1846–1852.

50. Remmers AE, Clark MJ, Liu XY, Medzihradsky F. Delta opioid receptor down-regulation is independent of functional G protein yet is dependent on agonist efficacy. *J Pharmacol Exp Ther* 1998; 287:625–632.

51. Keith DE, Murray SR, Zaki PA, et al. Morphine activates opioid receptors without causing their rapid internalization. *J Biol Chem* 1996; 271:19021–19024.

52. Keith DE, Anton B, Murray SR, et al. Mu-opioid receptor internalization: opiate drugs have differential effects on a conserved endocytic mechanism in vitro and in the mammalian brain. *Mol Pharmacol* 1998; 53:377–384.

53. Zhang J, Ferguson SS, Barak LS, et al. Role for G protein-coupled receptor kinase in agonist-specific regulation of mu-opioid receptor responsiveness. *Proc Nl Acad Sci U S A* 1998; 95:7157–7162.

54. Pei G, Kieffer BL, Lefkowitz RJ, Freedman NJ. Agonist-dependent phosphorylation of the mouse delta-opioid receptor: involvement of G protein-coupled receptor kinases but not protein kinase C. *Mol Pharmacol* 1995; 48:173–177.

55. Bot G, Blake AD, Li S, Reisine T. Fentanyl and its analogs desensitize the cloned mu opioid receptor. *J Pharmacol Exp Ther* 1998; 285:1207–1218.

56. Chakrabarti S, Wang L, Tang WJ, Gintzler AR. Chronic morphine augments adenylyl cyclase phosphorylation: relevance to altered signalling during tolerance/dependence. *Mol Pharmacol* 1998; 54:949–953.

57. Chakrabarti S, Rivera M, Yan SZ, Tang WJ, Gintzler AR. Chronic morphine augments G(beta)(gamma)/Gs(alpha) stimulation of adenylyl cyclase: relevance to opioid tolerance. *Mol Pharmacol* 1998; 54:655–662.

58. Ivarsson M, Neil A. Differences in efficacies between morphine and methadone demonstrated in the guinea pig ileum: A possible explanation for previous observations on incomplete opioid cross-tolerance. *Pharmacol Toxicol* 1989; 65: 368–371.

59. Paronis CA, Holtzman SG. Development of tolerance to the analgesic activity of mu agonists after continuous infusion of morphine, meperidine or fentanyl in rats. *J Pharmacol Exp Ther* 1992; 262:1–9.

60. Neil A. Morphine- and methadone-tolerant mice differ in cross-tolerance to other opiates. Heterogeneity in opioid mechanisms indicated. *Naunyn-Schmiedebergs Arch Pharmacol* 1982; 320:50–53.

61. Neil A. Studies on action mechanisms of morphine and 1-methadone in mice. *Neuropeptides* 1984; 5:189–192.

62. Duttaroy A, Yoburn BC. The effect of intrinsic efficacy on opioid tolerance. *Anesthesiology* 1995; 82:1226–1236.

63. Kissin I, Brown PT, Bradley EL, Jr. Magnitude of acute tolerance to opioids is not related to their potency. *Anesthesiology* 1991; 75:813–816.

64. Tiseo PJ, Cheng J, Pasternak GW, Inturrisi CE. Modulation of morphine tolerance by the competitive N-methyl-D-aspartate receptor antagonist LY274614: assessment of opioid receptor changes. *J Pharmacol Exp Ther* 1994; 268:195–201.

65. Mao J, Price DD, Phillips LL, Lu J, Mayer DJ. Increases in protein kinase C gamma immunoreactivity in the spinal cord of rats associated with tolerance to the analgesic effects of morphine. *Brain Res* 1995; 677:257–267.

66. Mao J, Price DD, Caruso FS, Mayer DJ. Oral administration of dextromethorphan prevents the development of morphine tolerance and dependence in rats. *Pain* 1996; 67:361–368.

67. Shimoyama N, Shimoyama M, Inturrisi CE, Elliott KJ. Ketamine attenuates and reverses morphine tolerance in rodents. *Anesthesiology* 1996; 85:1357–1366.

68. Cai YC, Ma L, Fan GH, Zhao J, Jiang LZ, Pei G. Activation of N-methyl-D-aspartate receptor attenuates acute responsiveness of delta-opioid receptors. *Mol Pharmacol* 1997; 51:583–587.

69. Fan GH, Zhao J, Wu YL, et al. N-Methyl-D-aspartate attenuates opioid receptor-mediated G protein activation and this process involves protein kinase C. *Mol Pharmacol* 1998; 53:684–690.

70. Mao J, Price DD, Mayer DJ. Mechanisms of hyperalgesia and morphine tolerance: a current view of their possible interactions. *Pain* 1995; 62:259–274.

71. Pasternak GW, Kolesnikov YA, Babey AM. Perspectives on the N-methyl-D-aspartate/nitric oxide cascade and opioid tolerance. *Neuropsychopharmacology* 1995; 13:309–313.

72. Herman BH, Vocci F, Bridge P. The effects of NMDA receptor antagonists and nitric oxide synthase inhibitors on opioid tolerance and withdrawal. Medication development issues for opiate addiction. *Neuropsychopharmacology* 1995; 13:269–293.

73. Vaccarino FM, Hayward MD, Nestler EJ, Duman RS, Tallman JF. Differential induction of immediate early genes by excitatory amino acid receptor types in primary cultures of cortical and striatal neurons. *Brain Res* 1992; 12:233–241.

74. Goelet P, Castellucci VF, Schacher S, Kandel ER. The long and the short of long-term memory—a molecular framework. *Nature* 1986; 322:419–422.

75. Feng J, Kendig JJ. The NMDA receptor antagonist MK-801 differentially modulates mu and kappa opioid actions in spinal cord in vitro. *Pain* 1996; 66:343–349.

76. Ebert B, Andersen S, Krogsgaard-Larsen P, Martin G, Nie Z, Siggins GR. Ketobemidone, methadone and pethidine are non-competitive N-methyl-D-aspartate (NMDA) antagonists in the rat cortex and spinal cord. *Neurosci Lett* 1995; 187:165–168.

77. Gorman AL, Elliott KJ, Inturrisi CE. The d- and l-isomers of methadone bind to the non-competitive site on the N-methyl-D-aspartate (NMDA) receptor in rat forebrain and spinal cord. *Neurosci Lett* 1997; 223:5–8.

78. Bruera E, Pereira J, Watanabe S, Belzile M, Kuehn N, Hanson J. Opioid rotation in patients with cancer pain. A retrospective comparison of dose ratios between methadone, hydromorphone, and morphine. *Cancer* 1996; 78:852–857.

79. Lawlor PG, Turner KS, Hanson J, Bruera ED. Dose ratio between morphine and methadone in patients with cancer pain: a retrospective study. *Cancer* 1998; 82:1167–1173.

80. Ripamonti C, Groff L, Brunelli C, Polastri D, Stavrakis A, De Conno F. Switching from morphine to oral methadone in treating cancer pain: what is the equianalgesic dose ratio? *J Clin Oncol* 1998; 16:3216–3221.

81. Mercadante S, Casuccio A, Agnello A, Serretta R, Calderone L, Barresi L. Morphine versus methadone in the pain treatment of advanced-cancer patients followed up at home. *J Clin Oncol* 1998; 16:3656–3661.

82. Cherny NI, Thaler HT, Friedlander-Klar H, et al. Opioid responsiveness of cancer pain syndromes caused by neuropathic or nociceptive mechanisms: a combined analysis of controlled, single-dose studies. *Neurology* 1994; 44:857–861.

83. Portenoy RK, Foley KM, Inturrisi CE. The nature of opioid responsiveness and its implications for neuropathic pain: new hypotheses derived from studies of opioid infusions *Pain* 1990; 43:273–286.

84. McQuay HJ, Jadad AR, Carroll D, et al. Opioid sensitivity of chronic pain: a patient-controlled analgesia method. *Anaesthesia* 1992; 47:757–767.

85. Arner S, Meyerson BA. Lack of analgesic effect of opioids on neuropathic and idiopathic forms of pain. *Pain* 1988; 33:11–23.

86. Paul D, Tran JG. Differential cross-tolerance between analgesia produced by alpha 2-adrenoceptor agonists and receptor subtype selective opioid treatments. *Eur J Pharmacol* 1995; 272:111–114.

87. Aley KO, Green PG, Levine JD. Opioid and adenosine peripheral antinociception are subject to tolerance and withdrawal. *J Neurosci* 1995; 15:8031–8038.

88. Aley KO, Levine JD. Multiple receptors involved in peripheral alpha 2, mu, and A1 antinociception, tolerance, and withdrawal. *J Neurosci* 1997; 17:735–744.

89. Goodchild CS, Guo Z, Freeman J, Gent JP. 5-HT spinal antinociception involves mu opioid receptors: cross tolerance and antagonist studies. *Br J Anaesth* 1997; 78:563–569.

90. Benoliel JJ, Becker C, Mauborgne A, Bourgoin S, Hamon M, Cesselin F. Interactions between central opioidergic and cholecystokininergic systems in rats: possible significance for the development of opioid tolerance. *Bull l Acad Natl Med* 1998; 182:311–324.

91. Idanpaan-Heikkila JJ, Guilbaud G, Kayser V. Prevention of tolerance to the antinociceptive effects of systemic morphine by a selective cholecystokinin-B receptor antagonist in a rat model of peripheral neuropathy. *J Pharmacol Exp Ther* 1997; 282: 1366–1372.

92. Zarrindast MR, Zabihi A, Rezayat M, Rakhshandeh H, Ghazi-Khansari M, Hosseini R. Effects of caerulein and CCK antagonists on tolerance induced to morphine antinociception in mice. *Pharmacol Biochem Behav* 1997; 58:173–178.

93. Vanderah TW, Bernstein RN, Yamamura HI, Hruby VJ, Porreca F. Enhancement of morphine antinociception by a CCKB antagonist in mice is mediated via opioid delta receptors. *J Pharmacol Exp Ther* 1996; 278:212–219.

94. Bernstein ZP, Yucht S, Battista E, Lema M, Spaulding MB. Proglumide as a morphine adjunct in cancer pain management. *J Pain Symp Manage* 1998; 15:314–320.

95. Martin JR, Takemori AE. Chronically administered morphine increases dopamine receptor sensitivity in mice. *Eur J Pharmacol* 1986; 121:221–229.

96. Gomaa AA, Mohamed LH, Ahmed HN. Modification of morphine-induced analgesia, tolerance and dependence by bromocriptine. *Eur J Pharmacol* 1989; 170:129–135.

97. Noble F, Cox BM. The role of dopaminergic systems in opioid receptor desensitization in nucleus accumbens and caudate putamen of rat after chronic morphine treatment. *J Pharmacol Exp Ther* 1997; 283:557–565.

98. Gutstein HB. The effects of pain on opioid tolerance: how do we resolve the controversy? *Pharmacol Rev* 1996; 48:403–407.

99. Askitopoulou H, Whitwam JG, Al-Khudhairi D, Chakrabarti M, Bower S, Hull CJ. Acute tolerance to fentanyl during anesthesia in dogs. *Anesthesiology* 1985; 63:255–261.

100. Stevens CW, Yaksh TL. Potency of infused spinal antinociceptive agents is inversely related to magnitude of tolerance after continuous infusion. *J Pharmacol Exp Ther* 1989; 250:1–8.

101. Huidobro F, Huidobro-Toro JP, Leong WE. Studies on tolerance development to single doses of morphine in mice. *J Pharmacol Exp Ther* 1976; 198:318–329.

102. Schug SA, Zech D, Grond S, Jung H, Meuser T, Stobbe B. A long-term survey of morphine in cancer pain patients. *J Pain Symp Manage* 1992; 7:259–266.

103. Sallerin-Caute B, Lazorthes Y, Deguine O, et al. Does intrathecal morphine in the treatment of cancer pain induce the development of tolerance? *Neurosurgery* 1998; 42:44–49.

104. Gutstein HB, Trujillo KA, Akil H. Does chronic nociceptive stimulation alter the development of morphine tolerance? *Brain Res* 1995; 680:173–179.

105. Collin E, Poulain P, Gauvain-Piquard A, Petit G, Pichard-Leandri E. Is disease pro-gression the major factor in morphine "tolerance" in cancer pain treatment? *Pain* 1993; 55:319–326.

106. Coyle N, Portenoy RK. Infection as a cause of rapidly increasing pain in cancer patients. *J Pain Symp Manage* 1991; 6:266–269.

107. Bruera E, MacDonald N. Intractable pain in patients with advanced head and neck tumors: a possible role of local infection. *Cancer Treat Rep* 1986; 70:691–692.

108. Bruera E, Schoeller T, Wenk R, et al. A prospective multicenter assessment of the Edmonton Staging System for cancer pain. *J Pain Symp Manage* 1995; 10:348–355.

109. McQuay HJ, Jadad AR. Incident pain. *Cancer Surv* 1994; 21:17–24.

110. Ferrante FM. Principles of opioid pharmacotherapy: practical implications of basic mechanisms. *J Pain Symp Manage* 1996; 11:265–273.

111. Coyle N, Adelhardt J, Foley KM, Portenoy RK. Character of terminal illness in the advanced cancer patient: pain and other symptoms during the last four weeks of life. *J Pain Symp Manage* 1990; 5:83–93.

112. Houde R, Wallenstein S, Beaver W. Clinical measurement of pain. In: de Stevens G, ed. *Analgetics*. New York, Academic Press, 1965:75–122.

113. Hanks GW, Hoskin PJ, Aherne GW, Turner P, Poulain P. Explanation for potency of repeated oral doses of morphine? *Lancet* 1987; 2:723–725.

114. Twycross RG. The therapeutic equivalence of oral and subcutaneous/intramuscular morphine sulphate in cancer patients. *J Palliat Care* 1988; 4:67–68.

115. Hasselstrom J, Sawe J. Morphine pharmacokinetics and metabolism in humans. Enterohepatic cycling and relative contribution of metabolites to active opioid con-centrations. *Clin Pharmacokin* 1993; 24:344–354.

116. Milne RW, Nation RL, Somogyi AA. The disposition of morphine and its 3- and 6-glucuronide metabolites in humans and animals, and the importance of the metabolites to the pharmacological effects of morphine. *Drug Metab Rev* 1996; 28:345–472.

117. Portenoy RK, Thaler HT, Inturrisi CE, Friedlander-Klar H, Foley KM. The metabo-lite morphine-6-glucuronide contributes to the analgesia produced by morphine infusion in patients with pain and normal renal function. *Clin Pharm Ther* 1992; 51:422–431.

118. Smith MT, Watt JA, Cramond T. Morphine-3-glucuronide—a potent antagonist of morphine analgesia. *Life Sci* 1990; 47:579–585.

119. Gong QL, Hedner J, Bjorkman R, Hedner T. Morphine-3-glucuronide may func-tionally antagonize morphine-6-glucuronide induced antinociception and ventilatory depression in the rat. *Pain* 1992; 48:249–255.

120. Ekblom M, Gardmark M, Hammarlund-Udenaes M. Pharmacokinetics and phar-macodynamics of morphine-3-glucuronide in rats and its influence on the antinoci-ceptive effect of morphine. *Biopharm Drug Dispos* 1993; 14:1–11.

121. Ouellet DM, Pollack GM. Effect of prior morphine-3-glucuronide exposure on morphine disposition and antinociception. *Biochem Pharmacol* 1997; 53:1451–1457.

122. Hagen N, Swanson R. Strychnine-like multifocal myoclonus and seizures in extremely high-dose opioid administration: treatment strategies. *J Pain Symp Manage* 1997; 14:51–58.

123. Sjogren P, Jonsson T, Jensen NH, Drenck NE, Jensen TS. Hyperalgesia and myoclonus in terminal cancer patients treated with continuous intravenous morphine. *Pain* 1993; 55:93–97.

124. De Conno F, Caraceni A, Martini C, Spoldi E, Salvetti M, Ventafridda. Hyperalgesia and myoclonus with intrathecal infusion of high-dose morphine. *Pain* 1991; 47:337–339.

125. MacDonald N, Der L, Allan S, Champion P. Opioid hyperexcitability: the application of alternate opioid therapy. *Pain* 1993; 53:353–355.

126. Lawlor P, Walker P, Bruera E, Mitchell S. Severe opioid toxicity and somatization of psychosocial distress in a cancer patient with a background of chemical dependence. *J Pain Symp Manage* 1997; 13:356–361.

127. Wright AW, Nocente ML, Smith MT. Hydromorphone-3-glucuronide: biochemical synthesis and preliminary pharmacological evaluation. *Life Sci* 1998; 63:401–411.

128. Smith GD, Smith MT. The excitatory behavioral and antianalgesic pharmacology of normorphine-3-glucuronide after intracerebroventricular administration to rats. *J Pharmacol Exp Ther* 1998; 285:1157–1162.

129. Bowsher D. Paradoxical pain. *BMJ* 1993; 306:473–474.

130. Faura CC, Olaso MJ, Garcia CC, Horga JF. Lack of morphine-6-glucuronide antinociception after morphine treatment. Is morphine-3-glucuronide involved? *Pain* 1996; 65:25–30.

131. Goucke CR, Hackett LP, Ilett KF. Concentrations of morphine, morphine-6-glucuronide and morphine-3-glucuronide in serum and cerebrospinal fluid following morphine administration to patients with morphine-resistant pain. *Pain* 1994; 56:145–149.

132. Faura CC, Collins SL, Moore RA, McQuay HJ. Systematic review of factors affecting the ratios of morphine and its major metabolites. *Pain* 1998; 74:43–53.

133. Ashby M, Fleming B, Wood M, Somogyi A. Plasma morphine and glucuronide (M3G and M6G) concentrations in hospice inpatients. *J Pain Symp Manage* 1997; 14:157–167.

134. Bartlett SE, Cramond T, Smith MT. The excitatory effects of morphine-3-glucuronide are attenuated by LY274614, a competitive NMDA receptor antagonist, and by midazolam, an agonist at the benzodiazepine site on the GABAA receptor complex. *Life Sci* 1994; 54:687–694.

135. Bartlett SE, Dodd PR, Smith MT. Pharmacology of morphine and morphine-3-glucuronide at opioid, excitatory amino acid, GABA and glycine binding sites. *Pharmacol Toxicol* 1994; 75:73–81.

136. Sjogren P, Dragsted L, Christensen CB. Myoclonic spasms during treatment with high doses of intravenous morphine in renal failure. *Acta Anaesthesiol Scand* 1993; 37:780–782.

137. Osborne R, Joel S, Grebenik K, Trew D, Slevin M. The pharmacokinetics of morphine and morphine glucuronides in kidney failure. *Clin Pharm Ther* 1993; 54: 158–167.

138. Milne RW, McLean CF, Mather LE, et al. Influence of renal failure on the disposition of morphine, morphine-3-glucuronide and morphine-6-glucuronide in sheep during intravenous infusion with morphine. *J Pharmacol Exp Ther* 1997; 282: 779–786.

139. Hagen NA, Foley KM, Cerbone DJ, Portenoy RK, Inturrisi CE. Chronic nausea and morphine-6-glucuronide. *J Pain Symp Manage* 1991; 6:125–128.

140. D'Honneur G, Gilton A, Sandouk P, Scherrmann JM, Duvaldestin P. Plasma and cerebrospinal fluid concentrations of morphine and morphine glucuronides after oral morphine. The influence of renal failure. *Anesthesiology* 1994; 81:87–93.

141. de Stoutz ND, Bruera E, Suarez-Almazor M. Opioid rotation for toxicity reduction in terminal cancer patients. *J Pain Symp Manage* 1995; 10:378–384.

142. Sjogren P, Jensen NH, Jensen TS. Disappearance of morphine-induced hyperalgesia after discontinuing or substituting morphine with other opioid agonists. *Pain* 1994; 59:313–316.

143. Smith MT, Wright AWE, Williams BE, Stuart G, Cramond T. Cerebrospinal fluid and plasma concentrations of morphine, morphine-3-glucuronide, and morphine-6-glucuronide in patients before and after initiation of intracerebroventricular morphine for cancer pain management. *Anesth Analg* 1999; 88:109–116.

144. Vermeire A, Remon JP, Rosseel MT, Belpaire F, Devulder J, Bogaert MG. Variability of morphine disposition during long-term subcutaneous infusion in terminally ill cancer patients. *Eur J Clin Pharmacol* 1998; 53:325–330.

145. McQuay HJ, Carroll D, Faura CC, Gavaghan DJ, Hand CW, Moore RA. Oral morphine in cancer pain: influences on morphine and metabolite concentration. *Clin Pharm Ther* 1990; 48:236–244.

146. Mikus G, Somogyi AA, Bochner F, Chen ZR. Polymorphic metabolism of opioid narcotic drugs: possible clinical implications. *Ann Acad Med, Singapore* 1991; 20:9–12.

147. Desmeules J, Gascon MP, Dayer P, Magistris M. Impact of environmental and genetic factors on codeine analgesia. *Eur J Clin Pharmacol* 1991; 41:23–26.

148. Eckhardt K, Li S, Ammon S, Schanzle G, Mikus G, Eichelbaum M. Same incidence of adverse drug events after codeine administration irrespective of the genetically determined differences in morphine formation. *Pain* 1998; 76:27–33.

149. Poyhia R, Seppala T, Olkkola KT, Kalso E. The pharmacokinetics and metabolism of oxycodone after intramuscular and oral administration to healthy subjects. *Br J Clin Pharmacol* 1992; 33:617–621.

150. Poyhia R, Olkkola KT, Seppala T, Kalso E. The pharmacokinetics of oxycodone after intravenous injection in adults. *Br J Clin Pharmacol* 1991; 32:516–518.

151. Poyhia R, Vainio A, Kalso E. A review of oxycodone's clinical pharmacokinetics and pharmacodynamics. *J Pain Symp Manage* 1993; 8:63–67.

152. Beaver WT, Wallenstein SL, Houde RW, Rogers A. Comparison of the analgesic effects of oral and intramuscular oxymorphone and morphine in patients with cancer. *J Clin Pharmacol* 1977; 17:186–198.

153. Maddocks I, Somogyi A, Abbott F, Hayball P, Parker D. Attenuation of morphine-induced delirium in palliative care by substitution with infusion of oxycodone. *J Pain Symp Manage* 1996; 12:182–189.

154. Walker P, Steiner N, Bruera E. Severe sedation and respiratory depression after rotation from oxycodone to hydromorphone (Unpublished data).

155. Galer BS, Coyle N, Pasternak GW, Portenoy RK. Individual variability in the response to different opioids: report of five cases. *Pain* 1992; 49:87–91.

156. Bruera E, Schoeller T, Wenk R, et al. A prospective multicenter assessment of the Edmonton staging system for cancer pain. *J Pain Symp Manage* 1995; 10:348–355.

157. Coyle N, Breitbart W, Weaver S, Portenoy R. Delirium as a contributing factor to "crescendo" pain: Three case reports. *J Pain Symp Manage* 1994; 9:44–47.

158. Houde RW, Wallenstein SL, Beaver W. Evaluation of analgesics in patients with cancer pain. In: Lasagna L, ed. *International Encyclopedia of Pharmacology and Therapeutics*. Oxford, Pergamon Press, 1966:59–67.

159. Cherny NI, Foley KM. Nonopioid and opioid analgesic pharmacotherapy of cancer pain. *Hematol-Oncol Clin North Am* 1996; 10:79–102.

160. Ripamonti C, De Conno F, Groff L, et al. Equianalgesic dose/ratio between methadone and other opioid agonists in cancer pain: comparison of two clinical experiences. *Ann Oncol* 1998; 9:79–83.

161. Bruera E, Watanabe S, Fainsinger RL, Spachynski K, Suarez-Almazor M, Inturrisi C. Custom-made capsules and suppositories of methadone for patients on high-dose opioids for cancer pain. *Pain* 1995; 62:141–146.

162. Thomas Z, Bruera E. Use of methadone in a highly tolerant patient receiving parenteral hydromorphone. *J Pain Symp Manage* 1995; 10:315–317.

163. Vigano A, Fan D, Bruera E. Individualized use of methadone and opioid rotation in the comprehensive management of cancer pain associated with poor prognostic indicators. *Pain* 1996; 67:115–119.

164. Manfredi PL, Borsook D, Chandler SW, Payne R. Intravenous methadone for cancer pain unrelieved by morphine and hydromorphone: clinical observations. *Pain* 1997; 70:99–101.

165. Fitzgibbon DR, Ready LB. Intravenous high-dose methadone administered by patient controlled analgesia and continuous infusion for the treatment of cancer pain refractory to high-dose morphine. *Pain* 1997; 73:259–261.

166. Morley JS, Makin MK. Comments on Ripamonti et al., Pain, 70 (1997) 109–115 *Pain* 1997; 73:114–115.

167. Beaver WT, Wallenstein SL, Rogers A, Houde RW. Analgesic studies of codeine and oxycodone in patients with cancer. I. Comparisons of oral with intramuscular codeine and of oral with intramuscular oxycodone. *J Pharmacol Exp Ther* 1978; 207:92–100.

168. Beaver WT, Wallenstein SL, Rogers A, Houde RW. Analgesic studies of codeine and oxycodone in patients with cancer. 2. Comparisons of intramuscular oxycodone with intramuscular morphine and codeine. *J Pharmacol Exp Ther* 1978; 207: 101–108.

169. Kalso E, Vainio A. Morphine and oxycodone hydrochloride in the management of cancer pain. *Clin Pharm Ther* 1990; 47:639–646.

170. Kalso E, Poyhia R, Onnela P, Linko K, Tigerstedt I, Tammisto T. Intravenous morphine and oxycodone for pain after abdominal surgery. *Acta Anaesthesiol Scand* 1991; 35:642–646.

171. Glare PA, Walsh TD. Dose-ranging study of oxycodone for chronic pain in advanced cancer. *J Clin Oncol* 1993; 11:973–978.

172. Silvasti M, Rosenberg P, Seppala T, Svartling N, Pitkanen M. Comparison of analgesic efficacy of oxycodone and morphine in postoperative intravenous patient-controlled analgesia. *Acta Anaesthesiol Scand* 1998; 42:576–580.

173. Bruera E, Belzile M, Pituskin E, et al. Randomized, double-blind, cross-over trial comparing safety and efficacy of oral controlled-release oxycodone with controlled-release morphine in patients with cancer pain. *J Clin Oncol* 1998; 16: 3222–3229.

174. Heiskanen T, Kalso E. Controlled-release oxycodone and morphine in cancer related pain. *Pain* 1997; 73:37–45.

175. Gagnon B, Bielech M, Watanabe S, Walker P, Hanson J, Bruera E. The use of intermittent subcutaneous injections of oxycodone for opioid rotation in patients with cancer pain. *Supp Care Cancer* 1999; 7:265–270.

176. Donner B, Zenz M, Tryba M, Strumpf M. Direct conversion from oral morphine to transdermal fentanyl: a multicenter study in patients with cancer pain. *Pain* 1996; 64:527–534.

177. Fainsinger RL, Bruera E. How should we use transdermal fentanyl (TF) for pain management in palliative care patients? *J Palliat Care* 1996; 12:48–53.

178. Hanks GW, Fallon MT. Transdermal fentanyl in cancer pain: conversion from oral morphine. *J Pain Symp Manage* 1995; 10:87.

179. Foley KM, Houde RW. Methadone in cancer pain management: individualize dose and titrate to effect. *J Clin Oncol* 1998; 16:3213–3215.

180. Dunbar PJ, Chapman CR, Buckley FP, Gavrin JR. Clinical analgesic equivalence for morphine and hydromorphone with prolonged PCA. *Pain* 1996; 68:265–270.

181. Babul N, Darke AC, Hagen N. Hydromorphone metabolite accumulation in renal failure. *J Pain Symp Manage* 1995; 10:184–186.

182. Paix A, Coleman A, Lees J, et al. Subcutaneous fentanyl and sufentanil infusion substitution for morphine intolerance in cancer pain management. *Pain* 1995; 63:263–269.

183. Watanabe S, Pereira J, Hanson J, Bruera E. Fentanyl by continuous subcutaneous infusion for the management of cancer pain: a retrospective study. *J Pain Symp Manage* 1998; 16:323–326.

16

Intraspinal Pain Therapy in Palliative Care

MAGNUS SJÖBERG AND NARINDER RAWAL

It has been suggested that the guidelines for treatment of cancer pain established by the World Health Organization[1] can control more than 90% of cancer-related pain syndromes.[2] The oral and parenteral routes of opioid therapy are favored for their simplicity and lower cost. Some patients do not respond adequately to these approaches, however, and more invasive techniques are needed.

The discovery that small doses of opioids administered in either the subarachnoid or epidural spaces provides profound and prolonged segmental analgesia represented a major breakthrough in pain management. Since their introduction into clinical practice in 1979, spinal opioids have achieved great international popularity, either as sole analgesic agents or in combination with a low-dose local anesthetic. Segmental analgesia induced by intraspinal opioids has a role in the management of a wide variety of surgical and nonsurgical painful conditions. The technique has been employed successfully to treat intraoperative, postoperative, traumatic, obstetric, chronic, and cancer pain.

About 2% of patients with cancer pain are candidates for spinal opioid treatment.[3,4] The indications are inadequate pain relief or intolerable side effects from other routes. The main advantages of spinal opioid analgesia are prolonged analgesic effect after a dose and a lower intensity of side effects such as sedation, drowsiness, emesis, nausea, and constipation. The unique feature of spinal opioid analgesia is the lack of sensory, sympathetic, or motor block, which allows a patient to ambulate without the risk of orthostatic hypotension or motor incoordination usually associated with local anesthetics administered epidurally or intrathecally.

In general, a good analgesic response to systemic opioids, compromised by intolerable side effects, appears to predict good pain relief with spinal opioids.[5] Some patients have pain syndromes that are relatively poorly responsive to spinal opioids (Table 16.1). The alternative treatments in the event of failed spinal opioid therapy include destructive methods (neurolytic blocks and neurosurgi-

Table 16.1. Likelihood of responsiveness to treatment with intraspinal opioids°

Continuous somatic pain
Continuous visceral pain
Intermittent somatic pain
Intermittent visceral pain
Neuropathic pain
Cutaneous, ulcer, and fistula

° From most to least likely.
Source: Arnér and Arnér, 1985.[5]

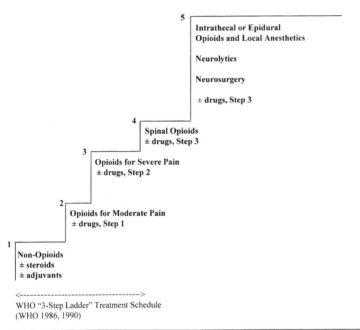

Figure 16.1. Horizontal axis: Increasing complexity and refractoriness of cancer pain. Vertical axis: Pain treatment ladder, including the WHO Analgesic Ladder (Steps 1–3), with additional methods of increasing invasiveness (4–5), adapted to the progress of cancer pain.[21]

cal interventions, both of which may cause irreversible side effects), or nondestructive methods using spinal infusion of non-opioids, with or without addition of opioids (Fig. 16.1, Step 5).

Intraspinal treatment provides reversible side effects and gives the patient the ability to control the pain treatment, both by close communication with the pain team and by patient-controlled analgesia (PCA). It encourages an acceptable balance between pain relief and side effects. A wide choice of drugs is, at least theoretically, possible. However so far, wide clinical use involves the choice between a combination of local anesthetics and opioids or clonidine and opioids. Treatment must choose between the epidural or intrathecal route and the use of technically well-functioning catheter systems with external or internal devices. Rational, safe routines in the care of the patients and the catheter systems are mandatory.

General Aspects of Intraspinal Infusion: Epidurally or Intrathecally?

The epidural and intrathecal routes for opioids, with or without addition of local anesthetics, are both useful to provide effective pain relief in severe cancer pain. Epidural treatment is familiar to every anesthesiologist and this may be advantageous. However, the intrathecal route has some potential advantages compared to the epidural route.

The main differences between the intrathecal and epidural modes are anatomical, biomechanical, and pharmacokinetic.[6–12] The epidural and intrathecal spaces are separated by the dura mater, which is difficult to penetrate by hydrophilic drugs, such as morphine, and more easily permeable to lipophilic drugs, such as sufentanil and fentanyl.[7,10] The epidural space is filled with loose connective tissue, fat, and blood vessels, which absorb a major part of the epidural drug. This results in enhanced risk of systemic opioid-related side effects by the epidural route compared to the intrathecal route. Opioid doses need to be increased rapidly during epidural treatment due to fibrosis and tolerance. The nerve roots in the epidural space are draped by a thick perineural tissue, which is also a thicker tissue barrier to drugs than the thin and easily permeable membrane that surrounds the rootlets in the intrathecal space.

There is often a rapid appearance of extensive fibrosis around an epidural catheter (Fig. 16.2a), whereas fibrosis around intrathecal catheters is scarce or nonexistent in humans (Fig. 16.2b).[13–15] Although animal studies have reported increased fibrous reaction with polyurethane,[16] polyethylene,[17] and silicone-elastomer[18] catheters, no fibrous reaction was noted when nylon[15,19] and polyamide catheters[19] were used in human studies. The difference in the rate of fibrosis results in more biomechanical complications, increased doses, and maldistribution of the drugs when the epidural route is used during long-term treatment.

Another anatomical cause of maldistribution of the spinal infusate is intraspinal tumor growth.[20] Epidural stenosis due to collapsed vertebrae and tumor growth are more frequent than intrathecal stenosis in cancer patients.[20] Furthermore, neuropathic pain induced by epidural metastases—a common mechanism of refractory cancer pain—must be blocked proximal to the epidural

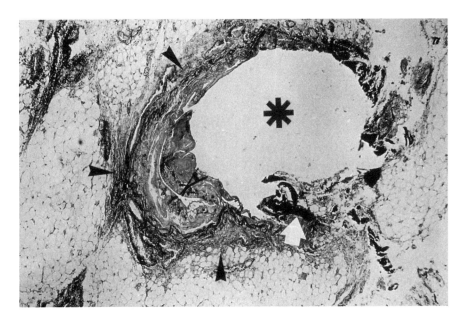

Figure 16.2a. Microscopic view. The epidural space after 188 days of intrathecal catheterization. Epidural tissue with fibrous capsule (small arrows) and calcifications (large arrow) around the catheter canal (*). (Stained by Van Gieson colour, bar, 1 mm.)

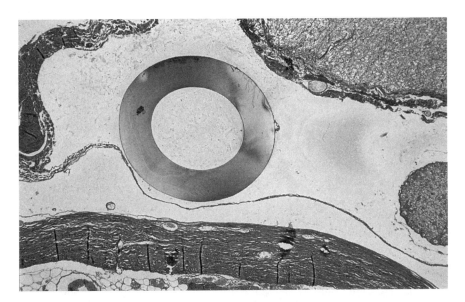

Figure 16.2b. Microscopic view. The catheter in the subarachnoid space after 274 days of intrathecal treatment by morphine and bupivacaine. There is no sign of reaction on its surface and adjacent spinal roots are normal. (Stained by Van Gieson colour. The diameter of the catheter is 1.1 mm.)

nerve damage. This is possible by an intrathecal catheter with its tip located above the stenosis.[20,21]

The considerable differences between the epidural and intrathecal routes regarding the fractions of morphine doses available for the spinal opioid receptors results in much higher doses of morphine and bupivacaine by the epidural compared to the intrathecal route. The epidural:intrathecal dose ratio suggested for morphine is 10–20:1 and for bupivacaine is ≈10:1. This results in larger volumes and more frequent exchange of drug cassettes or larger drug reservoirs when epidural therapy is used.[21,22] A 100 ml drug reservoir with mixture of morphine and bupivacaine usually lasts for 2–4 weeks when the intrathecal route is used, compared to 12–24 hours when epidural infusion is used.[11] To use bupivacaine and morphine storage in cassettes for several weeks seems to be possible, as the drugs have been reported to be stable for 30[23] and up to 90 days[24] with no bacterial contamination.

The technically more complicated procedure of insertion of intrathecal catheters[25] at a high thoracic or cervical level may favor the epidural route as the first choice when these procedures are needed. Lumbar or low thoracic insertion techniques seem to be more or less equally difficult.

Intrathecal Treatment for Cancer Pain

Combination of opioids and local anesthetics

The rationale for combining drugs intraspinally is that different types of drugs may eliminate pain by acting at different sites. Local anesthetics act at the nerve axon and opioids act at the receptor site in the spinal cord.

Local anesthetic and opioid combination techniques have been studied extensively in the obstetric population. If even an extremely low concentration of local anesthetic is added to the opioid, the quality of analgesia may be far superior. As might be expected, pain relief at rest is better than during movement. Spinal opioids alone provide good pain relief at rest but may not be adequate during physiotherapy and mobilization. Epidural local anesthetics alone are incapable of maintaining sensory anesthesia for a prolonged period due to tachyphylaxis.

Patient selection

Criteria for initiating trials of regional opioid analgesia, as well as for selecting a delivery system, remain ill-defined. In general, intraspinal opioids are considered in the presence of inadequate analgesia and/or persistent side effects despite careful trials of systemic analgesics titrated to effect. Relative contraindications include bleeding diathesis, severe immune dysfunction, local tumor infiltration, local or systemic infection, and lack of informed consent.

Table 16.2. Classification of drug delivery systems

Type I	Percutaneous epidural or intrathecal catheter (taped)
Type II	Percutaneous epidural or intrathecal catheter short-tunneled subcutaneously
Type III	Percutaneous epidural or intrathecal catheter long-tunneled subcutaneously with external, portable, PCA-programmable pump
Type IV	Totally implanted epidural or intrathecal catheter attached to a subcutaneous injection port
Type V	Totally implanted epidural or intrathecal catheter attached to implanted manually activated (patient-controlled) pump or a fixed rate infusion pump
Type VI	Totally implanted epidural or intrathecal catheter attached to implanted computer-programmed infusion pump

Patients with neuropathic pain because of plexus or peripheral nerve invasion, and those with movement-related pain, are more likely to require intraspinal therapy in which an opioid and local anesthetic are combined. This is independent of prognosis, although life expectancy is a major determinant of the selection of a drug delivery system.

Catheter and drug delivery systems

Intrathecal catheter systems can be either implantable or external percutaneous, tunneled devices (Table 16.2).

Percutaneous catheters
Untunneled or short-tunneled catheters should be used only for days or a week. For longer use, a percutaneous catheter should be tunneled subcutaneously for a longer distance. The drug is either administered manually by serial bolus injections or is infused via an external portable pump. Placement of the catheter is simple and undemanding for the patient, and this system is cost-effective for a very short-time use, for example, postoperatively. However, the short- or untunneled catheters are more prone to migration or dislodgement and, because they exit the skin near the spine, the risk of central nervous infection may be enhanced with prolonged use. Percutaneous, long-tunneled catheters with a firm fixation, herein termed *externalized long-tunneled systems,* can be used for long periods (months, years). This system is associated with a much lower rate of technical complications.[26]

Totally implantable systems
These systems consist of an internalized catheter system attached to a fully-implanted subcutaneous infusion pump (see Table 16.2.). A computer and special software are required to monitor and reprogram the devices. The cost ranges between $6000 and $10,000. The cost-effectiveness of these systems has been debated considerably. Proponents claim that by limiting pharmacy and

home care nursing costs, these techniques are cost-effective. It is generally agreed that these systems are indicated in highly functional, ambulatory patients and when therapy is anticipated for longer than 3–6 months.

Indications for intrathecal opioids and local anesthetics

Long-term infusion of intrathecal opioids and local anesthetics is indicated especially for pain that is poorly responsive to opioid drugs and when systemic or spinal opioids result in unacceptable side effects. The most common types of poorly responsive cancer pain include intermittent somatic pain, intermittent visceral pain, most types of neuropathic pain, and somatic pain due to large mucocutaneous ulcers. Experience to date is extensive enough to describe intrathecal administration as a safe and very effective method, and to use this method as an early choice in the clinical practice for long-term treatment of severe refractory cancer pain.[11,21,25,27–32]

Contraindications to treatment

Intrathecal catheterization is contraindicated in the setting of increased intracranial pressure (e.g., from intracranial metastases). Both epidural and intrathecal catheterization should be avoided in cases of infection in the catheterization area, septicemia, severe bleeding diathesis, severe immune dysfunction, local tumor infiltration, lack of informed consent, and severe mental disturbance or substantial lack of cooperation from the patient. When treatment at home is planned, cooperation is also needed from the family.[21,32] In cases with spinal stenosis because of epidural metastases, special consideration should be taken regarding the risk of neurologic complications and technical difficulties during the insertion of the intrathecal catheter. Epidural tumor and spinal stenosis are not absolute contraindications, however. Also debilitation is not a contraindication. At times, effective pain relief without heavy sedation can lead to a remarkable improvement.

Experience with long-tunneled intrathecal catheters

As previously discussed, the systems for long-term use should be either implanted or external long-tunneled devices. The following guidelines are based on experience using externalized long-tunneled intrathecal catheters in more than 330 patients during 27,600 treatment days, including more than 10,000 treatment days at home. The treatment lasted for between 2 and 755 days (median 40 days).[21,26]

Technique
The insertion of a long-tunneled catheter (intrathecal or epidural) should be performed under strictly sterile precautions in an operation theater. The procedure

is usually performed after infiltration of local anesthetics. In patients with multiple fractures or with other types of severe pain that complicate the positioning on the operation bed/table, spinal anesthesia can be given before the start of the insertion procedure. The use of different sizes of catheters has been described.[21,26,33–37] Up to 18G catheters can be used.[21,26] The dura mater is punctured by a Tuohy needle and the catheter is inserted. The tip of the catheter is placed in the middle of the segments of maximum pain. In cases with spinal stenosis, the catheter is usually placed immediately above the stenosis. To facilitate the location of the catheter, fluoroscopic imaging and soft steel mandrin can be used in the catheter.

The catheter is tunneled subcutaneously far from wounds and stomas. For example, the catheter can be tunneled paravertebrally over the shoulder with the exit at the level of the pectoral muscle. The catheter is fixed by a silicone muff and by two sutures at the exit. The catheter hub is fixed by two steel sutures. A reliable fixation of the catheter is a necessity for a long-term intrathecal catheter system used at home. An antibacterial Millipore filter (size 0.22 μM) is connected between the catheter hub and the drug tube.

Continuous infusion should be used preferably by a portable pump with PCA facility.[21,38] After catheter insertion, the patient is supervised in a postoperative ward for about 12 hours before admission to the ward. After another 2–5 days of dose adjustments, the patient is able to leave the hospital for home or hospice.

The infusate typically contains morphine without preservatives (0.5–1.0 mg/ml) and an isobaric solution of bupivacaine (4.5–4.75 mg/ml). A test dose of 0.75–1.0 ml of the mixture is injected. A starting dose of 4.5 ml/day is rapidly increased until acceptable pain relief is obtained. Further guidelines for dose adjustment are presented in Table 16.3.

Care
The dressing at the tunnel exit is changed within 48 hours after the catheter insertion and every 7–10 days thereafter. A compress protects the skin from pressure from the filter. The exit, the catheter hub, and the filter are covered by a transparent adhesive dressing. A label "intrathecal catheter" is recommended on the dressing. The antibacterial filter is changed once a month[23] This change carries a risk of bacterial contamination and meningitis. It should, therefore, be performed using strictly antiseptic precautions, including sterile gloves, and cleaning the catheter, hub, and filter with 0.5% chlorhexidine in 70% alcohol before the filter exchange. As chlorhexidine and alcohol are neurotoxic, the solution must not go into the catheter. The filter is primed with the drug mixture before connection of the hub. The filter is a protection against bacterial contamination. During the care on the pump side of the filter, the hands are cleaned by alcohol/chlorhexidine, and a strict antiseptic technique is used during filling and exchanging drug reservoirs. The drug reservoirs are exchanged when empty. When the tunnel exit is covered by an impermeable dressing, the patient may

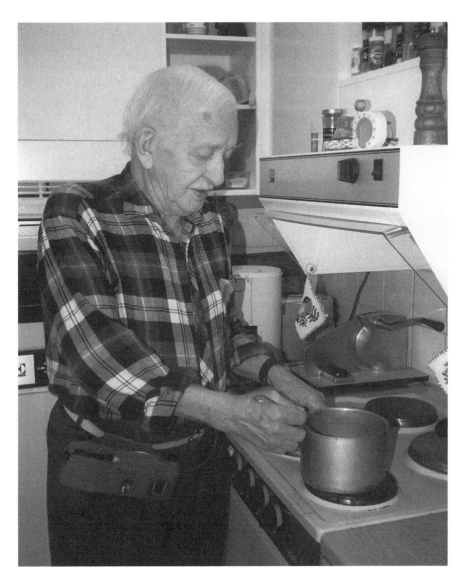

Figure 16.3. A patient with intrathecal pain treatment cooking his porridge at his home. He had a systemic morphine resistant pain. The catheter tip was placed at the segment of Th 8–9. He had a continuous intrathecal infusion of morphine and bupivacine by a portable pump, with patient-controlled analgesia-availability, and was treated at home for 8 months.

Table 16.3. Suggestions for starting intrathecal morphine or bupivacaine via lumbar and low thoracic catheters

---

These suggestions represent one of several different ways to start intrathecal treatment with mixtures of morphine and bupivacaine in refractory cancer pain. They are based on experience with >300 cancer patients during >25,000 days, including >9500 days that were at home. To make the dose adjustments more suitable, a mixture with fixed concentration of morphine and bupivacaine can be chosen. Bupivacaine is the more effective of the drugs, and a higher concentration and dose of bupivacaine is chosen to obtain good pain relief in severe morphine resistant pain.[49,58,62]

1. Place the tip of the catheter at the middle of the segments of maximum pain. In cases with spinal stenosis, the catheter is usually placed immediately above the stenosis.
2. Use continuous infusion, preferably by a volume-programmable pump with PCA facility.
3. The mixture contains morphine 0.5–1.0 mg/ml and isobaric solution of bupivacaine 4.5–4.75 mg/ml. After insertion, a test dose of 0.75–1.0 ml of the mixture is injected. The starting dose with this mixture is usually 0.2 ml/hour. The incremental dose is set to the dose corresponding to the infused dose of approximately 1 hour. The patient is supervised on the recovery unit for 12–14 hours before moving to the regular ward.
4. The volumes (doses) are increased gradually until adequate pain relief (VAS 0–2 out of 10) is obtained by adding the total infused dose with the sum of the incremental doses of the last 24 hours. This dose is set as the infused dose during the following 24 hours and the new incremental dose as described above.
5. The patient, family, and staff should be informed about the most common side effects. An incremental dose <1.25 mg bupivacaine/day does not usually result in side effects. Some of the side effects, for example, paresthesia, are transient within a few days despite the same dose.
6. Mostly high doses of bupivacaine per hour and on demand are required in patients with pain involving many spinal segments; deafferentation pain from spinal cord, nerve roots, or from the brachial, celiac, or lumbosacral plexus; and pain due to subileus and ileus or of ischemic origin or pain caused by large mucocutaneous ulcers from the tumor. In these cases, bupivacaine-related side effects are more common.
7. The systemic administration of opioids should be gradually decreased and not suddenly withdrawn. Opioid abstinence should be treated independently of the intrathecal morphine doses. An addition of oral clonidine may be used to treat withdrawal effects from systemic morphine. A dose of opioid by other routes with addition of peripheral and nonsteroidal analgesics are often needed to treat pain distant from the area treated by the intrathecal catheter.
8. Sedatives can gradually be reduced but not suddenly interrupted. The intrathecal pain treatment has no effect on anxiety, and many patients still have need for anxiolytics even during a well-functioning pain treatment.
9. Daily contact with the patient every day in the beginning of the treatment, for dose adjustments and recurrent pain analysis, is of great importance. A pain physician has to be easily available 24 hours/day in the event of breakthrough pain or complications. Psychosocial support is of great importance.

---

take a shower and change the dressing afterwards. The pump should be protected from water.

Results
Using these techniques, all patients with poorly responsive pain obtained acceptable pain relief during the major part of the rest of their lives. The pain score

on a 10 cm visual analogue scale declined to 0–2 from 6–10 before.[11,29] Other studies,[21,28] however, have shown temporary therapeutic failures when the catheter tip was not placed at the appropriate level, when the bupivacaine doses were too low and morphine doses too high, and when the pain was spread widely over, for example, over both upper/lower thoracic and lumbar segments.

Effective pain treatment was obtained at very different intrathecal doses (intrathecal morphine 1.0–25.0 mg/day, median 6 mg/day; bupivacaine 9.0–250.0 mg/day, median 50 mg/day, volumes 2–50 ml/day, median 10 ml/d). Therefore, the intrathecal doses must be individually titrated due to differences in spread and types of pain.[11,21,28,29]

There were large differences in doses required by patients with and without epidural or intraspinal metastases associated with spinal stenosis.[20] Epidural metastases obstruct epidural analgesia but intrathecal treatment can still be effective.[11] The largest doses were registered in cases with total spinal stenosis with paraplegia due to epidural tumor growth. After starting intrathecal treatment, the total opioid consumption could be reduced to a tenth of the systemic dose.[21,28,29] The patients' minds were clear and the use of sedatives[21,29] were reduced. The duration of undisturbed sleep improved from 2–3 hours to 4–6 hours per night in more than 90% of the patients.[11,21,28,29]

Intrathecal infusion did not significantly improve ambulation, but none of the patients became bedridden as a consequence of the treatment. Patients with impaired mobility could be moved more easily and spend more time out of bed because of less pain. Hospitalization was not because of the intrathecal treatment, but was needed because of the patient's general condition. In different reports, between 40%–79% of cancer patients with intrathecal infusion of morphine and bupivacaine were treated at home.[21,28,29,31]

Factors influencing intrathecal doses

The doses of intrathecal morphine and bupivacaine range widely, independent of age, sex, and weight. The only reported correlation between doses and pain types is an increased need of bupivacaine in cases with neuropathic pain.[21,29,30] Thus, the dose of morphine and bupivacaine have to be titrated individually.[21,28]

Eighty percent of patients with neuropathic pain required more than 60 mg/day of bupivacaine to obtain sufficient pain relief.[21,29] Increasing intrathecal morphine doses to more than 20–30 mg/day in combination with bupivacaine does not enhance pain relief in patients with refractory pain. In addition, intrathecal morphine infusion exceeding this limit may cause hyperalgesia, allodynia, and myoclonic jerking.[21,28,39–43] To keep the morphine doses low, the morphine concentration in the mixtures should be low, for example, 0.5–1 mg/ml.[11,28,29] The solution for infusion of morphine and bupivacaine in the literature ranges between morphine 0.2–5.0 mg/ml and bupivacaine 0.2–4.75 mg/ml.[11,21,27–32,36]

Side Effects

Drug-related side effects

The drug-related side effects and their management are similar when epidural and intrathecal morphine and bupivacaine solutions are used, but no studies have systematically presented the relationship between epidural dose and the rate of side effects. Therefore, intrathecal treatment with morphine and bupivacaine will be more extensively described. The drug-related side effects are dose-dependent and reversible.

Opioid-related side effects
When intrathecal morphine doses are kept below 10–15 mg/day, opioid-related side effects are kept to a minimum, except for a contribution to urinary retention. Pruritus is very rare. In the group of cancer patients who have previously received high opioid doses, respiratory depression during infusion of mixtures of intrathecal morphine and bupivacaine has not been reported.[11,21,27–32,36,44]

Bupivacaine-related side effects
The bupivacaine-related side effects consist mainly of urinary retention, paresthesias, and transient paresis. Urinary retention seems to be the earliest sign of the bupivacaine-related side effects in patients with lumbar catheters. During intrathecal bupivacaine infusion at doses >60–90 mg/day and morphine <10 mg day, urinary retention occurs in up to 33% and paresthesias in up to 23% of the patients. Transient paresis with gait impairment is reported by 3.5% of the patients who had 45–60 mg/day and in 15% of those who had >60 mg bupivacaine per day. The paresis, which is mostly transient, and the paresthesias appear sometimes after an intermittent extra-dose of >1.25 mg bupivacaine added to an infusion of >2–3 mg bupivacaine/hour or after a sudden large increase of the infused dose.[21,28,29] With infused bupivacaine doses of <30–45 mg/day and morphine doses of <5 mg/day, and incremental doses of ≤1.25 mg bupivacaine, the risk of urinary retention, paresthesia, or paresis is almost absent.[21,28,29,36] Postural hypotension is reported as a very rare side effect after large intermittent bupivacaine doses (3.75–5.0 mg) are added to infused doses of >85.0 mg/day.[21,28,29]

Factors potentially contributing to bupivacaine-related side effects are nerve lesions due to progression of tumor and polyneuropathy.[20,21] The margin for intrathecal doses causing motor disturbances and urinary retention is considerably reduced, often to 1.0 mg/hour of bupivacaine,[21,29] in patients with neurological disturbances in the lumbosacral segments before the start of intrathecal treatment. Compared to unaffected patients, the limit for this group may be 2–3 mg/hour of bupivacaine. The type of side effects is related to the site of catheter, for example, lumbar catheters more than thoracic catheters are associated with urinary retention.[21]

Management of the drug-related side effects

With reduction of the bupivacaine dose, the side effects decrease. An important point is to inform the patient, the family, and the staff about expected side effects to prevent unnecessary anxiety. Mostly, side effects are accepted by the patients when weighed against the very good pain relief. To keep side effects to a minimum and to obtain best control of the pain, continuous infusion is preferred. Intrathecal morphine and bupivacaine have mainly regional effects, which means that the catheter tip should be placed at the segment of maximum pain to avoid unnecessary high doses and to further reduce the side effects.[21,29,30] Gait impairment after intrathecal bolus doses mostly disappear spontaneously within 30–45 minutes.[21] Paresthesias and slight muscle weakness, which appear after dose adjustment, often disappear within 2–4 days despite the same infused intrathecal dose.[21] Urinary retention is managed by intermittent catheterization or indwelling catheter.[11,21,28,29]

Safety of intraspinal bupivacaine and morphine

The long-term intrathecal infusion of bupivacaine and morphine has, until recently, been considered hazardous due to anticipated risk of severe infections, cumbersome side effects, and neurological complications. However, no systemic toxicity has been reported despite long-term infusion of epidural bupivacaine up to 1800 mg/day and intrathecal infusion between 90 and 200 mg/day.[11,19,21,26–32,36,44–47]

Neurotoxicity of opioids

The use of opioid infusion with preservatives is a controversial subject. Despite negative outcomes in histopathological studies, there is an intuitive reluctance to administer preservative into the spinal space. However, no clinical or neuropathological signs of neurotoxicity were found by Nitescu et al.[48] in 125 cancer patients who received a mixture of morphine and bupivacaine intrathecally with sodium metabisulfite and edetate.

Hyperalgesia, allodynia, and myoclonic jerking have been reported in some cases during infusion of high doses of spinal morphine.[21,39–43] The mechanisms are unknown but Yaksh has suggested that the morphine-related allodynia could be because of the metabolite morphine-3-glucuronide, which has a glycine receptor antagonistic effect on spinal neurons. These side effects are extraordinarily painful and unpleasant. They can be reversed by stopping intrathecal morphine and starting again at a lower dose. Hyperalgesia, allodynia, and myoclonic jerking may be avoided when the daily intrathecal infusion of morphine is less than 20–30 mg/day. However, the risk of these morphine-related side effects appears to be individual, since several patients treated with more than 30 mg/day (including a patient receiving up to 215 mg/day) have been reported.

Neurotoxicity of local anesthetics

Based on multiple animal and clinical studies of diverse local anesthetics, it is clear that local anesthetics, per se, are neurotoxic to nerve.[49–52] However, in several animal studies, the doses and concentrations exceeded greatly the clinical doses in humans. The neurotoxic potential of local anesthetics has not been correlated clearly to pH, osmolality, dissociation constants, or lipid solubility in preservative-free solutions.[52,53] The toxicity seems to be dependent on the local anesthetic concentration in the tissue and not on the total dose.[52,54] In fact, their relative potency for nerve injury seems to be the same as their relative potency for producing nerve block.[52,54] The clinical reports of neurotoxic reaction during long-term infusion of local anesthetics is mainly related to the use of hyperbaric solutions and small-bore catheters, which might be related to catheter coiling in the most inferior aspects of the inferior intrathecal dural sac.[49,55–58] Drasner et al.[34] have reported from an in vitro model that repeated injections of hyperbaric solutions through a sacrally directed catheter result in continuously increasing CSF-concentration in the caudal segments to a level demonstrated to be neurotoxic. Thus, for long-term infusion of local anesthetics, hyperbaric solutions should not be used.

Clinically used concentrations (≤ 5.0 mg/ml) of plain bupivacaine produced no persistent neurologic damage in either rats[13] or rabbits.[59] Absence of abnormal neuropathological findings in dogs[60] or very discrete findings such as focal mononuclear cell infiltration (dog)[61] or focal slight neuronal vacuolation (rats)[62] are reported as well after long-term infusion of bupivacaine. Neuropathological studies on humans are rather few and performed on patients with disease (spinal metastasis or paramalignant phenomena), which may have influenced or concealed neuropathologic changes. However, none of these neuropathological[15,19,48] or clinical studies[11,28–32,36,48,63] have presented evidence of neurotoxicity attributed to plain bupivacaine during continuous infusion with concentrations <5 mg/ml.

Systemic toxicity

The risk of systemic and central nervous toxicity is presumably dependent on the level of the free (non-protein bound) bupivacaine fraction and not the total amount in plasma.[64] The level of bupivacaine-binding AAG (alpha-1-acid-protein) is enhanced in cancer patients and increases rapidly after a few days with spinal treatment with bupivacaine. This may explain the relative resistance to CNS toxicity.[12,64,65] Furthermore, the plasma threshold concentration for expressions of toxicity appear to be higher during infusion than during intermittent injections. Despite intrathecal bupivacaine doses between 90–200 mg/day for several months[11,21,28,29] and epidural infusion with doses of up to 1800 mg/day,[12] no cardiovascular, respiratory, or central nervous toxic symptoms are reported. No clinical signs of accumulation and uncontrolled rostral spread of the block affecting respiration and circulation after continuous intrathecal doses up to >250 mg/day of bupivacaine (>40 ml/day) are reported.[11,28,29] However, pharmacological data of the rostral spread of bupivacaine are still lacking.

Complications due to long-term epidural catheterization

Fibrosis
Epidural catheterization is associated with a high rate of epidural fibrosis around the catheter. Early clinical signs of epidural fibrosis (Fig. 16.2a) around a catheter are resistance and pain during injection. In some cases, the drugs will be maldistributed and there may be a backward leak of the injected drugs along the subcutaneous tunnel.[14] Subsequently, the analgesia tends to be patchy and insufficient and additional analgesics will be needed for satisfactory pain relief. Finally, infusion and injection will become impossible because of obstruction of the catheter.[14] Another mechanical complication by epidural catheters is a slight risk of inward migration of the catheter.

Complications due to fibrosis usually appear after 2–3 weeks of treatment and will increase with the duration of the use of the catheter. They often result in recatheterization. The rate of technical complications during long-term epidural catheterization, a major part of which is probably related to fibrosis, is reported to be up to 55%; this may be compared to 5%–7.5% after ≤3 weeks' use of an intrathecal catheter.[14,26] However, the complication rate during the first 3 weeks of catheterization is reported to be higher with the intrathecal (25%) than the epidural route (8%). The major part of these intrathecal complications is transient post-dural puncture headache. Thus, when the catheter is planned to be used more than a few weeks, the intrathecal route seems to be desirable.[14]

Infection
As the dura mater is a barrier, a deep infection associated with an epidural catheter will more likely be an epidural abscess rather than meningitis. An epidural abscess is not always sufficiently treated by antibiotics and surgery may be needed. The incidence of epidural abscess is reported to be 5%.[66]

Complications from long-term intrathecal catheterization

Cerebrospinal fluid leakage and post-dural puncture headache
Complications associated with intrathecal catheters seem to appear mostly during the first weeks after insertion. In contrast to the epidural route, these seem to be transient and do not usually cause abandonment of the treatment.[14] Within 2–3 weeks, the rate of complications is dramatically decreased and is thereafter reported to be not higher than 5%–7.5%.[14,26]

The most common complication is post-dural puncture headache (PDPH). The PDPH usually appears during the first days after the catheter insertion. It is mostly moderate and remits spontaneously within a week. It is often treated using analgesics, increased fluid intake, or intrathecal injection of isotonic sterile NaCl ≈10 ml 2–3 times a day during the first days. Only on rare occasions is a blood patch needed.[14,26,30]

The intrathecal technique had renewed interest after the introduction of small-bore catheters, for example, 24–32G. The reported rate of PDPH with microcatheters is 8%–13%.[34–36] With larger diameter catheters, for example, 18G and 22G, the rate of PDPH is 15%[21,26,36] and about 10%,[11,30] respectively. This advantage must be balanced against potential problems with microcatheters, including neurological complications,[57,67] kinking,[34–36] disconnection with loss between the connector and the catheter, or the obstruction of the catheter when the tube is screwed too tight. Finally, it can be difficult to place the catheter tip at the intended segment when the catheters are soft and weak.[57,67] These problems are minimized with the slightly larger diameter catheters.[21,26,30,36] There are probably other contributing factors to the appearance of PDPH, including the size of the needle and the number of dural punctures before successful insertion.

Chronic CSF leakage may result in prolonged post-spinal headache, CSF pseudomeningocele, catheter track infection, and epidural hematoma from the tearing of the subdural or epidural veins. Thus, CSF leakage should be treated in the early stages. To avoid infection, prophylactic antibiotics should be considered in these cases.[26] Cerebrospinal fluid leakage by external devices is usually not associated with removal the system. Leakage at the insertion site can be stopped by resuturing the skin in the cases of skin dehiscence and by local compression for 2–3 weeks. In cases of CSF leakage at the tunnel exit, the local compression at the insertion site should be combined with a purse-string suture around the tunnel outlet and a compressive, rolled dressing applied on the last part of the tunnel track (Fig. 16.4). When the CSF leakage has resulted in headache, an epidural blood patch should be considered.[26]

Infection
The occurrence of meningitis is probably the most feared complication, and the one which has contributed to the hesitation to use intrathecal treatment by many clinicians. Although deep infections such as meningitis probably cannot be avoided completely, they can be minimized by a careful routine, limitation of catheter interventions, and aseptic precautions during filling and exchanging the drug reservoirs and filters. With these precautions, the incidence of meningitis has been less than 1% (one case after a total of 6250 catheter days), despite cancer patients' predisposition to infections due to advanced age, malignancy, debility, diabetes, and infection sources (e.g., colostomy or catheters).[14,21,26,30,31,36,46]

An early sign of meningitis may be a rather rapid increase in pain with new distribution, sometimes generalized, and often intense and radiating in character. This may occur before septic symptoms such as neck stiffness, headache, fever, and unclear mind appear.[36] Intravenous antibiotics, sometimes in combination with intrathecal antibiotics during the first days before the intrathecal catheter is withdrawn, usually are sufficient.[21,36]

Overall, using the previously described approach to external long-tunneled intrathecal catheterization, the catheters were well functioning in 92% of the

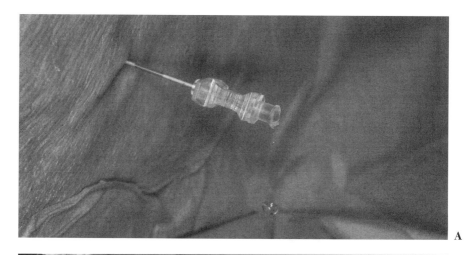

A

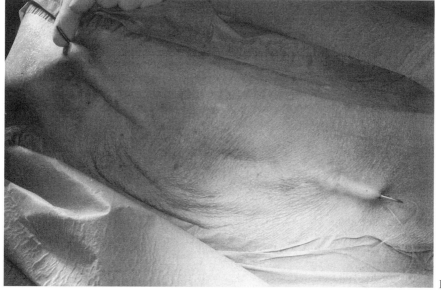

B

Figure 16.4. The procedure of insertion of an external long tunneled intrathecal catheter. *A*: The intrathecal space is identified and thereafter the catheter is introduced into the subarachnoid space. *B*: The catheter is subcutaneously tunneled by a Portex® tunneling instrument paravertebrally, over the shoulder, having the exit located at the level of the third condrocostal juntion. (*continued*)

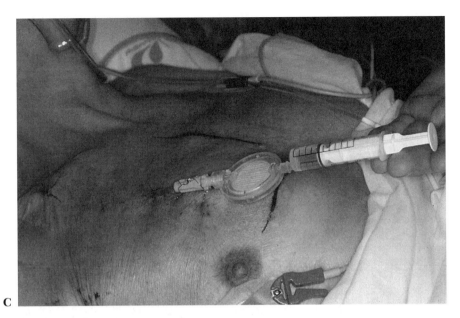

C

Figure 16.4. (*continued*) *C*: A = .22 μM Milliporefilter is connected to the catheter hub. The catheter hub is firmly fixed by steel sutures and an external portable pump with patient-controlled analgesia facilities is connected.

patients. Complications included transient leakage 1.5%; transient catheter obstruction 1%; dislocation of the catheter tip 1.5%; and unintended withdrawal 4%.[26]

Treatment failures during intrathecal morphine and bupivacaine

Beside technical failures of the catheter system and failure caused by psychological factors, other factors may be associated with a poor response to this therapy. As the effect of the intrathecal morphine and bupivacaine in opioid refractory pain is mainly regional, it is of great importance to place the catheter tip at the segment of maximum pain. Therefore, when widespread pain occurs or poorly responsive pain appears involving segments far from the catheter tip, insufficient pain relief may occur. A large increase in dose may be sufficient in some cases, but at an increased risk of side effects. Furthermore, large or widespread destruction or tumor compression of the spinal cord often results in transient failure due to an incomplete block of the neural axis proximal to the pain origin and incomplete spread of the drugs.[21,28–30]

Table 16.4. Long-term intrathecal catheters: external versus implanted devices

	Long-tunneled external intrathecal catheters (%)	Implanted intrathecal catheters (%)
Catheter obstruction	0–1–4	6
Catheter tip dislodgement	1.5–8	6
Accidental withdrawal	3	Not documented
External CSF leakage along the catheter or around the port	3.5–5–6	4
Removal of systems	4–6.5	5–50
CSF hygroma	1.5	4–6
Meningitis	<1–2	3
Port or pump pocket infection (implanted or local infection at catheter entry site (external)	0.5–4–6	11

CSF, cerebrospinal fluid.
Source: Nitescu et al., 1995.[26]

Devices for Long-Term Therapy

Decisive factors for the choice of device are the rate of technically well-functioning catheters, the safety, the convenience for the patient, the simplicity of the care, and finally, the cost of the method. A review of the advantages and disadvantages between external and implanted devices is presented in Table 16.4.

For long-term administration of intraspinal opioids and local anesthetics, internal (implanted) devices, with or without external or internal pumps and reservoirs,[68–71] generally have been recommended. It has been suggested that the externalized systems have a much higher rate of complications, such as local infections, meningitis or epidural abscess, accidental catheter withdrawal, and unmanageable CSF leakage. This conclusion is not definitive. Comparisons have been made between groups with implanted catheters on the one hand and a mixed group of patients with externalized non-tunneled, short-tunneled, and long-tunneled catheters on the other.[69] There is a great difference in the rate of complications between long-term intraspinal treatment with non-tunneled and long-tunneled catheters, with better outcomes in the latter group.[26] Several studies have reported the long-tunneled external devices to be just as safe and with a very high rate of well-functioning catheters compared to implanted devices for long-term intraspinal pain treatment.[11,21,26,28–31,36]

There are several options for externalized tunneled catheter systems.[11,28–30,32,36,66] Generally, the tunneled catheters are recommended to be long-tunneled and fixed firmly.[11,21,26,28,30,36,66] A closed catheter system is obtained by connecting the catheter and an antibacterial filter with an extension tubing to the drug reservoir. By exchanging the filter using strict hygienic precautions[26] once every 4th week, the risk of contamination of the system seems to be minimized.[21,26,30,36] The antibacterial filters have been reported to be used safely between 30[23] and 60 days[72] without bacterial contamination on the internal side of the filter and without clinical infection. Theoretically, the external systems are closed until the exchange of the filter once every fourth week.[21,26,36,72] Implanted ports and reservoirs that require frequent punctures have a risk of bacterial contamination from the skin around the port and further contamination of the port chamber, which may cause epidural abscess, systemic infection, or meningitis.

Using the precautions described previously with external long-tunneled catheters, complications mostly are kept equal or even lower than implanted devices for long-term infusion (Table 16.4).[26] The rates of CSF leakage or fistula and CSF hygroma are no higher with long-tunneled external intrathecal than with implanted devices. The main advantage of implanted systems is reduced risk of dislocation of the catheter by pull,[31] but some authors have reported spontaneous catheter tip dislodgement because of curling of the catheter with the implanted systems.[45] The risk of accidental withdrawal by external catheters can be reduced to minimum by firm fixation.[26]

Cost effectiveness

The completely implanted devices with implanted pumps are much more expensive and require more technically advanced programming equipment than a simple externalized catheter connected to a portable programmable pump with PCA.[26] This has to be weighed against the convenience of an implanted device, especially in young active patients.[69] It is probably more a matter of practical differences concerning insertion technique of catheters and the care of the pumps, the convenience for the patient, and, finally, the advantage of a simple device and simpler equipment, which can be handled by a large number of physicians.

Home Care

For many patients, it is of great worth to stay at home for at least a period of the last part of their lives (Fig. 16.3). This requires well-functioning catheter systems and drugs with predictable side effects. Long-term epidural and intrathecal infusion of morphine, with or without bupivacaine, is very effective and is reported to be safe and well-functioning for the home care setting, both with tunneled external and implanted devices.[11,12,21,29-32,36,45,73] The organization of the home care setting should be aimed at giving good pain relief, preventing complications, and recognizing and correcting them should they occur. To obtain a high rate of well-functioning catheters and a low infection rate, technical procedures and follow-up are of utmost importance.

In groups of patients with poorly responsive pain, up to 40%,[11,28,29,46] and in mixed groups with opioid-sensitive and non-sensitive pain, up to 70%[30,36] of the patients have been treated at home for shorter or longer periods. Several authors have reported succesful home care with intrathecal morphine and bupivacaine for a median time of 28–40 days, and single cases for up to more than 500 days.[11,28–32,36,46]

The staff who are responsible for the intraspinal treatment should have extensive experience with the technique and with intraspinal drugs. Follow-up is very important, with frequent and regular contact to ensure the patient's confidence. This will decrease anxiety and the experience of the pain as well. The patient and the family should have clear information about the contact staff person. A 24-hour consultation service by the pain doctors is desirable. Every event that could affect the results of the intraspinal pain treatment can, therefore, be immediately addressed and corrected. The most risky procedure in the care of the spinal catheters, such as, programming the pumps and exchanging the antibacterial filters of the external intrathecal catheter systems, should be performed only by a limited number of nurses and doctors with great experience with the method.[21,46]

Summary

Oral (and increasingly transdermal) opioid therapy remains the treatment of choice for uncomplicated cancer pain. However, spinal opioids with or without local anesthetics provide an important alternative for patients who cannot achieve acceptable pain control with simpler, conventional methods. Historically, cancer pain patients were the first group to receive spinal opioids. Although most patients with cancer pain have sufficient pain relief with standard drug treatment, 10%–30% of patients need alternative therapies because of persisting pain or side effects.

Intraspinal opioid analgesia is well adaptable to the home and home–hospice environment by virtue of the selective nature of pain relief and an absence of effects on sensory, motor, and autonomic functions. The administration of opioids in close proximity to their receptors in the central nervous system represents one of the most important recent advances in the management of chronic cancer pain. The chief advantage of regional opioid analgesia over systemic administration relates to the potential for achieving more analgesia with fewer attendant side effects. Reliable screening, together with reversibility, titratability, and suitability for generalized pains, have resulted in a preference for regional opioid therapies, with or without local anesthetics, over neurodestructive procedures.

Both epidural and intrathecal opioids provide very effective pain relief for opioid-sensitive pain. In cases with opioid refractory pain, a combination of opioids and local anesthetics (usually morphine and bupivacaine) provides a very effective option for long-term pain treatment. In poorly responsive cancer pain, the intrathecal route with opioids and local anesthetics, seems to be more effective, with smaller doses and smaller volumes, and fewer complications during long-term treatment compared to epidural administration. Furthermore, long-tunneled catheters connected to a portable programmable pump with PCA facilities seem to be equally safe as implanted devices for long-term pain treatment, both in home care and in hospital. However, as with all other invasive methods, long-term intraspinal infusion of opioids and/or bupivacaine is associated with risk, which should be weighed against the advantages and must be explained to the patient. Finally, the methods should be carefully handled and followed-up thoroughly.[1,26]

References

1. World Health Organization. *Cancer Pain Relief*. Geneva: World Health Organization, 1986.
2. Mercadante S. Problems of long-term spinal opioid treatment in advanced cancer patients. *Pain* 1999; 79:1–13.
3. Hogan Q, Haddox JD, Abram S, Weissman D, Taylor M, Janjan N. Epidural opiates and local anesthetics for the management of cancer pain. *Pain* 1991; 46:271–272.
4. Zech DFJ, Grond S, Lynch, Hertel D, Lehman A. Validation of World Health Organization guidelines for cancer pain relief: a 10-year prospective study. *Pain* 1995; 63:65–76.
5. Arnér S, Arnér B. Differential effects of epidural morphine in the treatment of cancer-related pain. *Acta Anaesthesiol Scand* 1985; 29:32–36.
6. Nordberg G, Hansdóttir V, Kvist L, Mellstrand T, Hedner T. Pharmacokinetics of different epidural sites of morphine administration. *Eur J Pharmacol* 1995; 33:499–504.
7. Nordberg G. Pharmacokinetic aspects of spinal morphine analgesia. *Acta Anaesth Scand* 1984; 28:Suppl:1–38.
8. Sjöström S, Tamsen A, Persson P, Hartvig P. Pharmacokinetics of intrathecal morphine and meperidine in humans. *Anesthesiology* 1987; 67:889–895.
9. Sjöström S, Hartvig P, Persson P. Pharmacokinetics of epidural morphine and meperidine in humans. *Anesthesiology* 1987; 67:877–888.
10. Hansdóttir V, Woestenborghs R, Nordberg G. Pharmacokinetics of epidural sufentanil and bupivacaine infusion after thoracotomy. In: *Epidural Sufentanil Analgesia: A Pharmacokinetic and Pharmacodynamic Study in Patients after Thoracotomy*. Academic thesis, Sahlgrenska University Hospital, University of Gothenburg, Sweden, 1995.
11. Nitescu P, Appelgren L, Linder L-E, Sjöberg M, Hultman E, Curelaru I. Epidural vs. intrathecal morphine-bupivacaine: assessment of consecutive treatment in advanced cancer pain. *J Pain Symp Manage* 1990; 5:18–26.
12. Du Pen SL, Karasch ED, Williams A, et al. Chronic epidural bupivacaine-opioid infusion in intractable cancer pain. *Pain* 1992; 49:293–300.
13. Bahar M, Rosen M, Vickers MD. Chronic cannulation of the intradural and extradural space in the rat. *Br J Anaesth* 1984; 56:405–410.

14. Crul BJP, Delhaas EM. Technical complications during long term subarachnoid or epidural administration of morphine in terminally ill cancer patients: a review of 140 cases. *Reg Anesth* 1991; 16:209–213.
15. Sjöberg M, Karlsson P-Å, Nordborg C, et al. Neuropathologic findings after long-term intrathecal infusion of morphine and bupivacaine for pain treatment in cancer patients. *Anesthesiology* 1992; 72:173–196.
16. Coombs DW, Colbum RW, Allen CD, Dero DB, Fratkin JD. Toxicity of chronic spinal analgesia in a canine model: neuropathologic observations with dezocine lactate. *Reg Anesth* 1990; 15:94–102.
17. James HE, Tibbs PA. Diverse clinical applications of percutaneous lumboperitoneal shunts. *Neurosurgery* 1981; 8:39–42.
18. Meir FA, Coombs DW, Saunders LR, Pageau MG. Pathologic anatomy of constant morphine infusion by intraspinal silastic catheter (abstract). *Anesthesiology* 1982; 47:A206.
19. Wageman MFM. Safety of long-term intrathecal administration of morphine or a morphine-bupivacaine mixture in cancer pain patients: a post mortem study. In: *Continuous Intrathecal Administration of Morphine and Bupivacaine for Cancer Pain Control at Home*. Academic Thesis, University of Vrije, Amsterdam, Netherlands, 1995:91–104.
20. Appelgren L, Nordborg C, Sjöberg M, Karlsson P-Å, Nitescu P, Curelaru I. Spinal epidural metastasis: An important cause of "refractory" cancer pain—its implications for intraspinal pain treatment. *J Pain Symp Manage* 1997; 13:25–42.
21. Sjöberg M. *Long-Term Intrathecal Morphine and Bupivacaine in Patients with Refractory Cancer Pain. Clinical, Technical and Neuropathological Aspects*. Academic thesis, Sahlgrenska University Hospital, University of Gothenburg, Sweden, 1994.
22. DuPen SL, Ramsey DH. Compounding local anesthetics and narcotics for epidural analgesia in cancer out-patients. *Anesthesiology* 1988; 69:No3A.
23. Nitescu P, Hultman E, Appelgren L, Linder L-E, Curelaru I. Bacteriology, drug stability and exchange of percutaneous delivery systems and antibacterial filters in long-term intrathecal infusion of opioid drugs and bupivacaine in "refractory pain." *Clin J Pain* 1992; 324–337.
24. Wulf H, Gleim M, Mignant C. The stability of mixtures of morphine hydrochloride, bupivacaine, and clonidine hydrochloride in portable pump reservoirs for the management of chronic pain syndromes. *J Pain Symp Manage* 1994; 9:308–311.
25. Appelgren L, Janson L, Nitescu P, Curelaru I. Continuous intracisternal and high cervical intrathecal bupivacaine analgesia in refractory head and neck pain. *Anesthesiology* 1996; 84:256–272.
26. Nitescu P, Sjöberg M, Appelgren L, Curelaru I. Complications of intrathecal opioids and bupivacaine in treatment of refractory cancer pain. *Clin J Pain* 1995; 11:45–62.
27. Mercadante S. Intrathecal morphine and bupivacaine in advanced cancer pain patients implanted at home. *J Pain Symp Manage* 1994; 9:201–207.
28. Sjöberg M, Appelgren L, Einarsson S, et al. Long-term intrathecal morphine and bupivacaine in refractory cancer pain. I. Results from the first series of 52 patients. *Acta Anaesthesiol Scand* 1991; 35:30–43.
29. Sjöberg M, Nitescu P, Appelgren L, Curelaru I. Long-term intrathecal morphine and bupivacaine in patients with refractory cancer pain. Results from a morphine : bupivacaine regimen of 0.5 : 4.75 mg/ml. *Anesthesiology* 1994; 80:284–297.

30. van Dongen RTM, Crul BJP, de Bock M. Long-term intrathecal infusion of morphine and morphine-bupivacaine mixtures in the treatment of cancer pain: a retrospective analysis of 51 cases. *Pain* 1993; 55:119–123.

31. van Dongen RTM, Crul JPB, van Egmond J, van Ee R. Combined intrathecal morphine-bupivacaine improves pain relief in patients unresponsive to intrathecal morphine; a prospective randomized double-blinded study in 43 cancer patients. pp 87–102. In: *Clinical Effects of Long-Term Intrathecal Morphine/Bupivacaine Administration In Cancer Patients*. Academic thesis, University of Nijmegen. The Netherlands.

32. van Dongen RTM. *Clinical Effects of Long-Term Intrathecal Morphine Versus Morphine/Bupivacaine Administration in Cancer Patients*. Academic thesis, University of Nijmegen, Nijmegen, The Netherlands, 1997.

33. Hurley RJ, Lambert DH. Continuous spinal anesthesia with a microcatheter technique. *Reg Anesth* 1990; 14(Suppl):3.

34. Drasner K, Connoly MT, Reece WM. Continuous spinal anesthesia: use of 28 gauge catheter passed through a 22 gauge needle. *Reg Anesth* 1990; 15(Suppl):34.

35. Hurley RJ, Lambert DH. Continuous spinal anesthesia with a micro catheter technique: preliminary experience. *Anesth Analg* 1990; 70:97–102.

36. Wageman MFM. Long-term intrathecal control of cancer pain comparing morphine/ bupivacaine and morphine/NaCl 0.9%: a prospective, randomized, double-blind study in 72 patients. In: *Continuous Intrathecal Administration of Morphine and Bupivacaine for Cancer Pain Control at Home*. Academic Thesis, University of Vrije, Amsterdam, Netherlands, 1995:53–70.

37. van Dongen RTM, Crul JPB, de Bock M. Efficacy of long-term intrathecal morphine administration. *Pain* 1993; 55:119–123.

38. Gourlay GK, Plummer J, Cherry DA, et al. Comparison of intermittent bolus with continuous infusion of epidural morphine in the treatment of severe cancer pain. *Pain* 1991; 47:135–140.

39. Krames SE, Gershow J, Glassberg A, et al. Continuous infusion of spinally administered narcotics for the relief of pain due to malignant disorders. *Cancer* 1985; 56:696–702.

40. Shohami E, Evron S, Weinstock M, Soffer D, Carmon A. A new animal model for action myoclonus. *Adv Neurol* 1986; 43:545–552.

41. Stillman MJ, Moulin DE, Foley KM. Paradoxical pain following high-dose spinal morphine. *Pain* 1987; 4(Suppl):389.

42. Woolf CJ. Intrathecal morphine for intractable pain secondary to cancer of pelvic organs. *Pain* 1985; 21:99–102.

43. Yaksh TL. Spinal opiate analgesia: characteristics and principles of action. *Pain* 1981; 11:293–346.

44. Berde CH, Sethna NF, Conrad L, Hershenson MB, Shillito J. Subarachnoid bupivacaine analgesia for seven months for a patient with spinal cord tumor. *Anesthesiology* 1990; 72:1094–1096.

45. Krames SE. The chronic intraspinal use of opioid and local anesthetic mixtures for the relief of intractable pain: when all else fails! Guest Editorial. *Pain* 1993; 55:1–4.

46. Sjöberg M. Treatment of cancer pain in home, with special reference to the use of intrathecal morphine and bupivacaine in severe refractory pain. In: van Zundert A, ed. *Scandinavian Perspectives in Regional Anaesthesia and Pain Control*. Proceedings of the ESRA Meeting, Stockholm, 1994.

47. Nitescu P, Appelgren L, Hultman E, Linder L-E, Sjöberg M, Curelaru I. Long-term, open catheterization of the spinal subarachnoid space for continuous infusion of opioid and bupivacaine in patients with "refractory" cancer pain: A technique of catheterization and its problems and complications. *Clin J Pain* 1991; 7:143–161.

48. Nitescu P, Karlsson P-A, Nordborg C, et al. No signs of local neurotoxicity in cancer pain patients treated with long-term subarachnoid infusions of morphine with preservatives (sodium metabisulfite and sodium edetate) and bupivacaine. *Eur J Pain* 1992; 13:76–88.

49. FDA Safety Alert. Cauda equina syndrome associated with the use of small-bore catheters in continuous spinal anesthesia, May 29, 1992.

50. Gentili F, Hudson AR, Hunter D, Kline DG. Nerve injection injury with local anesthetic agents: a light and electron microscopic, fluorescent microscopic, and horseradish peroxidase study. *Neurosurgery* 1980; 6:263–272.

51. Kalichman NM, Powell HC, Myers RR. Pathology of local anesthetic-induced nerve injury. *Acta Neuropathol* 1998; 75:583–589.

52. Kalichman M. Physiologic mechanisms by which local anesthetics may cause injury to nerve and spinal cord. *Reg Anesth* 1993; 18:448–452.

53. Kalichman NM, Powell HC, Myers RR. Quantitative histologic analysis of local anesthetic-induced injury to rat sciatic nerve. *J Pharmacal Exp Ther* 1989; 250:406–413.

54. Kalichman MW, Moorhouse DF, Powell HC, Myers RR. Relative neural toxicity of local anesthetics. *J Neuropathol Exp Neurol* 1993; 52:234–240.

55. Hassenbusch SJ, Stanton-Hicks M, Covington EC, Walsh JG, Guthry DS. Long-term intraspinal infusions of opioids in the treatment of neuropathic pain. *J Pain Symp Manage* 1995; 10:527–543.

56. Pitkanen M, Tuominen M, Rosenberg P, Wahlström T. Technical and light microscopic comparison of four different small-diameter catheters used for continuous spinal anesthesia. *Reg Anesth* 1992; 17:288–291.

57. Rigler M, Drasner K, Krejcie T, et al. Cauda equina syndrome after continuous spinal anesthesia. *Anesth Analg* 1991; 72:275–281.

58. Ross BK, Coda B, Heath CH. Local anesthetic distribution in a spinal model: a possible mechanism of neurologic injury after continuous spinal anesthesia. *Reg Anesth* 1992; 17:69–77.

59. Ready LB, Plumer MH, Haschke RH, Austin E, Sumi SM. Neurotoxicity of intrathecal local anesthetics in rabbits. *Anesthesiology* 1985; 63:364–370.

60. Ravindran RS, Bond VK, Tasch MD, Gupta CD, Luersen TG. Prolonged neural blockade following regional analgesia with 2-chloroprocaine. *Anesth Analg* 1980; 59:446–451.

61. Kroin JS, MacCarthy RJ, Penn RD, Kerns JM, Ivankovich AD. The effect of chronic subarachnoid bupivacaine infusion in dogs. *Anesthesiology* 1987; 66:737–742.

62. Li DF, Bahar M, Cole G, Rosen M. Neurological toxicity of the subarachnoid infusion of bupivacaine, lignocaine or 2-chloroprocaine in the rat. *Br J Anaesth* 1985; 57:424–429.

63. Coombs DW, Fratkin JD, Meier F, et al. Neuropathological lesions and CSF morphine concentrations during chronic continuous intraspinal morphine infusion: A clinical and postmortem study. *Pain* 1985; 22:337–351.

64. Denson DD, Myers JA, Hatrick CT, Pither CP, Coyle DE, Raj PP. The relationship between free bupivacaine concentration and central nervous system toxicity. *Anesthesiology* 1984; 61:A211.

65. Jackson PR, Tucker GT, Woods HF. Altered plasma drug binding in cancer: role of alpha-l-acid glycoprotein and albumin. *Clin Pharmacol Ther* 1982; 32:295–302.

66. Du Pen SL, Peterson DG, Williams A, Bogosian AJ. Infection during chronic epidural catheterization: diagnosis and treatment. *Anesthesiology* 1990; 73:905–909.

67. Myers RR, Kalichman MW, Reisner LS, Powell HC. Neurotoxicity of local anesthetics: altered perineural permeability, edema, and nerve fiber injury. *Anesthesiology* 1986; 64:29–35.

68. Coombs DW. Intraspinal narcotics for intractable cancer pain. In: Abram SE, ed. *Cancer Pain.* Boston: Kluwer Academic Publishers, 1989:77–96.

69. De Jong PC, Kansen PJ. A comparison of epidural catheters with or without subcutaneous injection ports for treatment of cancer pain. *Anesth Analg* 1994; 78:94–100.

70. Plummer JL, Cherry DA, Cousins MJ, Gourlay GK, Onley MM, Evans KHA. Long-term spinal administration of morphine in cancer and non-cancer pain: a retrospective study. *Pain* 1991; 44:215–220.

71. Rauck RL. Long-term intraspinal catheter. In: Abstracts of ASRA seventeenth annual meeting, II 8–23. Tampa Convention Center—Tampa, FL, March 26–29, 1992.

72. De Cicco M, Mativic M, Tarabini Castellani G, et al. Time-dependent efficacy of bacterial filters and infection risk in long-term epidural catheterization. *Anesthesiology* 1995; 82:765–771.

73. Samuelsson H. *Epidural Morphine in Cancer Pain.* Academic thesis, Department of Pharmacology, Sahlgrenska University Hospital, University of Gothenburg, 1993.

17

Diagnosis and Management of Delirium in the Terminally Ill

WILLIAM BREITBART

Delirium is a common and often serious medical complication in the patient with advanced illness. Cognitive disorders, and delirium in particular, have enormous relevance to symptom control and palliative care. Delirium is highly prevalent in cancer and AIDS patients with advanced disease, particularly in the last weeks of life. Depending on the population and assessment methods, prevalence rates range from 25% to 85%.[1–8]

Delirium is one of the most common mental disorders encountered in general hospital practice. Knight and Folstein[9] estimated that 33% of hospitalized medically ill patients have serious cognitive impairments. Massie and co-workers found delirium in 25% of 334 hospitalized cancer patients seen in psychiatric consultation and in 85% (11 of 13) of terminal cancer patients.[6] Pereira and co-workers found the prevalence of cognitive impairment in cancer inpatients to be 44%, and just prior to death, the prevalence rose to 62.1%.[10] Delirium also occurs in up to 51% of postoperative patients.[11,12]

The incidence of delirium is currently increasing, which reflects the growing numbers of elderly, who are particularly susceptible.[13] Studies of elderly patients admitted to medical wards estimate that between 30% and 50% of patients age 70 years or older showed symptoms of delirium at some point during hospitalization.[14–18] Elderly patients who develop delirium during a hospitalization have been estimated to have a 22%–76% chance of dying during that hospitalization.[19]

Delirium is associated with increased morbidity in the terminally ill, causing distress in patients, family members, and staff.[2,20,21] Delirium can interfere dramatically with the recognition and control of other physical and psychological symptoms, such as pain,[22–24] in later stages of illness. Often a pre-terminal event, delirium is a sign of significant physiologic disturbance, usually involving multiple medical etiologies, including infection, organ failure, medication side effects (including opioids), as well as extremely rare paraneoplastic syndromes.[8,25–28] Lawlor and colleagues[29] recently reported on their experience in the management of delirium in advanced cancer patients in a palliative care unit. While 42% of patients had delirium upon admission to their palliative care unit, terminal delirium occurred in 88% of the deaths.

Unfortunately, delirium is often under-recognized or misdiagnosed, and inappropriately treated or untreated in terminally ill patients. Impediments to progress in the recognition and treatment of delirium include confusion regarding terminology and lack of consistency in utilizing diagnostic classification systems. In addition, the signs and symptoms of delirium can be diverse and are sometimes mistaken for other psychiatric disorders, such as mood or anxiety disorders. Practitioners caring for patients with life threatening illnesses must be able to diagnose delirium accurately, undertake appropriate assessment of etiologies, and be knowledgeable about the benefits and risks of the pharmacologic and non-pharmacologic interventions currently available in managing delirium among the terminally ill.

Diagnosing Delirium

Clinical features

The clinical features of delirium are quite numerous and include a variety of neuropsychiatric symptoms that are also common to other psychiatric disorders such as depression, dementia, and psychosis.[30] Clinical features of delirium include prodromal symptoms (restlessness, anxiety, sleep disturbance, and irritability); rapidly fluctuating course; reduced attention (easily distractible); altered arousal; increased or decreased psychomotor activity; disturbance of sleep-wake cycle; affective symptoms (emotional lability, sadness, anger, and euphoria); altered perceptions (misperceptions, illusions, delusions [poorly formed], and hallucinations); disorganized thinking and incoherent speech; disorientation to time, place, or person; and memory impairment (cannot register new material). Neurologic abnormalities can also be present during delirium, including cortical abnormalities (dysgraphia, constructional apraxia, dysnomic aphasia); motor abnormalities (tremor, asterixis, myoclonus, and reflex and tone changes); and electroencephalogram (EEG) abnormalities (usually global slowing). It is this protean nature of delirious symptoms, the variability and fluctuation of clinical findings, and the unclear and often contradictory definitions of the syndrome that have made delirium so difficult to diagnose and treat.

Table 17.1 lists the DSM-IV[31] criteria for delirium. These criteria indicate that the essential defining features of delirium have shifted from the extensive list of typical symptoms and abnormalities described above to a focus on the two essential concepts of disordered attention (arousal) and cognition (while continuing to recognize the importance of acute onset and organic etiology). Associ-

Table 17.1. DSM-IV criteria for delirium

Delirium because of a general medical condition:

Disturbance of consciousness (that is, reduced clarity of awareness of the environment) with
  reduced ability to focus, sustain, or shift attention.

Change in cognition (such as memory deficit, disorientation, language disturbance, or perceptual
  disturbance) that is not better accounted for by a pre-existing, established, or evolving
  dementia.

The disturbance develops over a short period of time (usually hours to days) and tends to fluctuate
  during the course of the day.

There is evidence from the history, physical examination, or laboratory findings of a general
  medical condition judged to be etiologically related to the disturbance.

---

ated phenomena such as psychomotor behavioral changes, perceptual disturbances, hallucinations, or delusions are no longer viewed as essential to the diagnosis of delirium.

Delirium is now conceptualized primarily as a disorder of arousal and
cognition[32] in contrast to dementia, which is a disorder of cognition (with no
arousal disturbance). It is this disorder of the arousal system, with consequent disturbances in level of consciousness and attention, which is pathogno-
monic of delirium and is, in part, the basis for classifying delirium into several
subtypes.

Subtypes of delirium

Three clinical subtypes of delirium, based on arousal disturbance and psychomotor behavior, have been described. These subtypes included the *hyperactive* (hyperarousal, hyperalert, or agitated) subtype, the *hypoactive* (hypoarousal,
hypoalert, or lethargic) subtype, and a *mixed* subtype with alternating features
of hyperactive and hypoactive delirium.[8,33] Researchers[31] suggest (see Table 17.2)
that the hyperactive form is most often characterized by hallucinations, delusions, agitation, and disorientation, whereas the hypoactive form is characterized
by confusion and sedation, but is rarely accompanied by hallucinations, delusions, or illusions. In addition, there is evidence suggesting that specific delirium
subtypes may be related to specific etiologies of delirium, may have unique
pathophysiologies, and may respond differently to treatment.[34,35] It is estimated
that approximately two-thirds of deliria are either of the hypoactive or mixed
subtype; hence, the prototypically agitated delirious patient most familiar to clinicians is actually a minority of the deliria that occur.[33,34]

Differential diagnosis

Many of the clinical features and symptoms of delirium can also be associated
with other psychiatric disorders, such as depression, mania, psychosis, and

Table 17.2. Subtypes of delirium

	Hyperactive	*Hypoactive*	*Mixed*
Type	Hyperalert Agitated Hyperarousal	Hypoalert Lethargic Hypoarousal	Features of both hyperactive and hypoactive
Symptoms	Hallucinations Delusions Agitation	Sleepy Withdrawn Slowed	
Examples	Withdrawal syndromes (benzodiazepines, alcohol)	Encephalopathies (hepatic, metabolic) Benzodiazepine intoxication	
Pathophysiology	Elevated or normal cerebral metabolism EEG: fast or normal	Decreased global cerebral metabolism EEG: Diffuse slowing	

dementia. For instance, delirious patients may exhibit emotional (mood) disturbances such as anxiety, fear, depression, irritability, anger, euphoria, apathy, and mood lability. Delirium, particularly the hypoactive subtype, is often initially misdiagnosed as depression. Symptoms of major depression, including altered level of activity (hypoactivity), insomnia, reduced ability to concentrate, depressed mood, and even suicidal ideation, can overlap with symptoms of delirium, making accurate diagnosis more difficult.

In distinguishing delirium from depression, particularly in the context of advanced disease, an evaluation of the onset and temporal sequencing of depressive and cognitive symptoms is particularly helpful. Importantly, the degree of cognitive impairment in delirium is much more severe and pervasive than in depression, and has a more abrupt temporal onset. Also, the characteristic disturbance in arousal or consciousness is present in delirium but, usually is not a feature of depression.

A manic episode also may share some features of delirium, particularly a hyperactive or mixed subtype of delirium. Again, the temporal onset and course of symptoms, the presence of a disturbance of consciousness (arousal) as well as of cognition, and the identification of a presumed medical etiology for delirium are helpful in differentiating these disorders.

Delirium that is characterized by vivid hallucinations and delusions must be distinguished from a variety of psychotic disorders. In delirium, such psychotic symptoms occur in the context of a disturbance in consciousness or arousal, as well as memory impairment and disorientation, which is not the case in other psychotic disorders. Delusions in delirium tend to be poorly organized and of abrupt onset, and hallucinations are predominantly visual or tactile rather than auditory as is typical of schizophrenia. Finally, the development of these psychotic symptoms in the context of advanced medical illness makes delirium a more likely diagnosis.

The most common differential diagnostic issue is whether the patient has delirium, or dementia, or a delirium superimposed upon a pre-existing dementia. Both delirium and dementia are cognitive impairment disorders and so share such common clinical features as impaired memory, thinking, judgment, and disorientation. The patient with dementia is alert and does not have the disturbance of consciousness or arousal that is characteristic of delirium. The temporal onset of symptoms in dementia is more subacute and chronically progressive, and one's sleep-wake cycle seems less impaired. Most prominent in dementia are difficulties in short- and long-term memory, impaired judgment, and abstract thinking, as well as disturbed higher cortical functions (such as aphasia and apraxia).

Occasionally one will encounter delirium superimposed on an underlying dementia such as in the case of an elderly patient, an AIDS patient, or a patient with a paraneoplastic syndrome. Delirium, in contrast with dementia, is conceptualized as a reversible process. Reversibility of the process of delirium is often possible even in the patient with advanced illness; however it may not be reversible in the last 24 to 48 hours of life. This is most likely because irreversible processes such as multiple organ failure are occurring in the final hours of life. Delirium occurring in these last days of life is sometimes referred to as *terminal delirium* in the palliative care literature.

Delirium screening/diagnostic scales

A number of scales or instruments have been developed that can aid the clinician in rapidly screening for cognitive impairment disorders (dementia or delirium), or in establishing a diagnosis of delirium[36–44] (see Table 17.3). Such scales have been described and their relative strengths and weaknesses reviewed elsewhere.[35,45] Perhaps most helpful to clinicians are the Mini-Mental State Examination (a cognitive impairment screening tool) and several delirium diagnostic or rating scales, including the Delirium Rating Scale, the Delirium Rating Scale—Revised 98, The Confusion Assessment Method, the Abbreviated Cognitive Test for Delirium, and the Memorial Delirium Assessment Scale. These tools are described briefly below.

Mini-Mental State Examination

The Mini-Mental State Examination (MMSE)[43] is useful in screening for cognitive failure, but does not distinguish between delirium and dementia. The MMSE provides a quantitative assessment of the cognitive performance and capacity of a patient, and is a measure of severity of cognitive impairment. It is also most sensitive to cortical dementias, such as Alzheimer's disease, and less sensitive in detecting subcortical deficits such as those found in AIDS dementia. The Mini-Mental State Exam assesses five general cognitive areas including orientation, registration, attention and calculation, recall, and

Table 17.3. Assessment methods for delirium in cancer patients

---

Diagnostic classification systems
  DSM-IV
  ICD-9, ICD-10
Diagnostic interviews and instruments
  Delirium Symptom Interview[4] (DSI)
  Confusion Assessment Method[35] (CAM)
Delirium rating scales
  Delirium Rating Scale[76] (DRS)
  Delirium Rating Scale—Revised—98 (DRS-R-98)[46]
  Confusion Rating Scale[88] (CRS)
  Saskatoon Delirium Checklist[50] (SDC)
  Memorial Delirium Assessment Scale[13] (MDAS)
  Abbreviated Cognitive Test for Delirium (CTD)[48]
Cognitive impairment screening instruments
  Mini-Mental State Exam[29] (MMSE)
  Short Portable Mental Status Questionnaire[88] (SPMSQ)
  Cognitive Capacity Screening Examination[36] (CCSE)
  Blessed Orientation Memory Concentration Test[38] (BOMC)

---

language. Although a score of 23 or less has generally been considered the cutoff score for cognitive impairment, a three-tiered system is now often utilized suggesting that a score of 24–30: no impairment; 18–23: mild impairment; and 0–17: severe impairment.

Delirium Rating Scale
The Delirium Rating Scale (DRS), developed by Trzepacz et al.[42] is a 10-item clinician-rated symptom rating scale for diagnosing delirium. The scale is based on DSM-III-R diagnostic criteria for delirium and is designed to be used by the clinician to identify delirium, and distinguish it reliably from dementia or other neuropsychiatric disorders. Each item is scored by choosing one best rating and carries a numerical weight chosen to distinguish the phenomenological characteristic of delirium. A score of 12 or greater is diagnostic of delirium.

Delirium Rating Scale—Revised 98
The Delirium Rating Scale—Revised 98 (DRS-R-98) is a revision of the Delirium Rating Scale (DRS). The DRS-R-98 has 13 severity and 3 diagnostic items with descriptive anchors for each rating level. It includes more items than the DRS and was designed for phenomenological and treatment research, though it can be used clinically. The DRS-R-98 is a valid, sensitive, and reliable instrument for rating delirium severity. It has advantages over the original DRS for repeated measures and phenomenological studies because of its enhanced breadth of symptoms and separation into severity and diagnostic subscales.[46]

Confusion Assessment Method

The Confusion Assessment Method (CAM)[47] is a 9-item delirium diagnostic scale utilizing the DSM-III-R criteria for delirium, which can be administered rather quickly by a trained clinician. A unique and helpful feature of the CAM is that it also can be given using a simplified diagnostic algorithm, which includes only 4-items of the CAM. This algorithm is designed for rapid identification of delirium by non-psychiatrists. The 4-item algorithm requires the presence of (1) acute onset and fluctuating course, (2) inattention, and either (3) disorganized thinking, or (4) altered level of consciousness.

Abbreviated Cognitive Test for Delirium

The Abbreviated Cognitive Test for Delirium (CTD)[48] was recently developed as a tool to help identify delirium in patients in the intensive care unit setting who have limited ability to communicate verbally. This brief tool utilizes visualization span and recognition memory for pictures as 2 of 9 content scores that produces a total score that reliably identifies delirium and can discriminate delirium from dementia, depression, and schizophrenia.

Memorial Delirium Assessment Scale

The Memorial Delirium Assessment Scale (MDAS) is a 10-item delirium assessment tool, validated among hospitalized inpatients with advanced cancer and AIDS.[37] The MDAS is both a good delirium diagnostic screening tool as well as a reliable tool for assessing delirium severity among patients with advanced disease. A cut-off score of 13 is diagnostic of delirium. The MDAS has advantages over other delirium tools in that it is both a diagnostic and a severity measure, and is ideal for repeated assessments and for use in treatment intervention trials. Recently, Lawlor and colleagues[49] examined the clinical utility and validation of the MDAS in a population of advanced cancer patients in a palliative care unit. These investigators found the MDAS to be useful in this population, and found that a cutoff score of 7 out of 30 yielded the highest sensitivity (98%) and specificity (76%) for a delirium diagnosis in this palliative care population.

Management of Delirium in the Terminally Ill

The standard approach to managing delirium in the medically ill, and even in those with advanced disease, includes a search for underlying causes, correction of those factors, and management of the symptoms of delirium.[37,50,51] The desired and often achievable outcome is a patient who is awake, alert, calm, cognitively intact, not psychotic, and communicating coherently with family and staff. In the terminally ill patient who develops delirium in the last days of life (terminal delirium), the management of delirium is in fact unique, presenting a number of dilemmas, and the desired clinical outcome may be significantly altered by the dying process.

Assessment of etiologies of delirium

When confronted with a delirium in the terminally ill or dying patient, a differential diagnosis should always be formulated as to the likely etiology(ies). There is an ongoing debate as to the appropriate extent of diagnostic evaluation that should be pursued in a dying patient with a terminal delirium.[2,4,21,52] Most palliative care clinicians would undertake diagnostic studies only when a clinically suspected etiology can be identified easily, with minimal use of invasive procedures, and treated effectively with simple, interventions that carry minimal burden or risk of causing further distress. Diagnostic work-up in pursuit of an etiology for delirium may be limited by either practical constraints such as the setting (home, hospice) or the focus on patient comfort, so that unpleasant or painful diagnostics may be avoided.

Most often, the etiology of terminal delirium is multifactoral or not identifiable. Bruera et al.[2] report that an etiology is discovered in less than 50% of terminally ill patients with delirium. When a distinct cause is found for delirium in the terminally ill, it is often irreversible or difficult to treat.

Studies in patients with earlier stages of advanced cancer have demonstrated the potential utility of a thorough diagnostic assessment.[2,53] When such diagnostic information is available, specific therapy may be able to reverse delirium. One study found that 68% of delirious cancer patients could be improved, despite a 30-day mortality of 31%.[45] Another found that one-third of the episodes of cognitive failure improved following evaluation that yielded a cause for these episodes in 43%.[2]

In a recent prospective study of delirium in patients on a palliative care unit,[2] investigators reported that the etiology of delirium was multifactorial in the great majority of cases. Even though delirium occurred in 88% of dying patients in the last week of life, delirium was reversible in approximately 50% of episodes. Causes of delirium that were most associated with reversibility included dehydration and psychoactive or opioid medications. Hypoxic and metabolic encephalopathy were less likely to be reversed in terminal delirium.

The diagnostic work-up should include an assessment of potentially reversible causes of delirium. A physical examination should assess for evidence of sepsis, dehydration, or major organ failure. Medications that could contribute to delirium should be reviewed. A screen of laboratory parameters will allow assessment of the possible role of metabolic abnormalities, such as hypercalcemia, and other problems, such as hypoxia or disseminated intravascular coagulation. Imaging studies of the brain and assessment of the cerebrospinal fluid may be appropriate in some instances.

Delirium can have multiple potential etiologies. In patients with advanced cancer, for instance, delirium can be because of the direct effects of cancer on the central nervous system (CNS), or to indirect CNS effects of the disease or treatments (medications, electrolyte imbalance, failure of a vital organ or system, infection, vascular complications, and preexisting cognitive impairment or dementia).[2] Given the large numbers of drugs cancer patients require, and the fragile state of their physiologic functioning, even routinely ordered hypnotics are enough to tip patients over into a delirium. Opioid analgesics such as levorphanol, morphine sulfate, and meperidine, are common causes of confusional states, particularly in the elderly and terminally ill. Chemotherapeutic agents known to cause delirium include methotrexate, fluorouracil, vincristine, vinblastine, bleomycin, BCNU, cis-platinum, asparaginase, procarbazine, and the glucocorticosteroids.[25,54-58] Except for the steroids, most patients receiving these agents will not develop prominent CNS effects.

The spectrum of mental disturbances related to steroids includes minor mood lability, affective disorders (mania or depression), cognitive impairment (reversible dementia), and delirium (steroid psychosis). The incidence of these disorders ranges from 3% to 57% in non-cancer populations, and they occur most commonly at higher doses. Symptoms usually develop within the first 2 weeks of treatment, but in fact can occur at any time, on any dose, even during the tapering phase.[53] These disorders are often rapidly reversible upon dose reduction or discontinuation.[53]

Non-pharmacologic interventions

In addition to seeking out and potentially correcting underlying causes for delirium, symptomatic and supportive therapies are important.[3,4,21,37,52] In the dying patient, these interventions may be the only steps taken. Fluid and electrolyte balance, nutrition, vitamins, measures to help reduce anxiety and disorientation, and interactions with and education of family members may be useful. Measures to help reduce anxiety and disorientation (i.e., structure and familiarity) may include a quiet, well-lit room with familiar objects, a visible clock or calendar, and the presence of family. Judicious use of physical restraints, along with one-to-one nursing observation may also be necessary and useful.

Recently, Inouye and colleagues[59] reported on a successful multicomponent intervention program to prevent delirium in hospitalized older patients. This program focuses on a set of risk factors that were highly predictive of delirium in the elderly, including: pre-existing cognitive impairment, visual impairment, hearing impairment, sleep deprivation, immobility, dehydration, and severe illness. Interventions directed at constant reorientation, correction of hearing and visual impairment, reversal of dehydration and early mobilization appeared to significantly reduce the number and duration of episodes of delirium in hospitalized older patients. The applicability of these interventions and the likelihood that they would prevent delirium in the terminally ill, particularly in the last days of life, is likely minimal.

Table 17.4. Medications for managing delirium in terminally ill patients

Generic name	Approximate daily dosage Range route
Neuroleptics	
Haloperidol	0.5–5 mg every 2–12 hour, PO, IV, SC, IM
Thiorodazine	10–75 mg every 4–8 hour PO
Chlorpromazine	12.5–50 mg every 4–12 hour PO, IV, IM
Molindone	10–50 mg every 8–12 hour PO
Risperidone	1–3 mg every 12 hour PO
Olanzapine	2.5–10 mg every 12 hour PO
Methotrimeprazine	12.5–50 mg every 4–8 hour IV, SC, PO
Benzodiazepines	
Lorazepam	0.5–20 mg every 1–4 hour PO, IV, IM
Midazolam	30–100 mg every 24 hour IV, SC
Anesthetics	
Propofol	10–70 mg every hour IV, titrated up to 200–400 mg/hr

PO, Perorum; IV, Intravenously; SC, Subcutaneously; IM, Intramuscularly.

Pharmacologic interventions in delirium

Supportive techniques alone are often not effective in controlling the symptoms of delirium, and symptomatic treatment with neuroleptics or sedative medications are necessary (Table 17.4). Neuroleptic drugs (dopamine-blocking drugs) such as haloperidol, are utilized frequently as antiemetics in the medical setting, but only 0.5%–2% of hospitalized cancer patients, for instance, receive haloperidol for the management of the symptoms of delirium.[60,61] In terminally ill populations, as many as 17% receive an antipsychotic for agitation or psychological distress, despite an estimated prevalence of delirium ranging from 25% in the hospitalized cancer patient to 85% in the terminally ill.[62,63]

Haloperidol, a neuroleptic drug that is a potent dopamine blocker, is often the drug of choice in the treatment of delirium in patients with advanced disease.[7,37,54,64–70] Haloperidol in low doses, 1–3 mg/day, is usually effective in targeting agitation, paranoia, and fear. Typically 0.5–1.0 mg haloperidol [perorum (PO), intravenously (IV), intramuscularly (IM), subcutaneously (SC)] is administered, with repeat doses every 45–60 minutes titrated against target symptoms.[6,71,72] Parenteral doses are approximately twice as potent as oral doses. An intravenous route can facilitate rapid onset of medication effects. If intravenous access is unavailable, one can start with intramuscular or subcutaneous administration and switch to the oral route when possible. Although the majority of delirious patients can be managed with oral haloperidol, the subcutaneous route is utilized by many palliative care practitioners.[66,73]

Low doses of neuroleptic medication are usually sufficient in treating delirium in elderly terminally ill patients. In general, doses need not exceed 20 mg of haloperidol in a 24-hour period; however, there are those that advocate high doses (up to 250 mg/24 hour of haloperidol usually intravenously) in selected cases.[66]

A common strategy in the management of symptoms related to delirium is to add parenteral lorazepam to a regimen of haloperidol.[51,54,64,71,73,74] Lorazepam (0.5–1.0 mg q 1–2 hour PO or IV), along with haloperidol may be more effective in rapidly sedating the agitated delirious patient, and may help minimize extrapyramidal side effects associated with haloperidol.[75] In a double-blind, randomized comparison trial of haloperidol versus chlorpromazine versus lorazepam, Breitbart and colleagues demonstrated that lorazepam alone, in doses up to 8 mg in a 12 hour period, was ineffective in the treatment of delirium and in fact contributed to worsening delirium and cognitive impairment.[1] Both neuroleptic drugs however, in low doses (approximately 2 mg of haloperidol equivalent/per 24 hours), were highly effective in controlling the symptoms of delirium (dramatic improvement in DRS scores) and improving cognitive function (dramatic improvement in MMSE scores). In addition, both haloperidol and chlorpromazine were demonstrated to significantly improve the symptoms of delirium in both the hypoactive as well as the hyperactive subtypes of delirium.[76]

Methotrimeprazine, a phenothiazine neuroleptic with properties similar to chlorpromazine is often utilized parenterally (intravenously or by subcutaneous infusion) to control confusion and agitation in terminal delirium.[77] Dosages range from 12.5 mg to 50 mg every 4–8 hours, up to 300 mg per 24 hours for most patients. For the elderly, doses at the lower end of the range are preferable. Hypotension and excessive sedation are potential limitations of this drug. Methotrimeprazine has the advantage of also being an analgesic.[76]

Several new antipsychotic agents with less or more specific dopamine-blocking effects (less risk of extrapyramidal side effects or trade-off dyskinesia) are now available. These include such agents as clozaril, risperidone, and olanzapine.[26,78] Risperidone has been useful in the treatment of dementia and psychosis in AIDS patients at doses of 1–6 mg per day, suggesting safe use in patients with delirium.[69] There are a limited number of published studies of the use of these agents in the treatment of delirium.[79–81] Many palliative care clinicians are using risperidone in low doses (e.g., 0.5–1.0 mg twice a day, orally) or olanzapine (2.5–20 mg/day in divided doses) in the management of delirium in terminally ill patients, particularly in those who have a demonstrated intolerance to the extrapyramidal side effects of the classic neuroleptics.[82] Currently, a limitation on the use of these new agents is the lack of availability of these agents in parenteral formulations. Figure 17.1 illustrates an algorithm that has been developed for use by the Memorial Sloan-Kettering Cancer Center Psychiatry Service, for the management of delirium in hospitalized cancer patients.

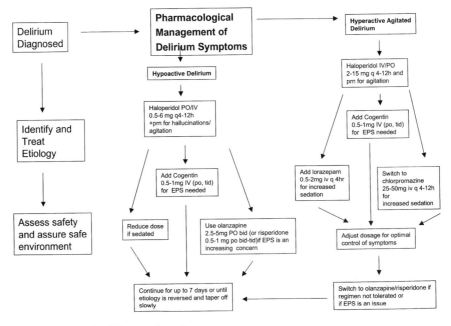

Figure 17.1. The delirium algorithm.

While neuroleptic drugs such as haloperidol are most effective in diminishing agitation, clearing the sensorium and improving cognition in the delirious patient, this is not always possible in a delirium that complicates the last days of life. Processes causing delirium may be ongoing and irreversible during the active dying phase. Ventafridda et al.[19] and Fainsinger et al.[24] have reported that a significant group (10%–20%) of terminally ill patients experience delirium that can only be controlled by sedation to the point of a significantly decreased level of consciousness. Lawlor and colleagues[29] report that at least 50% of terminal delirium is reversible. The goal of treatment with such agents as midazolam, propofol, and to some extent methotrimeprazine, is quiet sedation only. Midazolam, given by subcutaneous or intravenous infusion in doses ranging from 30 to 100 mg/24 hours can be used to control agitation related to delirium in the terminal stages.[83,84] Propofol, a short-acting anesthetic agent, has also begun to be utilized primarily as a sedating agent for the control of agitated patients with terminal delirium. In several case reports of propofol's use in terminal care, an intravenous loading dose of 20 mg of propofol was followed by a continuous infusion of propofol with initial doses ranging from 10 mg/hour to 70 mg/hour, and with titration of doses up to as high as 400 mg/hour over a period of hours to days in severely agitated patients.[85,86] Propofol has an advantage over midazolam in that the level of sedation is more easily controlled and recovery is rapid upon decreasing the rate of infusion.[84]

Controversies in the management of terminal delirium

Several aspects of the use of neuroleptics and other pharmacologic agents in the management of delirium in the dying patient remain controversial. Some have argued that pharmacologic interventions with neuroleptics or benzodiazepines are inappropriate in the dying patient. Delirium is viewed by some as a natural part of the dying process that should not be altered. In particular, there are clinicians who care for the dying and view hallucinations and delusions that involve dead relatives communicating with, or in fact welcoming dying patients to heaven, as an important element in the transition from life to death. Clearly, there are many patients who experience hallucinations and delusions during delirium that are pleasant and in fact comforting, and many clinicians question the appropriateness of intervening pharmacologically in such instances.

Another concern that is often raised is that these patients are so close to death that aggressive treatment is unnecessary. Parenteral neuroleptics or sedatives may be mistakenly avoided because of exaggerated fears that they might hasten death through hypotension or respiratory depression. Some clinicians are unnecessarily pessimistic about the possible results of neuroleptic treatment for delirium. They argue that since the underlying pathophysiologic process often continues unabated (such as hepatic or renal failure), no improvement can be expected in the patient's mental status. There is concern that neuroleptics or sedatives may worsen a delirium by making the patient more confused or sedated.

Clinical experience in managing delirium in dying patients suggests that the use of neuroleptics in the management of agitation, paranoia, hallucinations, and altered sensorium is safe, effective, and often quite appropriate.[75] Management of delirium on a case-by-case basis seems wisest. The agitated, delirious dying patient should probably be given neuroleptics to help restore calm. A wait-and-see approach, prior to using neuroleptics, may be appropriate with some patients who have a lethargic, or somnolent presentation of delirium, or those who are having frankly pleasant or comforting hallucinations. Such a wait-and-see approach must however be tempered by the knowledge that a lethargic or hypoactive delirium may very quickly and unexpectedly become an agitated or hyperactive delirium that can threaten the serenity and safety of the patient, family, and staff. An additional rationale for intervening pharmacologically with patients who have a lethargic or hypoactive delirium is recent evidence that neuroleptics (i.e., haloperidol, chlorpromazine) are effective in controlling the symptoms of delirium in both hyperactive as well as hypoactive subtypes of delirium.[1] In fact neuroleptics improved both the arousal disturbance, as well as cognitive functioning in patients with hypoactive delirium. Also, some clinicians suggest that hypoactive delirium may respond to psychostimulants or combinations of neuroleptics and stimulants.[27] Similarly, hallucinations and delusions during a delirium that are pleasant and comforting can quickly become menacing and terrifying. It is important to remember that by their nature, the symptoms of delirium are unstable, and fluctuate over time.

Finally, perhaps the most challenging of clinical problems is management of the dying patient with a terminal delirium that is unresponsive to standard neuroleptic interventions (the 10%–20% of patients described by Ventafridda et al.[19] and Fainsinger et al.[87]), whose symptoms can only be controlled by sedation to the point of a significantly decreased level of consciousness. Before undertaking interventions, such as midazolam or propofol infusions, where the best achievable goal is a calm, comfortable, but sedated and unresponsive patient, the clinician must first take several steps. The clinician must have a discussion with the family (and the patient if there are lucid moments when the patient appears to have capacity), eliciting their concerns and wishes for the type of care that can best honor their desire to provide comfort and symptom control during the dying process. The clinician should describe the optimal achievable goals of therapy as they currently exist. Family members should be informed that the goal of sedation is to provide comfort and symptom control, and not to hasten death. They should also be told to anticipate that sedation may result in a premature sense of loss, and that they may feel their loved one is in some sort of limbo state, not yet dead, but yet no longer alive in the vital sense. The distress and confusion that family members can experience during such a period can be ameliorated by including the family in the decision-making and emphasizing the shared goals of care. Sedation in such patients is not always complete or irreversible; some patients have periods of wakefulness despite sedation, and many clinicians will periodically lighten sedation to reassess the patient's condition. Ultimately, the clinician must always keep in mind the goals of care and communicate these goals to the staff, patients, and family members. The clinician must weigh each of the issues outlined above in making decisions on how to best manage the dying patient who presents with delirium in a manner that preserves and respects the dignity and values of that individual and family.

Several interesting clinical questions in this area exist, and more research could helpfully inform clinical management. Must we always treat delirium in the terminally ill or dying patient? What are appropriate goals for treatment? What is the impact of delirium on patients, family, staff? What are effective pharmacologic and non-pharmacologic interventions?

Summary

The clinician caring for patients with life threatening illnesses is likely to encounter delirium as a common major psychiatric complication of advancing illness, particularly in the elderly and during the last weeks of life when up to 85% of patients may develop a delirium. Proper assessment, diagnosis, and management are important in minimizing morbidity and improving quality of life.

Acknowledgments

Dr. Breitbart's work is supported by grants from the Faculty Scholar's Program—Open Society Institute Project on Death in America, and the Lucy and Henry Moses Foundation.

References

1. Breitbart W, Marotta R, Platt M, et al. A double-blind trial of Haloperidol, Chlorpromazine, and Lorazepan in the treatment of delirium in hospitalized AIDS patients. *Am J Psychiatry* 1996:231–237.
2. Bruera E, Miller MJ, McCallion J, et al. Cognitive failure in patients with terminal cancer: a prospective study. *J Pain Symp Manage* 1992; 7:192–195.
3. Fainsinger R, Young C. Cognitive failure in a terminally ill patient. *J Pain Symp Manage* 1991:492–494.
4. Leipzig R, Goodman H, Gray G, et al. Reversible narcotic associated mental status impairment in patients with metastatic cancer. *Pharmacology* 1987; 35:47–54.
5. Levine PM, Silberfarb P, Lipowski ZJ. Mental disorders in cancer patients. *Cancer* 1978; 42:1385–1391.
6. Massie MJ, Holland J, Glass E. Delirium in terminally ill cancer patients. *Am J Psychiatry* 1983; 140:1048–1050.
7. Murray GB. Confusion, delirium, and dementia. In: Hackett TP, Cassem NH, eds. *Massachusetts General Hospital Handbook of General Hospital Psychiatry* (2nd ed.). Littleton, Massachusetts: PSG Publishing Company, 1987:84–115.
8. Posner JB. Delirium and exogenous metabolic brain disease. In: Beeson PB, McDermott W, Wyngaarden JB, eds. *Cecil Textbook of Medicine*. Philadelphia: W.B. Saunders, 1979:644–651.
9. Knight EB, Folstein MF. Unsuspected emotional and cognitive disturbance in medical patients. *Ann Intern Med* 1977; 87:723–724.
10. Pereira J, Hanson J, Bruera E. The frequency and clinical course of cognitive impairment in patients with terminal cancer. *Cancer* 1997:835–841.
11. Lipowski ZJ. *Delirium: Acute Confusional States*. New York: Oxford, 1990.
12. Tune LE. Post-operative delirium. Int Psychogeriatr 1991; 3:325–332.
13. Lipowski ZJ. Transient cognitive disorders (delirium, acute confusional states) in the elderly. *Am J Psychiatry* 1983; 140:1426–1436.
14. Gillick MR, Serrel NA, Gillick LS. Adverse consequences of hospitalization in the elderly. *Soc Sci Med* 1982; 16:1033–1038.
15. Warsaw GA, Moore J, Friedman SW, et al. Functional disability in the hospitalized elderly. *JAMA* 1982; 248:847–850.
16. Berman K, Eastham EJ. Psychogeriatric ascertainment and assessment for treatment in an acute medical ward setting. *Aging* 1974; 3:174–188.

17. Seymour DJ, Henschke PJ, Cape RDT, et al. Acute confusional states and dementia in the elderly: the role of dehydration/volume depletion, physical illness and age. *Aging* 1980; 9:137–146.

18. Hodkinson HM. Mental impairment in the elderly. *J R Coll Physicians Lond* 1973; 7:305–317.

19. Varsamis J, Zuchowski T, Maini KK. Survival rates and causes of death in geriatric psychiatric patients: A six year follow-up study. *Can Psychiatr Assoc J* 1972; 17:17–22.

20. Stiefel F, Holland J. Delirium in cancer patients. *Int Psychogeriatr* 1991; 3:333–336.

21. Trzepacz PT, Teague GB, Lipowski ZJ. Delirium and other organic mental disorders in a general hospital. *Gen Hosp Psychiatry* 1985; 7:101–106.

22. Bruera E, Fainsinger R, Miller MJ, Kuehn N. The assessment of pain intensity in patients with cognitive failure: a preliminary report. *J Pain Symp Manage* 1992; 7:267–270.

23. Coyle N, Breitbart W, Weaver S, Portenoy R. Delirium as a contributing factor to "Crescendo" pain: three case reports. *J Pain Symp Manage* 1994; 9:44–47.

24. Fainsinger R, MacEachern T, Hanson J, et al. Symptom control during the last week of life in a palliative care unit. *J Palliat Care* 1991; 7:5–11.

25. Bruera E, Macmillan K, Hanson J, MacDonald RN. The cognitive effects of the administration of narcotic analgesics in patients with cancer pain. *Pain* 1989; 39:13–16.

26. Silberfarb PM. Chemotherapy and cognitive defects in cancer patients. *Annu Rev Med* 1983; 34:35–46.

27. Stiefel F, Breitbart WS, Holland JC. Corticosteroids in cancer: Neuropsychiatric complications. *Cancer Invest* 1989; 7:479–491.

28. Stiefel F, Fainsinger R, Bruera E. Acute confusional states in patients with advanced cancer. *J Pain Symp Manage* 1992; 7:94–98.

29. Lawlor PG, Gagnon B, Mancini IL, Pereira JL, Hanson S, Suarez-Almazor ME, Bruera ED. The occurrence, causes and outcomes of delirium in advanced cancer patients: a prospective study. *Arch Intern Med* 2000; 160:786–794.

30. Wise MG, Brandt GT. Delirium. In: Yudofsky SC, Hales RE, eds. *Textbook of Neuropsychiatry*, 2nd ed. Washington, DC. American Psychiatric, 1992.

31. American Psychiatric Association. *Diagnostic and Statistical Manual of Mental Disorders*, Fourth Edition, Washington, D.C., American Psychiatric Association, 1994.

32. Ross CA. CNS arousal systems: possible role in delirium. *Int Psychogeriatr* 1991; 3:353–371.

33. Lipowski ZJ. *Delirium: Acute Brain Failure in Man*. Springfield, IL. Charles C Thomas, 1980.

34. Breitbart W, Bruera E, Chochinov H, Lynch M. Neuropsychiatric Syndromes and Psychological Symptoms in Patients with advanced cancer. *J Pain Symp Manage* 1995; 10:131–141.

35. Ross CA, Peyser CE, Shapiro I, Folstein MF. Delirium: Phenomenologic and etiologic subtypes. *Int Psychogeriatr* 1991; 3:135–147.

36. Albert MS, Levkoff SE, Reilly C, et al. The delirium symptom interview: an interview for the detection of delirium symptoms in hospitalized patients. *J Geriatr Psychiatry Neurol* 1991; 5:14–21.

37. Breitbart W, Rosenfeld B, Roth A, et al. The Memorial Delirium Assessment Scale. *J Pain Symp Manage* 1997; 13:128–137.
38. Folstein MF, Folstein SE, McHugh PR. "Mini-mental status:" A practical method for grading the cognitive state of patients for clinicians. *J Psychiatr Res* 1975; 12:189–198.
39. Jacobs JC, Bernhard MR, Delgado A, Strain JJ. Screening for organic mental syndromes in the medically ill. *Ann Int Med* 1977; 86:40–46.
40. Katzman R, Brown T, Fuld P, et al. Validation of a short orientation-memory-concentration test of cognitive impairment. *Am J Psychiatry* 1983; 140:734–739.
41. Levkoff S, Liptzin B, Cleary P, et al. Review of research instruments and techniques used to detect delirium. *Int Psychogeriatr* 1992; 3:253–272.
42. Trzepacz PT, Baker RW, Greenhouse J. A symptom rating scale for delirium. *Psychiatric Res* 1988; 1:89–97.
43. Williams MA. Delirium/acute confusional states: evaluation devices in nursing. *Int Psychogeriatr* 1991; 3:301–308.
44. Wolber G, Romaniuk M, Eastman E, Robinson C. Validity of the short Portable Mental Status Questionnaire with elderly psychiatric patients. *J Consult Clin Psychol* 1984; 52:712–713.
45. Smith MJ, Breitbart WS, Platt MM. A critique of instruments and methods to detect, diagnose, and rate delirium. *J Pain Symp Manage* 1995; 10:35–77.
46. Trzepacz PT, Mittal D, Torres R, Norton J, Kanary K, Jimerson N. *Validity of the Delirium Rating Scale—Revised—98 (DRS-R-98)* Abstract #41. Proceedings of the 46th Annual Meeting of the Academy of Psychosomatic Medicine. November 18–21, 1999, New Orleans, LA.
47. Inouye BK, Vandyck CH, Alessi CA, et al. Clarifying confusion: the confusion assessment method, a new method for detection of delirium. *Ann Int Med* 1990; 113:941–948.
48. Hart RP, Best AM, Sessler CN, Levenson JL. Abbreviated cognitive test for delirium. *J Psychosom Res* 1997; 43:417–423.
49. Lawlor PG, Nekolaichuk C, Gagnon B, Mancini IL, Pereira JL, Bruera ED. Clinical utility, factor analysis and further validation of the Memorial Delirium Assessment Scale (MDAS). *Cancer* 2000; 88:2859–2867.
50. American Psychiatric Association. Practice Guidelines for the Treatment of Patients with Delirium. *Am J Psychiatry* 1999; 156:S1–S20.
51. Bruera E. Case Report. Severe organic brain syndrome. *J Palliat Care* 1991; 7:1:36–38.
52. Lichter I, Hunt E. The last 24 hour of life. *J Palliat Care* 1990; 6(4):7–15.
53. Tuma R, DeAngelis L. Acute encephalopathy in patients with systemic cancer. *Ann Neurol* 1992; 32:288.
54. Adams F, Wuesada JR, Gutterman JU. Neuropsychiatric manifestations of human leukocyte interferon therapy in patients with cancer. *JAMA* 1984; 252:938–941.
55. Denicoff KD, Rubinow Dr, Papa MZ, et al. The neuropsychiatric effects of treatment with interleukin-w and lymphokine-activated killer cells. *Ann of Int Med* 1987; 107(3):293–300.
56. Holland JC, Fassanellows, Ohnuma T. Psychiatric symptoms associated with L-asparaginase administration. *J Psychiatr Res* 1974; 10:165.
57. Weddington WW. Delirium and depression associated with amphotericin B. *Psychosomatics* 1982; 23:1076–1078.

58. Young DF. Neurological complications of cancer chemotherapy. In: Silverstein A, ed. *Neurological Complications of Therapy: Selected Topics*. New York: Futura Publishing, 1982:57–113.

59. Inouye BK, Bogardus Jr. ST, Charpentier PA, Leo-Summers L, Acampora D, Holford TR, Cooney J & LM. A multicomponent intervention to prevent delirium in hospitalized older patients. *NEJM* 1999:669–676.

60. Derogatis LR, Feldstein M, Morrow G, et al. A survey of psychotropic drug prescriptions in an oncology population. *Cancer* 1979; 44:1919–1929.

61. Steifel F, Kornblith A, Holland J. Changes in prescription patterns of psychotropic drugs for cancer patients during a 10-year period. *Cancer* 1990:1048–1053.

62. Goldberg G, Mor V. A survey of psychotropic use in terminal cancer patients. *Psychosomatics* 1985; 26:745–751.

63. Jaeger H, Morrow G, Brescia F. A survey of psychotropic drug utilization by patients with advanced neoplastic disease. *Gen Hosp Psychiatry* 1985; 7:353–360.

64. Akechi T, Uchitomi Y, Okamura H, et al. Usage of haloperidol for delirium in cancer patients. Supp Care Cancer 1996; 4:390–392.

65. Fernandez F, Holmes VF, Adams F, Kavanaugh JJ. Treatment of severe refractory agitation with a Haldol drip. *J Clin Psychiatry* 1988; 49:239–241.

66. Fernandez F, Levy JF, Mansell PWA. Management of delirium in terminally ill AIDS patients. *Int J Psychiat Med* 1989; 19:165–172.

67. Rosen JH. Double-blind comparison of haloperidol and thioridazine in geriatric outpatients. *J Clin Psychiatry* 1979; 40:17–20.

68. Smith GR, Taylor CW, Linkons P. Haloperidol versus thioridazine for the treatment of psychogeriatric patients: A double-blind clinical trial. *Psychosomatics* 1974; 15:134–138.

69. Thomas H, Schwartz E, Petrilli R. Droperidol versus haloperidol for chemical restraint of agitated and combative patients. *Ann Emerg Med.* 1992; 21:407–413.

70. Tsuang MM, Lu LM, Stotsky BA, Cole JO. Haloperidol versus thioridazine for hospitalized psychogeriatrics patients: Double-blind study. *J Am Geriatr Soc* 1971; 19:593–600.

71. Breitbart W. Psychiatric complications of cancer. In: Brain MC, Carbone PP, eds. *Current Therapy in Hematology Oncology-3*. Toronto and Philadelphia: B.C. Decker Inc., 1988:268–274.

72. Breitbart W. Psychiatric management of cancer pain. *Cancer* 1989; 63:2336–2342.

73. Twycross RG, Lack SA. *Symptom Control in Far Advanced Cancer: Pain Relief*. London: Pitman Brooks, 1983.

74. Stiefel F, Bruera E. Psychostimulants for hypoactive hypoalert delirium? *J Palliat Care* 1991; 3:25–26.

75. Menza M, Murray G, Holmes V. Controlled study of extrapyramidal reactions in the management of delirious medically ill patients: Intravenous haloperidol versus intravenous haloperidol plus benzodiazepines. *Heart Lung* 1988; 17:238–241.

76. Perry SW. Organic Mental disorders caused by HIV: update on early diagnosis and treatment. *Am J Psychiatry* 1990; 147:696–710.

77. Oliver DJ. The use of Methotrimeprazine in terminal care. *Br J Clin Pract* 1985; 39:339–340.

78. Baldessarini R, Frankenburg F. Clozapine: A novel antipsychotic agent. *N Eng J Med* 1991; 324:746–752.

79. Passik SD, Cooper M. Complicated delirium in a cancer patient successfully treated with olanzipine. *J Pain Symp Manage* 1999; 17:219–223.
80. Sipahimalani A, Massand PS. Olanzipine in the treatment of delirium. *Psychosomatics* 1998; 39:422–430.
81. Sipahimalani A, Sime RM, Masand PS: Treatment of delirium with risperidone. *Int J Geriatr Psychopharmacol* 1997; 1:24–26.
82. Breitbart W, Chochinov HM, Passik S. Psychiatric aspects of palliative care. In: Doyle D, Hanks GEC, MacDonald N, eds. *Oxford Textbook of Palliative Medicine*, Second Edition. New York: Oxford University Press, 1998:933–954.
83. Bottomley DM, Hanks GW. Subcutaneous midazolam infusion in palliative care. *J Pain Symp Manage* 1990; 5:259–261.
84. De Sousa E, Jepson A. Midazolam in terminal care. *Lancet* 1988; 1:67–68.
85. Mercadante S, DeConno F, Ripamonti. Propofol in terminal care. *J pain Symp Mange* 1995; 10:639–642.
86. Moyle J. The use of propofol in palliative medicine. *J Pain Symp Manage* 1995; 10:643–646.
87. Fainsinger R, Bruera E. Treatment of delirium in a terminally ill patient. *J Pain Symp Manage* 1992; 7:54–56.

Index